CANCER BIOLOGY

R J B KING

SCHOOL OF BIOLOGICAL SCIENCES, UNIVERSITY OF SURREY

Prentice
Hall

An imprint of **Pearson Education**

Harlow, England · London · New York · Reading, Massachusetts · San Francisco · Toronto · Don Mills, Ontario · Sydney
Tokyo · Singapore · Hong Kong · Seoul · Taipei · Cape Town · Madrid · Mexico City · Amsterdam · Munich · Paris · Milan

Pearson Education Limited
Edinburgh Gate
Harlow
Essex CM20 2JE
England

and Associated Companies throughout the world

Visit us on the World Wide Web at:
www.pearsoneduc.com

First published under the Longman imprint 1996
Second edition 2000

ISBN 0582 40432 0

British Library Cataloguing-in-Publication Data
A catalogue record for this book is available from the British Library

Library of Congress Cataloging-in-Publication Data
King, R. J. B. (Roger John Benjamin)
  Cancer biology / Roger J. B. King.–2nd ed.
    p. cm
  Includes bibliographical references and index.
    1. Cancer. 2. Carcinogenesis. I. Title.
  [DNLM: 1. Neoplasms–physiopathology. 2. Neoplasms-etiology. 3.
  Neoplasms-therapy. QZ 200 K54c 2000]
  RC254.6. K54 2000
  616.99'4 21–dc21

10 9 8 7 6 5 4 3
05 04 03 02 01

Typeset in 10/12 Bembo by 35
Produced by Pearson Education Asia Pte Ltd
Printed in Singapore (COS)

Cancer Biology *2nd edition*

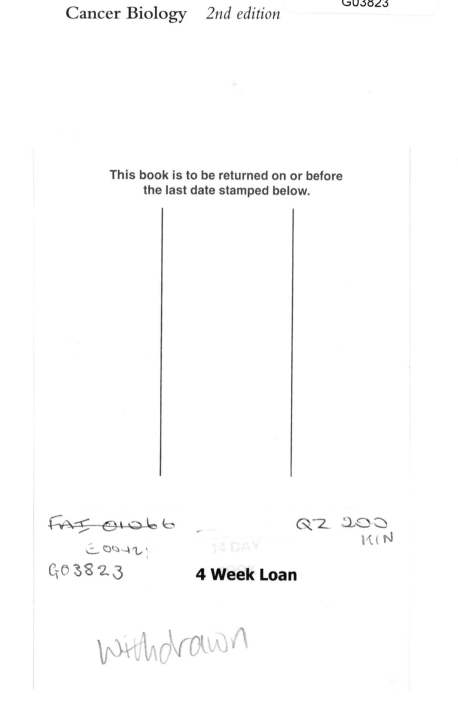

This book is to be returned on or before
the last date stamped below.

We work with leading authors to develop the
strongest educational materials in biology,
bringing cutting-edge thinking and best learning
practice to a global market.

Under a range of well-known imprints, including
Prentice Hall, we craft high quality print and
electronic publications which help readers to
understand and apply their content,
whether studying or at work.

To find out more about the complete range of our
publishing please visit us on the World Wide Web at:
www.pearsoneduc.com

CONTENTS

4. Epidemiology: identifying causes for human cancers

5. Tumour immunology and immunotherapy

6. Oncogenes, repressor genes and viruses

7. Chemical and radiation carcinogenesis

8. Mutations, DNA repair and genetic instability

9. Familial cancers

10. Growth: a balance of proliferation, death and differentiation

11. Responding to the environment: growth regulation and signal transduction

12. Invasion and metastasis

13. Principles of cancer treatment

14. Approaches to cancer prevention

PREFACE

In collecting the information to revise this book, I was impressed by the advances that have been made over the four years since the first edition was written. When one is actively involved in specific areas of cancer research, it is possible to get frustrated at periods of limited progress. However, when one takes a broader perspective, as I have done here, it is clear that substantial progress continues on many fronts: I congratulate the workers involved and I hope they will get 'the cure' before I need it! This will be my last substantial piece of scientific writing, so I would like to conclude with special thanks to four scientists from whose guidance I have benefited enormously: Professor Guy Marrian FRS, Professor Sir Michael Stoker FRS, Professor Sir Walter Bodmer FRS and Dr Veronica King. The first three were successive directors of research at the Imperial Cancer Research Fund and without them I would not have got very far; without the last person, my wife, I would have got nowhere.

PREFACE TO THE FIRST EDITION

This book is intended to provide information, at undergraduate level, on the biological principles underlying the causes and treatments of cancer. It is structured to illustrate those principles with specific examples taken wherever possible from human cancers. The human emphasis is supplemented with data from other species wherever appropriate.

The basis for the book is a 20 lecture module I give to final year students in the School of Biological Sciences, University of Surrey. The students are mostly following a biochemistry and molecular biology based course but include microbiologists with minimal knowledge of mammalian cell function. The microbiologists cope well with the mammalian information and most difficulties arise with the section on how cells communicate with their environment (Chapter 11). There are no medical students at Surrey but the course would be well tailored to their requirements.

The stimulus for preparing the book came from the realisation that a modern, affordable book at the appropriate level did not exist. There are good multi-author volumes whose expense precludes widespread student use. The academic level of this book has been pitched somewhat higher than that required for a good degree at this university. The offering of information more detailed than required, particularly in molecular detail, is intentional so as to cater for the wide range of abilities among the students and, hopefully, to lead the more adventurous students to further study.

In addition to the Surrey students, other sources of help in compiling this book should be acknowledged. Veronica King, Tony Avades, Jack Salway, Brian Stace, Ron Hubbard, Maurice Coombes, Ian Hart, Margaret Green and Wynne Aherne contributed greatly to the generation of an understandable text. The Imperial Cancer Research Fund is to be thanked for providing me with a lifetime's working environment in which I learned the basics encompassed by this book and then for giving me the freedom to write it.

This book is dedicated to
the students of SBS310 in the
School of Biological Sciences
University of Surrey

ACKNOWLEDGEMENTS

The following are reproduced by kind permission of the copyright holders:

Figure 1.1: Adapted from Fig. 9.6 in DeVita, V.T., Hellman, S. and Rosenburg, S.A. (eds) (1993) *Cancer: Principles and Practice of Oncology*, 4th edn, J.B. Lippincot, Philadelphia PA.

Figure 1.4: Based on data in *Cancer Statistics* (1989), American Cancer Society, Philadelphia PA.

Figure 2.3: Graph adapted from Tannock, I.F. (1968) *British Journal of Cancer*, **22**, 258–73.

Figure 2.4: Based on data in Muller, W.J. *et al.* (1988) *Cell*, **54**, 105–15.

Figure 2.8: Based on data in Anderson, M.J. and Stanbridge, E.J. (1993) *FASEB Journal*, **7**, 826–33.

Figure 2.9: Reproduced from Fig. 24-3 in, Alberts, B., Bray, D., Lewis, J., Raff, M., Roberts, K. and Watson, J.D. (1994) *Molecular Biology of the Cell*, 3rd edn, Garland Publishing, New York.

Figure 2.11: Adapted from Fearon, E.R. and Vogelstein, B. (1990) *Cell*, **61**, 759–67.

Table 4.1: Adapted from Table 9.5 in DeVita, V.T., Hellman, S. and Rosenburg, S.A. (eds) (1993) *Cancer: Principles and Practice of Oncology*, 4th edn, J.B. Lippincot, Philadelphia PA.

Table 4.2: Based on data in Bosch, F.X. *et al.* (1992) *International Journal of Cancer*, **52**, 750–58.

Tables 4.4 and 4.5: Adapted from data in DeVita, V.T., Hellman, S. and Rosenburg, S.A. (eds) (1993) *Cancer: Principles and Practice of Oncology*, 4th edn, J.B. Lippincot, Philadelphia PA, Section 20.6.

Tables 4.6, 14.1 and Figures 4.9, 4.11: Based on data in *Food, nutrition & the Prevention of Cancer: a Global Perpective* (1997) World Cancer Research Fund/ American Institute for Cancer Research. American Institute for Cancer Research, Washington.

Table 4.9: Adapted from Wynder, E.L. (1977) *Nature*, **268**, 284.

Tables 5.3 and 5.4: Based on data in Van den Eynde, B.J. & van der Bruggen, P. (1997) T cell defined tumor antigens. *Current Opinion in Immunology*, **9**, 684–693.

Figure 4.3: Adapted from data in *Cancer Facts and Figures* (1995), American Cancer Society, Philadelphia PA.

Figure 4.5: Adapted from data in Crawford, F.G. *et al.* (1994) *Journal of the National Cancer Institute*, **86**, 1398–1402.

Figure 4.6: Adapted from Greenblatt, M.S. *et al.* (1994) *Cancer Research*, **54**, 4855–4878.

Figure 4.7: Reproduced from Fig. 3 in Greenblatt, M.S. *et al.* (1994) *Cancer Research*, **54**, 4855–78.

Figure 4.8: Adapted from Fig. 2.8 in Tannock, I.F. and Hill, R.P. (eds) (1992) *The Basic Science of Oncology*, 2nd edn. McGraw-Hill, New York.

Figure 4.10: Adapted from Fig. 9 in Hirayama, T.J. (1992) *National Cancer Institute Monograph*, **12**, 65–74.

Figure 5.4: Adapted from Fig. 8.7 in Roitt, I., Brostoff, J. and Male, D. (1993) *Immunology*, 3rd edn. Mosby, London.

Figure 6.12: Based on data in Kinzler, K. W. and Vogelstein, B. (1996) Lessons from hereditary colorectal cancer. *Cell*, **87**, 159–170.

Table 7.7: Adapted from Table 12.2 in DeVita, V.T., Hellman, S. and Rosenburg, S.A. (eds) (1993) *Cancer: Principles and Practice of Oncology*, 4th edn, J.B. Lippincot, Philadelphia PA.

Table 7.9: Adapted from Table 1 in Greenblatt, M.S. *et al.* (1994) *Cancer Research*, **54**, 4855–78.

Table 7.9: Adapted from Table 2 in Greenblatt, M.S. *et al.* (1994) *Cancer Research*, **54**, 4855–78.

Figure 7.12: Adapted from Fig. 4 in Levine, A.J. *et al.* (1994) *British Journal of Cancer*, **69**, 409–16.

Table 8.1: Based on data in Simpson, A.J.G. (1997) The natural somatic mutation frequency and human carcinogenesis. *Advances in Cancer Research*, **71**, 209–240.

Figure 10.5: Adapted from Fig. 1 in Peters, G. (1994) *Nature*, **371**, 204–5.

Figure 10.20: Based on data in Sieweke, M.H. and Graff, T. (1998) A transcription factor party during blood cell differentiation. *Current Opinion in Genetics & Development*, **8**, 545–551.

Table 11.3: Based on data in Sawyers, C.L. and Denny, C.T. (1994) *Cell*, **77**, 171–73.

Figure 12.4: Adapted from Fig. 4 in Maemura, M. and Dickson, R.B. (1994) *Breast Cancer Research and Treatment*, **32**, 239–60.

Figure 13.2: Adapted from Fig. 1 in Galea, M.H. *et al.* (1992) *Breast Cancer Research and Treatment*, **22**, 207–19.

Figure 13.3: Adapted from Fig. 28.2 in Jordan, V.C. (ed.) (1986) *Estrogen/ Antiestrogen Action and Breast Cancer Therapy*, University of Wisconsin Press, Madison WI.

Figure 13.4: Based on data in McPherson, A. (1985) *Cervical Screening: A Practical Guide*, Oxford University Press, Oxford.

Figure 13.7: Reproduced from Fig. 17.2 in Franks, L.M. and Teich, N.M. (eds) (1991) *Introduction to the Cellular and Molecular Biology of Cancer*, 2nd edn, Oxford University Press, Oxford.

Figure 13.14: Based on data in Lobell, R.B. and Kohl, N.E. (1998) Pre-clinical development of farnesyltransferase inhibitors. *Cancer & Metastasis Reviews*, **17**, 203–210.

Figure 13.15: Based on data in Klohs, W.D., Fry, D.W. and Kraker, A.J. (1997) Inhibitors of tyrosine kinase. *Current Opinion in Oncology*, **9**, 562–568.

Figure 14.2: Based on data in Stanford, J.L. (1991) Oral contraceptives and neoplasia of the ovary. *Contraception*, **43**, 543–546.

Figure 14.3: Based on data in Thun, M.J., Namboodri, M.M. & Heath, C.W. (1991) Aspirin use and reduced risk of fatal colon cancer. *New England Journal of Medicine*, **325**, 1593–1596.

Figure 14.4: based on data in Omenn, G.S., Goodman, G.E., Thornquist, M.D., Balmes, J., Cullen, M.R. *et al.* (1996) Risk factors for lung cancer and for intervention effects in CARET: the beta-carotene and retinol efficacy trial. *Journal of the National Cancer Institute,* 88, 1550–1559.

Whilst every effort has been made to trace the owners of copyright material, in a few cases this has proved impossible and we take this opportunity to offer our apologies to any copyright holders whose rights we may have unwittingly infringed.

BASIC SCIENCE, TERMINOLOGY AND ABBREVIATIONS

To describe the biology of cancer it is necessary to cover all aspects of cell function. To do this a decision has to be made on how much basic science is included in a book of this type. I have adopted the approach of providing the pertinent information in boxes and placed each box in the chapter where it is most relevant; the Box number refers to the chapter in which it appears. This approach has also been used for molecular biology, genetics and cell biology, which have broad relevance and which may create cross reference problems. The following chapters contain general details of such topics.

Molecular biology
Gene regulation: Box 6.1
DNA structure and synthesis: Box 6.1 and Box 10.1
Genetic terminology and chromosone structure: Box 9.1, Table 6.1
Cell and animal biology
Chapter 2
Transgenic, knock-out, immunodeficient mice: Box 2.1
Cytoskeleton, cell adhesion, cell migration: Box 11.1
Classification of tumours
Box 3.1
Epidemiology
Box 4.1
Immunology
Box 5.1

Abbreviations can be confusing, especially as illogical names are often used. No one could reasonably expect to know that 'son of sevenless' is a gene involved in signal transduction! To clarify the situation as far as is possible, where an abbreviation is used for the first time, I have put in bold type the letters that contribute to the abbreviation, although there are cases where this approach is not possible. Thus, SOS first appears in the text as **s**on **o**f **s**evenless. The literature often uses multiple terminologies for a single entity. As far as possible, I have mentioned the alternates for the more common abbreviations. Box 6.1 describes abbreviations relevant to oncogenes and repressors.

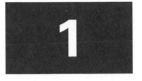

WHAT IS CANCER?

Key points

- Cancer is a collection of diseases with the common feature of uncontrolled growth.
- There are multiple causes but 'lifestyle' factors are a major influence.
- Several cellular changes are required to generate a cancer.
- All cell types are susceptible but epithelial cells are most prone to change.
- Cell changes continue to occur after a cancer has formed.
- Mutations in repressor genes and oncogenes are important.
- Invasion and metastasis distinguish cancers from benign growths.
- Cancers are not always lethal.
- It is possible to prevent cancer formation.

Introduction

The most common question asked of cancer specialists is 'are you making progress?' This begs the question 'progress towards what?' To answer that, one has to know what cancers are. The use of the plural is deliberate because cancer is really a collection of different diseases with three common features: uncontrolled growth is their core property and they are life-threatening but the third feature is a more philosophical one. It is that generalisations about cancer are invalid because there are always exceptions that disprove the generalisation. Despite this, generalisations are essential in order to convey an understanding of the topic, otherwise one would end up with a jungle of confusing statements. Thus, although cancer has multiple causes, an acceptable clinical definition would be: a set of diseases characterised by unregulated cell growth leading to invasion of surrounding tissues and spread (metastasis) to other parts of the body. This definition would be considered too narrow by experimentalists who would not require evidence of invasion and metastasis. The variable use of definitions sometimes results in confusion, with cancer, tumour and neoplasm being used in an interchangeable way. This is not correct as 'neoplasm' means new growth without qualifying the nature of that growth whereas 'tumour' can be applied to both benign and malignant growths.

Carcinogenesis requires several cellular changes

Cancer is an ancient condition and was known to the early Egyptians. Despite this ancient lineage, two modern components, longevity and lifestyle, have major impacts

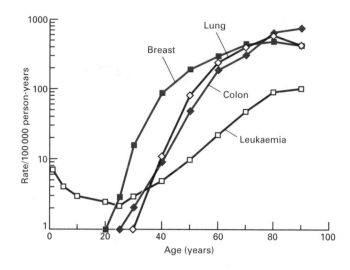

Figure 1.1

Influence of age on cancer incidence (USA).

on both the type and number of cancers encountered. Carcinogenesis, the process by which cancers are generated, is a multistep mechanism resulting from the accumulation of errors in vital regulatory pathways. It is initiated in a single cell which then multiplies and acquires additional changes that give it a survival advantage over its neighbours. The altered cells must be amplified to generate billions of cells that constitute a cancer. As it takes time to generate these errors and cell numbers, it follows that the longer one lives, the more likely one is to get cancer. Figure 1.1 shows the age distribution of several cancers indicating their increase with age, but sadly the dictum that cancer is a disease of old age has exceptions in that some cancers are characterised by onset in childhood: cancers of the eye and certain leukaemias fall into this category. This explains the initial high incidence of leukaemia followed by a dip and then a rise in older people (Figure 1.1).

Lifestyle and family influences on cancer

The impact of lifestyle is illustrated by the prevalence of certain cancers in different countries (Figure 1.2); breast and prostate cancer are common in Western countries whilst cancers of the cervix and stomach are more prevalent in nations such as China. As lifestyles change, so do the types of cancer; these geographical differences are due to more than just genetic variations between races. Environmental influences are important even though they exert their effects via the genetic machinery of the cells.

In the majority of situations, the accumulation of errors in the cellular machinery occurs after birth in somatic cells. Important exceptions are those defects inherited via the germ cells (sperm, egg) that contribute to a minority of cancers like those of the eye and kidney. Even some of the major cancers include a small proportion of patients who inherit a predisposition for that cancer. Such situations illustrate the diverse nature of cancers even if they have the same name. Thus, the majority of colon cancers have no inherited features but at least three different types of inherited genetic defects have

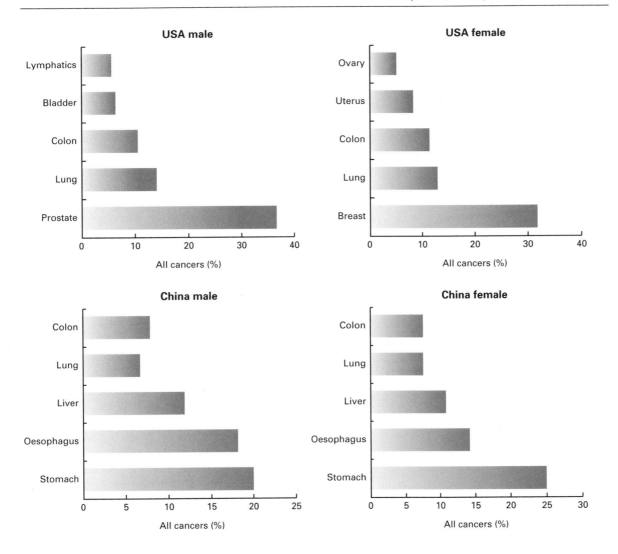

Figure 1.2

Comparison of the five commonest cancers in the USA and China.

been identified in a minority of cases. This requirement for error generation introduces the linked questions: what agents cause cancer and how do they generate mutations? Laboratory tests show that an enormous range of products can generate cancers but the emphasis is on the word 'can' rather than 'do' because such tests are not always relevant to the human situation. The laboratory tests were designed around the idea that cancers were generated by environmental chemicals, a view that was fully justified on the basis of occupational cancers in humans (such as bladder cancers in dye-workers, lung cancers in smokers) and chemical induction of cancers in animals. However, the word 'environmental' conjures up the impression of synthetic, unnatural agents and, with the exception of smoking, these types of reagent have minor impact on the prevalence of human cancers. Diet and lifestyle changes are of much greater importance and the feeling is growing that natural events such as free radical generation or hormonal proliferation stimuli, may be the driving force for common human cancers such as those of the colon and breast. This is coupled with the realisation that initial cellular changes accelerate the appearance of subsequent mutations and so carcinogenesis involves the generation of genetic instability.

Changes continue to accumulate after cancer formation

It is not always appreciated that the generation of errors does not stop once a cancer has been formed; cancers continue to change their behaviour as they progress, a fact that creates problems when it comes to treating patients. For example, a breast cancer may initially be sensitive to the same hormones as influence normal breast but then become hormone insensitive. This progression or dedifferentiation of cancers reflects the genetic instability of the cells involved, resulting in more and more of the cells' economy being diverted towards growth.

Cancers are most common in epithelial cells

Figure 1.2 shows that some tissues are more prone to develop cancer than others and that men and women have different cancer patterns. This is emphasised in Table 1.1, which presents data from one country, the USA. Men do not have ovaries or uteri or women prostate glands so the reason for the absence of these cancers in the relevant sexes is clear, but the big sex difference in breast cancer points to sex-related influences. In fact, it is not always realised that men do get breast cancer. On the other hand, colon cancer is similar in men and women. The three most common cancers in both sexes are of epithelial origin but mesenchymal cells are affected to a lesser degree (leukaemias/lymphomas in Table 1.1, sarcomas not shown) and thus most cell types are susceptible. The data in Table 1.1 are repeated in Figure A.1 to indicate sites in the body of these cancers.

Table 1.1 Types of cancer in men and women as percentage of all cancers (USA, 1995).

Site	Men		Women	
	New cancers	Death	New cancers	Death
Breast	<1	<1	32	18
Lung	14	33	13	24
Colon/rectum	10	9	12	11
Mouth	3	2	2	1
Skin melanoma	3	1	3	1
Pancreas	2	7	2	5
Leukaemia/lymphoma	7	8	6	8
Prostate	36	14	–	–
Ovary	–	–	5	6
Uterus/cervix	–	–	9	4

Cancer results from uncontrolled growth

No single explanation accounts for these differences in susceptibility of cells to cancer formation but proliferation is correctly ascribed to being a core feature of cancer. This is often erroneously linked with faster rather than uncontrolled proliferation. It is true that in experimental systems such as cell culture or animals, faster proliferation is common but it is not always so in humans. Mouth and skin cancers, which only account for 5% of all cancers, both contain rapidly proliferating cells whereas breast cancer, the most common female cancer (Table 1.1), proliferates slowly. Many normal cells hyperproliferate on occasions (hyperplasia, Chapter 3) but otherwise retain their normal appearance and behaviour. The crucial feature of cancer cells is that they are antisocial and have a degree of autonomy not enjoyed by their normal counterparts. Normal cells are subject to internal and external inhibitory signals that, to varying degrees, are lost during carcinogenesis. Identification of these regulatory signals is therefore important to our understanding of how the extracellular environment can influence cell function, how a cancer cell can manipulate its environment and what determines the overall behaviour of a mass of cells (Figure 1.3). A decreased rate of cell death is at least as important as increased proliferation in determining the size of a cancer, and supply of nutrients by the generation of new blood vessels is essential if a tumour mass is to exceed a critical size. As cells differentiate they divide more slowly. Thus, blocking differentiation (as occurs in some leukaemias) or causing dedifferentiation (as in many advanced cancers) increases growth. Contact with other cells or with the extracellular matrix is growth inhibitory for normal cells but not for cancer cells, whereas some cancers are seen as 'foreign' and therefore subject to influence by the host immune system.

Figure 1.3

Behaviour of a cell mass: influential factors.

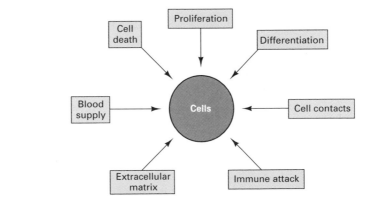

Cancer genes

In the area of cell regulation, the concept of cancer genes or oncogenes has borne fruit with the realisation that the activities of key regulatory genes involved in normal signal pathways can be increased by qualitative or quantitative changes and thereby change cell function. A fascinating twist to this story is that many cancers are generated by loss rather than increase of gene function and this loss of normal inhibitory influence, repression, is particularly evident in events related to cell proliferation and death. Once again, the diversity of cancer changes is seen in the fact that different cancers change different signalling pathways to achieve the same end result – uncontrolled growth.

Invasion and metastasis

Increased cell mass on its own generates what a clinician would consider to be a benign, easily controllable growth and not a cancer. Additional changes are required that enable those cells to invade the surrounding tissue and metastasise to other parts of the body. This ability of cancer cells to overcome the normal containment mechanisms reflects membrane modifications resulting in diminished cell–cell interactions as well as the production of proteases that facilitate movement through the extracellular matrix. Additionally, cancer cells can use chemical messengers to signal normal cells to help them. Thus, they promote the appearance of new blood vessels, thereby ensuring an adequate supply of essential nutrients. The acquisition of invasive properties is what distinguishes malignant cells from benign cells, whilst metastasis to other parts of the body is the primary cause of clinical problems and death.

Some cancers are curable

The fear of cancer is probably the biggest medical concern of people living in affluent societies. This is understandable but it is important to put that concern in perspective to other causes of death (Figure 1.4). Death from cancer is second to death from heart disease, with other individual causes being far behind. Another way of looking at this is to consider the years of life lost through death from heart disease and cancer. As heart disease affects younger people more than cancer, cancer

Figure 1.4

Causes of death in the USA.

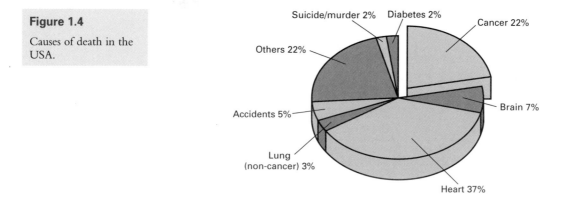

could be considered less dangerous than heart disease by this criterion. In most people's minds, cancer is linked to death but this is not the invariable situation because, although only 3% of people are alive 5 years after diagnosis of pancreatic cancer, the figure is 91% for testicular cancer and can almost be considered a cure. At present, the major cancers cannot be cured in their entirety but comparison of the numbers of people developing specific cancers with those dying therefrom indicates that something beneficial is happening with some cancers (Table 1.1). In women, 32% of all cancers arise in the breast but they account for only 18% of cancer deaths. The same pattern is seen for cancers of the uterus, but unfortunately the converse pattern of incidence and death occurs with lung cancer. However, some cancers can be cured, e.g. choriocarcinoma in the placenta.

Death is an all too frequent consequence of cancer but we do not always know how cancer kills. Most frequently this is due to disruption of vital organs such as brain or liver but it is not immediately apparent why bone metastases should be so lethal. The wasting (cachexia) commonly seen in cancer patients may be due to toxins released into the circulation.

Treatment

The best form of treatment is prevention and ideas along this line are being put into practice with initiatives such as smoking control and recommendations on dietary habits. The next best approach is early detection. The smaller the number and less malignant the nature of the cancer cells, the greater the probability of achieving a cure. With this objective in mind, screening programmes are in place for early detection of cervical, breast and colon cancers.

Treatment of cancer is based on the removal and/or killing of the tumour cells while minimising unwanted side effects on normal cells. Surgery is often the first line of attack but it is becoming increasingly the practice to consider cancer as a systemic disease at the time of first detection and to give additional (adjuvant) medical treatment such as chemotherapy and radiotherapy at the same time. Medical rather than surgical attack is used because of the inaccessibility or unknown site of metastatic spread. The majority of treatments are based on inhibiting cell proliferation whilst targeted X-radiation is effective in some cases.

NATURAL HISTORY: THE LIFE OF A CANCER

Key points

- The life history of a cancer can be divided into stages. Carcinogenesis, the process of cancer development from a normal cell, is divided into initiation and promotion stages. Progression describes the additional changes occurring after a cancer has formed.
- Most characteristics identified by laboratory models have counterparts in human cancers but initiation is difficult to define in some human cancers.
- Altered DNA bases (mutations) are the basis of cellular changes that cause cancer. This can involve chemical alteration of individual bases or the order in which the bases occur.
- Several mutations are required for carcinogenesis. This involves genes that either gain (dominant) or lose (recessive) function as a result of mutation.
- Multiple pathways exist by which a cancer in one cell type is generated.
- Different cancers have different aetiologies although they may have some common features.
- Cancers arise in single cells (clonal origin).
- Cancers detected by clinical means are at an advanced stage of their natural history.

Introduction

The sequence of events involved in carcinogenesis and the data on which our knowledge of these events are based have been derived from sources ranging from animal studies through cell and molecular biology to clinical experiences. Therefore, it is not surprising that different perspectives and terms exist to describe the various stages in the natural history or pathogenesis of cancer development. Four representations are given in Figure 2.1 which, with varying degrees of overlap, illustrate models derived from animal experiments (1,4), cell biology (2), molecular biology (2,3) and clinical data (4). This chapter will look at the overall process of carcinogenesis and tumour progression from the separate perspectives of the experimental biologist and the medical practitioner. These two broad categories have been chosen because they provide different insights into the processes involved that reinforce each other in some situations but raise doubts about the relevance of animal data to human cancer in others. By their nature, experimental approaches are capable of providing more clear-cut answers than data derived from clinical experiences, but clinical experiences are more relevant to the human situation. The

Figure 2.1

Cancer development: four models. Each connecting arrow represents several events and multiple pathways can exist between each stage.

Model 1 Animal experiments

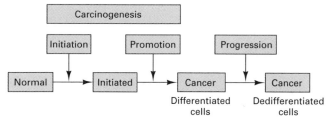

Model 2 Cell biology

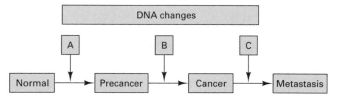

Model 3 Molecular biology

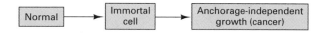

Model 4 Clinical and animal data

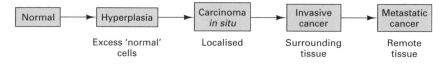

concluding part of the chapter will bring the two perspectives together with some general comments plus a discussion of their relevance to two human cancers, colon cancer and chronic myeloid leukaemia (CML).

Clonal origins of cancer

Regardless of viewpoint, cancers arise by expansion of cell numbers from a single cell (clonal origin). Clinical data derived from analysis of enzymes such as glucose-6-phosphate dehydrogenase have provided good evidence for such a model. Some people are heterozygous for this X chromosome-linked enzyme and have cells that contain either type A or B enzyme but not both, so that normal tissues are a mosaic of cells with different phenotypes (Figure 2.2). The A and B enzymes differ by one amino acid and can be distinguished electrophoretically. Normal myeloid cells in the blood from a heterozygous individual display both A and B forms of the dehydrogenase whereas CML cells contain only one form; individuals with CML display either A or B forms but not both. Another striking example of clonal origins are the benign, smooth muscle tumours of the uterus, leiomyoma or fibroids, several

Figure 2.2

Cancers arise from single cells: clonal origin.

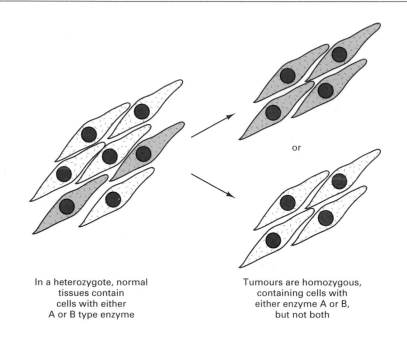

In a heterozygote, normal
tissues contain
cells with either
A or B type enzyme

or

Tumours are homozygous,
containing cells with
either enzyme A or B,
but not both

of which can occur in the same uterus. Normal muscle cells from a heterozygous individual express either A or B forms in a random manner but all cells within individual fibroids express only one enzyme type, with separate fibroids within one uterus exhibiting either an A or B phenotype but not both. Although glucose-6-phosphate dehydrogenase mutations illustrate clonal origins of growth, the enzyme is not a causal component of that growth. The repressor gene p53 fulfils that criterion (Chapter 6) and mutations in this gene also indicate clonal origins. Sun-induced skin lesions carry mutations in the p53 gene; all regions from a single lesion contain the same mutation but this is different from mutations elsewhere in the same patient.

Experimental biology

The main feature of models derived from experimental systems is of a discrete, ordered series of changes to which terms such as initiation, promotion, progression and immortality can be applied. Animal experiments generated terms like 'carcinogenesis', which covers events leading up to the generation of a cancer, whereas 'progression' is the term applied to changes after a tumour has formed (Figure 2.1, model 1). Progression includes invasion and metastasis but these fundamental features of human cancer occur infrequently in primary animal tumours. Cell culture experiments tend to be described in terms of immortalisation or prolonging the lifespan of cells plus an altered ability to recognise adjacent cells and extracellular components. These properties often result in anchorage-independent growth (ability to proliferate without attachment to the plastic culture dish) (model 2). Molecular biologists think in terms of discrete mutational events (model 3). Progression would be equated to change C in model 3. Model 4 describes the sequence of histological changes observed in human and animal tumours, with progression referring to stages beyond *in situ* carcinoma. Data so derived have emphasised the multifactorial nature of cancer aetiology, the multiple changes required to generate a cancer and the fact that changes continue to occur in established tumours.

Animal studies

Carcinogenesis: initiation and promotion

It was the surgeon Sir Percival Potts who first showed that cancer could be caused by an external agent when he identified soot as the cause of scrotal cancer in young, male chimneysweeps in the eighteenth century. This observation led to the testing of chemicals on animals, and the resultant subdivision of carcinogenesis into two stages, initiation and promotion, arose from mouse skin painting experiments. By itself dimethylbenzanthracene (DMBA), a carcinogenic polycyclic hydrocarbon, will not generate skin cancers; it requires subsequent treatment with another agent, croton oil. There can be an appreciable time interval (weeks) between exposure to the two reagents. The hydrocarbon initiates a cancer but additional events, generated by the croton oil and termed promotion, are also required in order for a cancer to develop (Figure 2.1). We now know that, in this example, initiation involves the formation of a covalent adduct of an epoxide metabolite of DMBA to a guanine base in DNA, thereby generating inheritable mutations (Chapter 7). The active ingredient of croton oil is the phorbol ester, **t**etradecanoyl **p**horbol **a**cetate (TPA), which by binding to a membrane receptor, protein kinase C, activates a cytoplasmic serine/threonine protein kinase cascade resulting in increased gene transcription and cell proliferation (Chapter 11). The genetic alterations brought about by the initiating agent require cell proliferation, triggered by the promoting agent, to transform a single potential cancer cell into a multicellular tumour. However, additional cellular changes are required over and above simply expanding a pool of initiated cells. The promoting agent on its own can generate proliferative changes but not cancers.

Promotion can occur by different pathways in different cells, but two common features highlighted by animal studies are altered cell proliferation and the formation of new blood vessels (Figure 2.3). Proliferation rate is discussed later in this chapter but angiogenesis will be dealt with here. Tumours will grow to about 1 mm diameter in the absence of new capillaries (angiogenesis) but further expansion requires the production of angiogenic growth factors by the cancer cells. The need for new blood vessels is reflected in the rapid proliferation of cells adjacent to the vessel and the progressive decrease in this proliferation with increasing distance from the vessel (Figure 2.3b).

Hormones are promoters Carcinogenic polycyclic hydrocarbons were widely used in early experiments because of their availability and the fact that their high potency generated clear-cut results. Two additional features are illustrated in another example of their use – in rat mammary carcinogenesis.

Figure 2.3

New blood vessels are required for cancer growth.

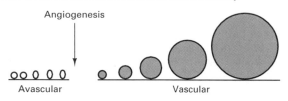

Cancer size remains small until blood vessels develop

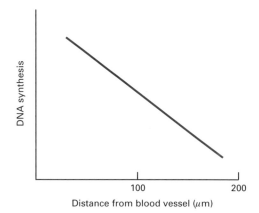

DNA synthesis decreases with distance from a blood vessel

A single oral dose of DMBA generates breast cancers but only under specific conditions. Removal of the ovarian hormone oestradiol immediately after DMBA treatment blocks carcinogenesis, an effect that is reversed by readministration of oestradiol. This is analogous to the skin model but with the hormone rather than TPA acting as the promoter. However, in intact animals, DMBA only works when given at a specific age – when the mammary gland is developing – indicating that cells are only susceptible to initiating agents at certain stages of their development. There is thus a link between carcinogenesis and cell development (differentiation status).

The second feature is that cancers other than breast cancer are rarely caused by DMBA in this model system, indicating different sensitivities of cells to a carcinogen.

Conceptual problems with the term 'initiation'   Important as the concepts of initiation and promotion are, conceptual problems arise if they are applied too widely. Carcinogenicity studies indicate that active agents can be classified into genotoxic and non-genotoxic categories depending on whether or not they damage DNA (Chapter 7). Compounds like DMBA are genotoxic, although they must be metabolised to compounds that react with DNA. The reactive metabolite is referred to as the ultimate carcinogen, which is the actual initiator. Non-genotoxic agents act by diverse mechanisms, some of which raise conceptual problems. Ovarian hormones like oestradiol are non-genotoxic but can generate breast and ovarian cancers in rodents without additional treatments probably by virtue of their mitogenic effect. Ovarian hormones are usually described as tumour promoters, but what is the initiator in this model? A similar situation occurs in humans with cancers generated by a single hormone. This is discussed in the section linking laboratory and clinical results.

On the other hand, the antilipotrophic drug clofibrate acts as a hepatic carcinogen by increasing the number of intracellular organelles, peroxisomes. This increases reactive oxygen, free radical production which, in turn, can damage DNA. It is not certain that clofibrate is an initiating agent.

It is a recurring theme throughout cancer research that definitions resulting from early discoveries are useful but, because of the many aetiologies of cancers, those definitions become too restrictive. The oestradiol and clofibrate problems may be examples where a discrete step under the heading 'initiation' may not always be necessary. This conceptual difficulty does not arise with the term 'promotion' because the molecular changes involved are more diverse and can be accommodated within a multiple change model. These points are also relevant to human carcinogenesis and are further elaborated on p. 23.

Progression

A second set of animal experiments showed that tumours, once formed, underwent further changes (progression) as demonstrated by dedifferentiation, increasingly autonomous growth and aggressive behaviour (Figure 2.1). The original work, using spontaneous mouse mammary tumours still serves as a good model for tumour progression. Initially, the tumours grow only when the animals become pregnant, regress at parturition and regrow at the next pregnancy. The hormonal changes accompanying pregnancy stimulate growth of the tumour, which is therefore defined as being hormone dependent because the cells are completely dependent on the hormones; cessation of hormone production is accompanied by disappearance of the tumour. However, small numbers of tumour cells remain and at the next pregnancy, the tumour regrows at the same place but almost invariably its behaviour changes with time, becoming first hormone responsive (partial regression at parturition) and then hormone independent (no regression). Histological examination indicates that loss of hormone sensitivity is accompanied by cellular dedifferentiation and increased mitotic activity. This irreversible sequence of changes does not always occur in the order just stated, as hormone-responsive or hormone-independent tumours can arise without prior detection of the dependent stage. This illustrates the variability of the development pathways that can exist even within one tumour type.

Progression reflects multiple changes in growth regulatory mechanisms. These include altered sensitivity to adjacent cells, local growth factor production, changes in receptors that initiate signal transduction and alterations to the downstream transduction pathways. The culmination of these events is autonomous cell growth, an ability to grow outside their normal environment and to metastasise to other parts of the body.

Special mice

Two types of mice have facilitated dissection of the steps involved in tumour development (pathogenesis). The first set are strains in which specific genes have been altered in all cells within the animal, whilst the second set are animals with defective immune systems.

The availability of engineered mice in which all cells have a specific gene that has either been activated (transgenic mice) or inactivated (knock-out mice) has facilitated analysis of the biological consequences of altered gene function (Box 2.1).

Box 2.1   Special mice used in cancer research

Transgenic studies   If a gene, a *transgene*, is injected into a unicellular egg that is then transplanted into a mother, all the cells in the offspring contain that gene and the mice are said to be *transgenic*. Frequently the gene to be studied is joined to a strong promoter (Box 6.1) from another gene to ensure adequate expression. This manipulation allows analysis of *potential* function of the gene in question but, in the absence of the normal promoter, quantitative differences in expression do not permit the conclusion that the gene actually generates the observed effects in normal animals. The animal can be monitored to see what biological changes result from having this gene engineered; this technique is widely used to study oncogene function. Alternatively, DNA base changes can be engineered in a gene and the immediate consequences monitored by introduction into cultured cells with a technique called *transfection*. However, cultured cells have different regulatory restraints to those encountered in animals so use of transgenic animals overcomes that problem.

Knock-out mice   Repressor genes are important in carcinogenesis when their normal inhibitory function is lost. Somatic cells are diploid; they contain two copies of each allele. Both copies have to be deleted before the consequences of their loss can be determined, although exceptions do exist (Chapter 6). This approach requires a complex combination of methodologies. An inactivating mutation is engineered in a repressor gene such as that coding for the 53 kDa protein, p53, and transfected into cultured cells. If recipient cells are from an early stage of egg development (a blastocyst), they have the ability to develop into any type of adult cell – they are said to be *totipotent* – so the introduced mutant p53 has the potential for modifying all the adult cells. *Homologous recombination* (Box 9.1) of chromosomes during mitosis will generate some *heterozygous* cells with one normal allele and one mutant allele. Reintroduction of these cells into the blastocyst followed by implantation into a mother will result in some heterozygous offspring. By cross-breeding two heterozygotes, some of their embryos will be *homozygous* (both alleles the same) for mutant (inactive) p53. These embryos are known as *knock-out, null/ null or −/− mice*.

Immunodeficient mice   Strains of mice have been developed with immune system defects. One strain has no thymus gland, the consequent absence of T-cells leads to loss of that cell-mediated immunity, so the mice do not reject foreign cells (Chapter 5). Such animals can be hairless and they are known as *nude mice*. A different group of mice, known as SCID (Severe Combined Immuno Deficiency) mice have no B or T lymphocytes of their own. Transplantation of stem cells from human bone marrow repopulates the mouse with human lymphocytes that protect SCID mice from opportunistic infections but will not reject human cells. SCID mice can be used to analyse effects of drugs and growth factors on human samples whose cellular architecture is maintained. Additionally, many normal tissues will not survive in immunodeficient mice whereas cancers will survive; changes related to carcinogenesis can thus be monitored. It is not known why normal cells have difficulty in surviving this environment but presumably it is related to their more complex growth requirements.

Transgenic mice   Genes in which mutations activate function (oncogenes, Chapter 6) can be analysed by inserting that gene (a transgene) into mouse cells. Thus, ras, myc and neu oncogenes code for proteins involved in signal transduction, gene transcription and cell membrane receptor respectively. The transgenic approach showed that the ras gene generated breast tumours in some but not all mice and that other cell types did not become cancerous (Figure 2.4). In the context of tumour pathogenesis, this indicates that single gene changes can inefficiently generate cancers and that cell-specific influences exist that determine which cells can be transformed into cancers. Myc had a similar effect to that of ras but the two together were synergistic. This cooperation between oncogenes fits well with multistage models of carcinogenesis. The third oncogene, neu, generated breast cancers in all the female offspring. This example illustrates the multiple ways a cancer type can be generated.

Knock-out mice   To define effects of genes whose normal function is inhibitory, it is more informative to delete the inhibitory factor. Repressor genes are studied in this way; inactivation of both alleles is usually necessary because of their recessive characteristics (Chapter 6). Thus, p53 $-/-$ mice appear normal at first, indicating that p53 is not required for early development but in later life about three-quarters then develop cancers such as lymphomas and sarcomas. This indicates that normal p53 is not required for early development but that in its absence, errors accumulate that lead to cancers. This is compatible with its normal role in inhibiting cell proliferation when damaged DNA is present (Chapter 8). It also highlights the

Figure 2.4

Transgenic mice are used to analyse oncogene effects.

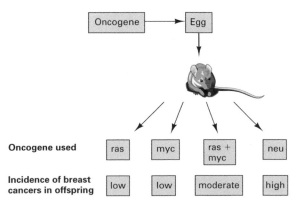

existence of cell-specific factors because only certain cells develop into cancers. Another example is mice in which both alleles of the **a**denomatous **p**olyposis **c**oli (APC) gene have been knocked-out (*Min* mice) and which develop multiple polyps in the colon (see below).

Immunodeficient mice The response of solid human tissues or cultured human cells to growth manipulation *in vivo* can be studied in such mice as the host immune mechanisms are lost (Box 2.1). The *in vitro* carcinogenesis example described in the next section provides an illustration of their use.

Cell and molecular biology

When methods became available to culture single cells, less complex and therefore more readily interpretable experiments were possible. It was noted that, in the media available, cancer cells grew more readily than their normal counterparts, which gave rise to the notion that carcinogenesis was accompanied by the need for less stringent growth conditions. This has developed into the autocrine/paracrine model of growth regulation whereby cancer cells produce or respond, via altered receptors, to locally synthesised growth factors (Figure 11.3). It was further noted that cultured cancer cells often lose a normal property called density or contact inhibition (Figure 2.5). As the name implies, when normal cells become crowded and contact adjacent cells they stop and will not overgrow their neighbours, whereas many cancer cells continue to proliferate. This antisocial behaviour is a reflection of altered interactions between the cell membranes in contact with other cells and with the plastic substrates on which they were growing. Normal cells must attach to plastic in order to grow (monolayer culture); free-floating normal cells do not proliferate. But some cancer cells grow without attachment, a phenomenon known as suspension culture or anchorage independence. Cultured cells are said to be transformed if they exhibit these behavioural changes, which are often accompanied by morphological alterations as well.

Figure 2.5

Proliferation characteristics of cultured cells.

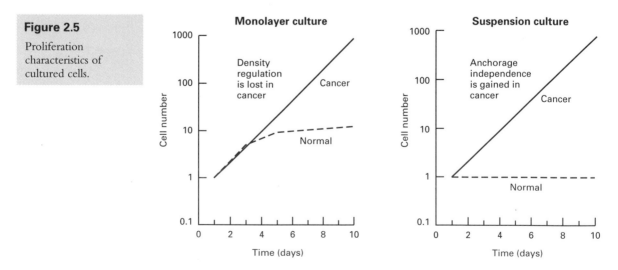

Carcinogenesis can be mimicked in culture

Comparison of various cell biological properties with ability to grow as tumours in immunodeficient animals indicated that anchorage independence was the best, but not invariate indication that the cell in question was cancerous. This was demonstrated by an *in vitro* carcinogenesis experiment in which cultured, normal fibroblasts were briefly treated with the carcinogen benzopyrene and the subsequent behaviour of the cells in culture monitored. The cultured cells were periodically injected into immunodeficient mice to see whether they formed tumours (Figure 2.6). By analogy with *in vivo* animal studies, carcinogen treatment was equivalent to initiation and additional changes in culture to promotion. Several post-initiation events were observed such as changed morphology and secretion of proteases like plasminogen activator, but it was not until the cells acquired the ability to grow in suspension culture that they also behaved as cancer cells when injected into mice. As these promotional events did not occur without prior benzopyrene exposure, the benzopyrene must have set in train a series of changes leading to cells capable of an autonomous existence. Several inheritable changes are required before cultured cells can grow as tumours in mice so, in this respect, the experimental model mimics the situation seen in patients and animals. However, differences also exist. In culture, benzopyrene acts as both initiator and promoter whereas in animals it often requires a promoter as well. The different pattern of behaviour probably reflects the strong proliferative environment in culture. Culture conditions have been deliberately established to maximise proliferation and minimise inhibitory influences, whereas in animals there exists an equilibrium between positive and negative controls. The culture medium with its plentiful supply of growth factors may be equivalent to the promotional agent needed *in vivo*.

Are cancer cells immortal?

Normal, cultured cells have a lifespan of about 40 generations (cell doublings) by which time the build-up of errors results in senescence and death (Figure 2.7). A component of the carcinogenic process is disruption of these events so that cells live longer and there is greater probability of error accumulation. The term 'immortal' (Figure 2.1, model 2) is sometimes used but it is inappropriate, because cancer cells do die even in fast-growing tumours. It is better to think in terms of extended life rather than immortality, although 'immortal' is firmly embedded in the literature. Senescent cells are viable but have lost the ability to replicate. Increasing numbers of

Figure 2.6

Carcinogenesis in cell culture: changes over time.

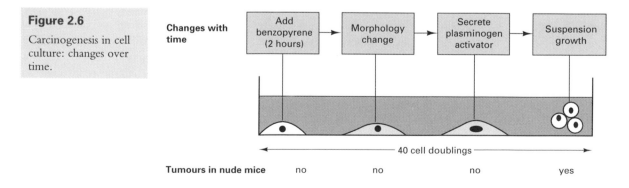

Changes with time

| Add benzopyrene (2 hours) | → | Morphology change | → | Secrete plasminogen activator | → | Suspension growth |

←———————————— 40 cell doublings ————————————→

Tumours in nude mice   no   no   no   yes

Figure 2.7

The life cycle of normal cultured cells.

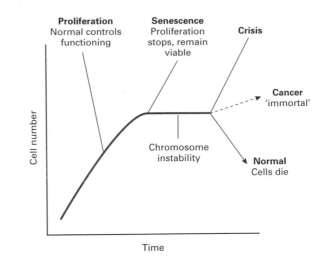

abnormal chromosomes accumulate, and eventually 'crisis' occurs, a loosely defined set of events at which most cells undergo programmed cell death (Chapter 10). A few cells may restart proliferating during the crisis period and become immortal cell lines. Cancer cells *in vivo* may have acquired some of the properties of these post-crisis, cultured cells. Little is known about causative events linked to senescence and crisis except that chromosome instability and the enzyme telomerase are involved (Chapter 10).

Genes involved in carcinogenesis are sometimes classified into those that influence the lifespan of cells and those that have other effects such as altering sensitivity to external stimuli. The former group tend to code for nuclear repressor proteins such as p53 and Rb, whereas the latter category code for extranuclear oncogene proteins such as ras and erbB2. The functions of these gene products are described in Chapter 6. This generalisation should not be taken too far; one exception is the mitochondrial protein Bcl2. Loss of Bcl2 effectively extends lifespan by decreasing cell death (Chapter 10). Immortalisation of cultured cells has been equated with initiation.

Any discussion on build-up of errors in cell DNA (see above) must involve mutation rates. Mutation rates for normal cells increase with age; in culture this means the number of cell doublings, and the same phenomenon occurs with normal human cells *in vivo*. Biological age of cells is related to the number of divisions they have undergone; the higher the number of divisions, the 'older' the cell. This behaviour in culture equates with the clinical picture of cancer being more common in older people (Figure 1.1). Mechanisms must exist in normal cells to generate and accelerate mutations with age. The same applies in cancer cells but there is unresolved debate as to whether or not the normal picture is adequate to explain the mutator phenotype ascribed to cancer cells (Chapter 8). The mutation rate varies according to cell type and it may be that the rate in embryonic cells determines the rate in normal adult cells, which in turn influences cancer risk for that cell type. This is only a hypothesis but the inference would be that high incidence sites such as breast would have higher mutation rates than low incidence sites such as brain.

Genes can be carcinogenic: oncogenes

Cell culture provides a means of growing cells whose genetic complement has been manipulated by molecular techniques and analysing the biological effects of those manipulations. The technique of transfection (introducing foreign DNA into intact cultured cells) was initially used to compare DNA fragments from normal and cancer cells. The carcinogenic potential of the ras gene from bladder cancer was identified in this way (Chapter 6). This experiment indicated that a single gene, ras, was capable of generating cancers whereas animal biologists (see above), epidemiologists and clinical geneticists (see below) had shown a requirement for multi-hit mechanisms. This was resolved when it was realised that the host cells were not truly normal but had already undergone genetic changes prior to transfection. Similar experiments with different oncogenes showed that, although a few like Rb and neu could generate cancers on their own, in the majority of cases at least two were required.

Transfection experiments are also used to test the effects of specific mutations on gene function. For example, mutations engineered in codon 12 of the ras oncogene increased its transforming potential and decreased its guanosine triphosphatase (GTPase) activity thus providing a cause-and-effect link between these two functions.

Loss of gene function can be carcinogenic

The above results indicate that cancers can result from acquisition of genetic information, but loss of such information is at least as important. If a normal fibroblast is fused with a cancer cell in culture, the hybrid behaves not as a cancer but as a normal cell when transplanted into nude mice (Figure 2.8). Thus, the normal phenotype is dominant as it generates a product capable of inhibiting the cancer phenotype. Several such inhibitory genes have been identified, many of which are involved in regulating cell proliferation and death. Terms such as 'repressor', 'anti-oncogene', 'recessive' and 'loss of function' have been used to describe this phenomenon (Chapter 6). When these 'normal' hybrids are further cultured, they lose chromosomes and revert to a cancer-like behaviour because a repressor gene on a normal chromosome is lost.

Figure 2.8

Cell hybrids show that inhibitory factors are lost in cancers.

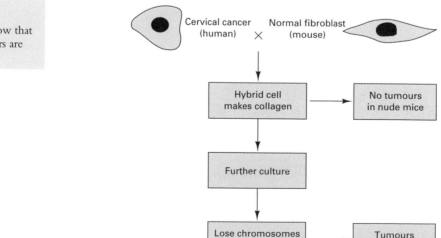

This type of experiment also demonstrates the inverse link between differentiation and carcinogenesis. Normal fibroblasts synthesise collagen (an index of differentiation) and this property is retained by the hybrid but lost when cells become tumorigenic.

DNA sequences that do not code for proteins are important

The above discussion about DNA changes conveys the impression that only coding sequences or their immediate regulatory regions are altered during carcinogenesis. This is not correct as mutations in microsatellite DNA may also participate. This type of DNA is made up of multiple 2 to 4 oligonucleotide repeats of $C:A/G:T$ whose functions are unknown. Currently the important relevance of microsatellite DNA is that an increased size is a marker for one type of DNA repair defect (mismatch repair). Such defects contribute to accelerated accumulation of mutations (Chapter 8). A second situation where non-coding sequences are relevant to carcinogenesis is in the replication of telomeric termini of chromosomes. These are composed of tandem TTAGGG repeats which require a special replication process. Chromosome instability occurs if telomere replication is disrupted (Chapter 10).

Clinical data

Data relevant to pathogenesis of cancers can be obtained from several sources.

Epidemiology

Age at which cancers occur indicates the number of changes required for carcinogenesis

Cancers most commonly arise in older people (Figure 1.1) because time is needed to accumulate the multiple changes required. It follows that the more changes (hits, errors) required, the greater the age at which that cancer is likely to occur. Most cancers show a linear relationship between log (age) and log (incidence):

$$\text{probability of getting cancer} = \text{age}^n$$

where n = number of changes. For colon cancer (Figure 1.1) $n = 3$–6, which is gratifyingly close to the number of genetic changes actually identified thus far in this cancer (see below).

A limited number of cancers arise at an earlier age because fewer changes are required. Retinoblastoma (eye cancer) is one such example that results from the loss of both alleles of the **r**etino**b**lastoma (Rb) gene. In the familial form of this cancer, one hit is inherited through the germ cells and one acquired after birth. The early age of onset of retinoblastoma (before age 2) is due to only two hits being required, one for each Rb allele (Chapter 9). The Rb gene codes for a protein that normally blocks cell division (Chapters 6 and 10).

The changes identified by the above mean values represent the number of rate-limiting mutations required and does not imply that additional mutations cannot contribute to the overall process of carcinogenesis.

Rate of error accumulation accelerates: genetic instability

In the retinoblastoma example, acquisition of the first hit invariably leads to the second one, which would be unexpected if it were a random event. Something about the first hit increases the probability of the second one occurring. Similarly, the mutation rates measured in young, normal cells are too low to explain the observed age–incidence data for many common cancers (Chapter 8); something happens to accelerate change. This genetic instability, also called mutator phenotype or **r**eplication **e**rror **r**epair (RER) phenotype, occurs in many cancers.

Risk factors characterise carcinogenic events

The changes identified by the above methods do not indicate their relationship to the stages of carcinogenesis identified by experimental biologists. Other types of epidemiological study can provide such data. The causes of occupational cancers associated with certain industries have been identified through epidemiological studies and the causative agents equated with initiation. Thus, the genotoxic chemical β-naphthylamine previously used in the rubber industry caused bladder cancer, whereas ionising radiation from atomic bombs had widespread carcinogenic effects due to the DNA damage it caused (Chapter 8). Clear-cut as these examples are, it is difficult to prove an initiation and promotion requirement for common cancers like those of colon, prostate and breast. In these situations, the strength of epidemiological data is in identifying risk factors that influence human carcinogenesis without necessarily showing the stage at which those factors work. For example, people who have a diet high in saturated fats have an elevated probability of developing one of several types of cancer but why this should be is unclear (Table 4.7). The increasing linkage of molecular and epidemiological studies will help resolve this type of problem. With cervical cancer, comparison of specific types of human papilloma virus by polymerase chain reaction in normal and abnormal cervical tissues implicates this virus as an early and possible initiating influence in this cancer (Chapter 6).

Pathology

The judgements made by pathologists as to the nature, malignant or otherwise, of tissue samples are largely based on the divergence from normal appearance of the material being examined. It is therefore logical that the more abnormal a sample, the more likely it is to have progressed towards malignancy. This conclusion is substantiated by clinical observation of the behaviour of such abnormalities such that simple hyperproliferation (hyperplasia) is less dangerous than more complex types of hyperproliferation accompanied by additional cellular changes. This equates with model 4 in Figure 2.1. Thus, in one series of endometrial (lining of the uterus) analyses, untreated patients with simple (cystic) hyperplasia had <1% chance of developing cancer as compared to 27% and 82% for those with the more complex histologies of adenomatous and atypical hyperplasia respectively; carcinoma *in situ* invariably became invasive if treatment was withheld.

For glandular epithelial cancers such as those of breast and endometrium the sequence shown in Figure 2.1, model 4 would be a typical description of their natural history but variations do occur, e.g. colon and thyroid adenocarcinomas progress through stages known as adenomas.

Progression is monitored histologically according to degree of differentiation and of tumour spread. Various grading protocols are used to assess differentiation and increasingly, immunohistochemical, biochemical or molecular markers are used to better define this feature. Thus, good morphological data have been crucial in generating information on where specific pathological changes are sited within the carcinogenic sequence and have provided the material that biologists can use to identify molecular changes. This is compatible with either models 3 or 4 in Figure 2.1. Molecular data from colon cancers indicate that the sequence in which changes occur is less important than the number accumulated, which is difficult to reconcile with model 1 (Figure 2.1) in which initiation must precede progression (see below).

Clinical evidence

Clinicians come into contact with a cancer at a relatively late stage in its development and therefore deal mainly with progression rather than carcinogenesis. A growth detected in a clinic has already passed the halfway stage in its life (Figure 2.9). Earlier detection identifies smaller cancers, e.g. by the presence of haemoglobin in faeces for colon cancer or X-rays for breast cancer (mammography).

Figure 2.9

Clinical symptoms related to cancer size.

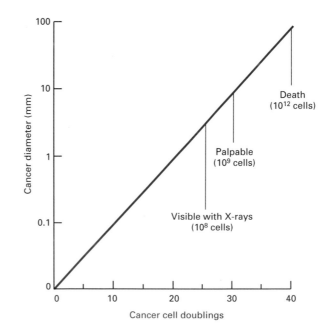

Histological data indicates that such cancers tend to be at an earlier stage in their progression than those detected by symptom appearance.

Clinicians have to deal with progression rather than carcinogenesis, and to select a patient's treatment, they must determine how advanced that progression might be (Chapter 13).

Linking laboratory and clinic

Initiation and promotion

The various mechanisms described above all refer to the same entity, a specific cancer, so it is necessary to relate the various terms and descriptions used in laboratory experiments to human conditions. The initiation and promotion model is especially relevant as it has been so influential. This is more than an exercise in semantics because the concept of initiation has generated an industry devoted to the identification of agents that cause it. This is valid if it results in better health but questionable if natural processes such as metabolic free radical generation, diet and endogenous hormone changes account for the majority of human cancers. There are clear examples with lung cancer (tobacco smoke), bladder cancer and leukaemia (ionising radiation) where initiating agents have been identified. However, with the exception of smoking and lung cancer, these are not of the first importance. Of greater relevance are the common cancers. It is difficult to define initiating events in colon cancer, leukaemias unrelated to radiation or hormone-related breast and prostate cancers. The main feature of hormones, which are usually defined as promotional agents, is that they are mitogenic for the cells whose risk they increase and proliferation alone might generate sufficient errors to cause a breast or prostate cancer. This idea has attractions for other cancers − brain cells (slow growth) rarely develop into cancers whereas colon epithelium (fast growth) frequently becomes neoplastic. However, the inevitable exceptions exist, such as the mucosal epithelium of the mouth (fast growth) which is not a major cancer. It might be explained by the continual loss (exfoliation) of both normal and damaged cells during eating. If the 'proliferation alone' model has merit, a discrete early step under the heading 'initiation' may not be necessary. It might clarify conceptual problems about the word 'initiation' (see Animal studies above) if it were dropped in favour of 'DNA damage' or 'mutation'. It may be that for some human tumours, the clear-cut distinction between an initiating event followed by promotion (Figure 2.1, model 1) should be modified (Figure 2.10). Continual exposure of cells to mutational events (DNA damage), linked with proliferative pressure (promotion) could generate the cellular changes required for carcinogenesis. Cancer progression to a more dedifferentiated state would be a continuation of these events.

Mutation rate increases with cell age (Chapter 8) in both normal and cancer cells, so it is not clear whether there is anything special about cancer cells in this respect. Based on the data from normal cells, it has been hypothesised that carcinogenesis is a natural consequence of getting old. Acceleration in the mutation rate can be

Figure 2.10

Initiation and
promotion: modified
model.

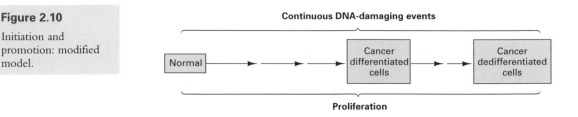

caused by defective DNA repair, increased proliferation, decreased apoptosis or combinations of these processes (Chapter 10).

As depicted in Figure 2.10, both damaging and proliferative influences are continuous. This would be correct for damaging events of endogenous origin, such as free radical formation or incomplete repair of misaligned bases, but it does not preclude additional exposures to exogenous carcinogens such as ultraviolet light or drugs (Chapter 8). Proliferative signals could derive from exogenous factors such as diet, virus infection or hormones (contraceptive pills, hormone replacement therapy) or endogenous sources such as hormonal changes. In the case of hormones, they fluctuate on a monthly basis (menstrual cycle) and at different stages of development (puberty, menopause).

No single model will explain the pathogenesis of all human cancers but it is important to have appropriate models against which data can be tested.

Angiogenesis

Animal studies identified angiogenesis as a crucial event in cancer growth; the same is true in humans, both in the transition from *in situ* to invasive growth and for metastasis. In the case of transition from *in situ* to invasive growth, an angiogenic switch is activated at the start of invasive growth of breast cancer and in the transition from CIN II to CIN III (**c**ervical **i**ntraepithelial **n**eoplasia, stages II or III) of cervical cancer prior to invasion of the surrounding tissue.

Conclusions

At the molecular level, animal and cell biological experiments have identified DNA sequences and proteins directly relevant to human cancers. The ras oncogene and p53 repressor genes were first identified by combinations of molecular and cell biological techniques, and numerous other examples are provided throughout this book. Molecular analysis is also helping to identify causative agents for specific human cancers (Chapter 4). Knowledge is accumulating about types of mutation generated by different carcinogens (mutational spectral analysis) so that it is becoming possible to predict the type of agent causing a mutation (see Chapter 8).

No single model will explain the pathogenesis of all human cancers. Two specific examples – a solid tumour (colon cancer) and a blood cancer (chronic myeloid leukaemia) – will be used to illustrate the relevance of the terms and features derived from experimental systems to these very different human cancers. More detailed molecular descriptions of the events to be described will be found in subsequent chapters.

Colon cancer

Clinical picture

Adenocarcinoma of the colon is a common cancer accounting for about 15% of all cancers in Western countries and occurs equally in men and women, mainly between the ages of 55 and 70; Appendix A gives more clinical details. About half of all patients survive for five years after first detection but this depends on the degree of spread (stage) when the cancer is first detected. A commonly used staging system (Dukes') divides degree of spread into three categories depending on whether the cancer is localised (A), has invaded through the colon wall (B) or has spread outside the colon (C). The cancer metastasises by several routes. Direct invasion through the colonic mucosa results in peritoneal outgrowths whereas liver is the major site of blood-borne spread. Lymph nodes become involved via the lymphatic vessels.

Presenting symptoms include irregular and problematic bowel movements and the appearance of blood in the faeces. Blood in the faeces has been developed as a method for early detection of abnormal changes based on the detection of faecal iron derived from haemoglobin. Surgery is the main treatment together with chemotherapy and radiotherapy.

Several types of colon cancer can be identified according to the degree and type of familial involvement. About 80% are sporadic but the remaining 20% exist in two hereditary forms: **f**amilial **a**denomatous **p**olyposis **c**oli (FAP) and **h**ereditary **n**on-**p**olyposis **c**olon **c**ancer (HNPCC) or Lynch's syndrome. As the names imply, FAP is characterised by thousands of benign, adenomatous polyps at an early age (about 20), that if untreated progress to invasive cancer. Cancers appear in HNPCC cases without passing through this intermediate stage. Both familial types occur before age 50, earlier than the sporadic cancers.

Figure 2.11

Gene changes during colon carcinogenesis.

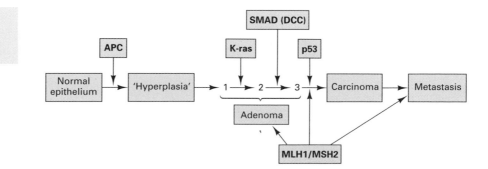

Cellular changes

Colon cancers have clonal origins in the epithelial stem cells at the base of the crypt (Figure 15.3). The subsequent sequence of events defined from pathology samples is analogous to model 4 in Figure 2.1 although some of the names are different (Figure 2.11). Benign adenomas are largely classified by size and degree of cellular abnormality whilst 'carcinoma *in situ*' is not a term that is applied to colon cancer. The availability of tissue from each of these stages has allowed analysis of DNA alterations at each stage, and a picture has been built up to describe which DNA changes contribute to different stages of development. The mutations identified in familial cancers also occur in sporadic cases, but to different extents. APC mutations occur in most sporadic colon cancers (Table 2.1) and alteration of this gene is the rate-limiting step in colon carcinogenesis. Because of its importance, the gene has been called a gatekeeper gene. The difference between FAP familial cancers and sporadic forms is that the sporadic forms result from somatic cell mutations whereas germline mutations contribute to the familial connection. This difference in source of mutational events is compatible with the earlier appearance of the familial cancers as fewer errors have to be generated. In contrast to FAP, HNPCC mutations have only been identified in a minority of sporadic cancers (Table 2.1).

Additional DNA alterations have been identified by their loss of heterozygosity (Chapter 9), whereas more general defects occur during progression that increase the DNA content per nucleus (ploidy).

DNA mutations can result in loss or gain in function of the base sequences affected. Both loss and gain are required for colon carcinogenesis (Table 2.1) with the loss predominating. Loss of function is characteristic of repressor genes whereas gain of function occurs with oncogenes (Chapter 7).

Mechanisms

The functions of the genes listed in Table 2.1 can be related to general behavioural changes discussed earlier. The normal adenomatous polyposis coli (APC) gene codes for a protein that mediates signal transduction from a cell membrane adhesion molecule (a cadherin) to the cytoskeleton and nucleus (Chapter 11). Loss of this function disrupts the tight linkage of epithelial cells in normal colon and represents

Table 2.1 Gene changes identified in colon cancers.

Gene	Type of change	Chromosome	Function	Cancers showing that change (%)
APC	loss	5	Cell adhesion	>70
K–ras	gain	11	Signal transduction	50
SMAD (DCC)	loss	18	Proliferation, differentiation	>70
p53	loss	17	DNA repair, apoptosis	>70
MSH2	loss	2	DNA repair	5
MLH1	loss	3	DNA repair	35

an early step in the process of invasion. Its gatekeeper role might suggest that it functions as an initiator but this creates conceptual problems for the classical model (Figure 2.1, model 1) in that it is not always the first gene to be altered (see below) in sporadic cancers. However, it is compatible with a promotional or proliferative role in either that model or its modified form (Figure 2.10).

The original model of gene changes associated with colon carcinogenesis included one gene called DCC (**d**eleted in **c**olon **c**ancer), sometimes called MCC (**m**utated in **c**olon **c**ancer). It was initially described as coding for a cell adhesion molecule (N–CAM) and then for a membrane receptor for polypeptides (netrins) responsible for directional movement of cells (Chapter 12). It now appears that, due to an error in mapping the chromosomal location of DCC, the real culprit is a nearby gene, SMAD4, involved in the signalling pathway for **t**ransforming **g**rowth **f**actor **β** (TGF-β). TGF-β is a growth inhibitory, differentiation-inducing cytokine (Chapters 10 and 11) so loss of signal transduction from this factor could mediate tumour promotion. In mice containing an APC deletion on one allele, knocking out SMAD4 increased the size and invasiveness of adenomas whereas DCC deletions had no effect. The relevance of these mice experiments to human colon remains to be established, but in this book the original DCC terminology has been changed to SMAD.

The K-ras mutation activates signal transduction from membrane to nucleus by virtue of the loss of its GTPase activity (Chapter 11) whilst DNA repair defects (MSH2 and MLH1) increase the probability of accumulating further errors in the DNA (Chapter 8). The p53 protein links three cellular functions: proliferation, death and DNA repair (Chapter 10). In normal cells, p53 blocks proliferation and enables completion of DNA repair before DNA synthesis takes place. If repair is incomplete, the cell dies. Loss of p53 function therefore contributes to propagation of damaged DNA to daughter cells. A minority of cancers exhibit gene changes not listed in Table 2.1. These include various cyclins (4% of cancers), myc (2%) and erbB2 (2%).

The functions listed in Table 2.1 embrace many cell functions and indicate the varied nature and chromosomal involvement of the multiple changes required for carcinogenesis and progression. The sequence of the changes shown in Figure 2.11 is highly simplified. Not all colon cancers pass through all stages (Table 2.1); the order in which changes occur can vary and any one gene can have mutations in different bases.

One signalling pathway not shown in Figure 2.11 is the pathway for prostaglandins. Clinical trials on the beneficial effects of aspirin, a **n**on-**s**teroidal **anti-**inflammatory **d**rug (NSAID), in patients with heart and rheumatism problems also indicated a marked protective effect against colon carcinogenesis; aspirin markedly decreased the risk of getting both cancer and polyps (Chapter 14). Aspirin inhibits **c**ycl**o****o**xygenase (COX) enzymes responsible for prostaglandin synthesis, although the mechanisms by which COX enzymes influence colon carcinogenesis are unclear (Chapter 11).

The multiple pathways are most clearly seen by comparing FAP and HNPCC; FAP involves polyp formation whereas HBPCC does not. Variation in sequence or requirement for specific events is demonstrated by the fact that of colon cancers exhibiting changes in four of the genes in Table 2.1 (K-ras, APC, p53, SMAD) 10%

had all four, 40% three and 80% only two alterations. The overall accumulation of errors rather than their sequence may be important. The late involvement of p53 in this cancer contrasts with that seen in other tumours and accentuates the point about variable routes of carcinogenesis. This diversity is even seen at the single gene level. Most germline mutations of the APC gene generate stop codons and a truncated protein is therefore produced. However, amino acid substitutions and frameshifts have also been identified. Somatic cell mutations in the APC gene show a lower proportion of stop codons with a more localised distribution than seen with germline mutations (Chapter 11).

Relevance to models of carcinogenesis

The histological picture fits with model 4 in Figure 2.1 with the caveats that colon adenoma and polyps should be considered as stages between hyperplasia and carcinoma. Also the term 'carcinoma *in situ*' is not used with colon cancer. The sequence of gene changes is compatible with model 3. Initiation (model 1) is usually shown as the first event in carcinogenesis; thus if the APC gene is that event, it is difficult to reconcile changes in cell–cell contact with initiation, and the modified model in Figure 2.10 might be more appropriate. DNA repair defects resulting from MSH2 and MLH1 mutations on the other hand, by generating a mutator phenotype, would be prime candidates as an initiating event but they only occur in a minority of sporadic cancers.

It is important to identify the causes of the genetic alterations. Chemical carcinogens can generate colon cancers in rodents but, in humans, one is largely confined to talking about environmental or dietary carcinogens with minimal definition of what that means. There is a 19-fold difference between countries with the highest incidence (USA) and lowest incidence (India) of colon cancer; this indicates a lifestyle effect, probably dietary. High meat and animal fat plus low-fibre diets increase risk but the mechanism remains to be established. Production of carcinogens during cooking of meat is one possibility; animal and cell culture experiments indicate that fat can be a promoter (Chapter 4). Activated ras would increase cell proliferation and play a promotional role.

Chronic myeloid leukaemia

Clinical picture

CML is characterised by the progressive replacement of normal bone marrow cells by mature myeloid cells that have altered sensitivity to normal regulatory mechanisms (Figure 2.12). The ratio of leukaemic to normal cells gradually increases to a critical level when a 'blast crisis' occurs. If uncorrected, this leads to blast cell invasion of vital organs such as the brain. These abnormal blast cells have variable phenotypes but myeloblasts are commonly seen in about two-thirds of cases and lymphoblasts in one-third, although the phenotypes can change with time or even be a mixture (Figure 2.12). The acute phase rapidly results in death due to haemorrhage in the invaded organ. It takes about 4 years from first detection to death.

Figure 2.12

Development of chronic myeloid leukemia.

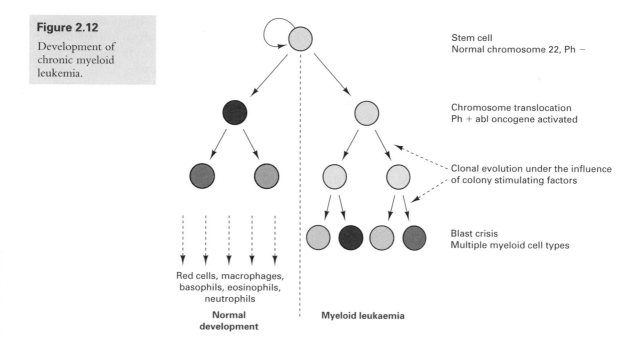

Stem cell
Normal chromosome 22, Ph −

Chromosome translocation
Ph + abl oncogene activated

Clonal evolution under the influence
of colony stimulating factors

Blast crisis
Multiple myeloid cell types

Red cells, macrophages,
basophils, eosinophils,
neutrophils

**Normal
development**

Myeloid leukaemia

Cellular changes

CML is characterised by the possession of an abnormally small chromosome 22, the **Ph**iladelphia chromosome (Ph), caused by the translocation of part of its genetic material to chromosome 9. This brings the abl oncogene from chromosome 9 under the regulatory influence of oncogene bcr on chromosome 22, increasing the tyrosine kinase activity of abl (Chapter 6). Different breakpoints occur in the bcr gene in different patients although the biochemical end result is the same − elevated tyrosine kinase activity in the myeloid cells that renders them hyperresponsive to growth factors. This variability in breakpoints with the same end result illustrates the multiple pathways to cancer evident from experimental models. When CML progresses to the terminal acute phase, additional chromosome abnormalities can be detected such that the chromosome number changes from the normal 46 (diploid) to a modal number of 47–50. Cell proliferation rates of CML do not increase in the acute phase so progression involves more than simply increasing growth rate.

Analysis of chromosomes and of isoenzymes such as glucose-6-phosphate dehydrogenase indicates that clonal selection occurs at least twice: the original generation of Ph and during events leading up to blast crisis.

Mechanisms

CML results from blocked differentiation and continued proliferation of immature myelocytes (Figure A.4). The chromosome translocation resulting in increased tyrosine kinase activity is a crucial event as transfection of the abl cDNA into normal cells generates leukaemias. This is probably not equivalent to initiation because, although the protein product of the translocation has the properties of an initiating agent as defined in experimental models, it begs the question of what causes the translocation. Whatever causes the chromosome change would have a better claim to be the initiator. Candidates identified through animal experiments include viruses, radiation, immune deficiency and carcinogenic chemicals. Of these, only radiation has been identified as a causal influence in humans.

Little is known about promotional events other than the increased activity of growth factors such as **c**olony-**s**timulating **f**actor (CSF). Animal experiments show that continuous exogenous or autocrine production of CSF will produce hyperplasia in normal cells but not leukaemias. On the other hand, if the cells are first immortalised with a virus, overproduction of CSF will generate leukaemias. Similar changes may occur with human CML, but as none of the observed chromosome changes involve CSF genes, more subtle changes must be happening.

Transition to the acute phase, characterised by the blast crisis, is equivalent to progression. Multiple events are required for each stage, much as in the experimental models, but apart from the chromosome changes, the nature of these events is obscure. The only other identified agent is a family of growth factors, CSFs. As their name implies, these glycoproteins are required for proliferation of CML colonies, analogous to anchorage-independent growth. CML cells will survive but not grow if suspended in agar but addition of CSF stimulates this anchorage-independent growth; they are therefore CSF-dependent for growth, a property that is retained by most, but not all blast cells. As in the experimental models, human CML can progress by more than one pathway.

PATHOLOGY: DEFINING A NEOPLASM

3

Key points

- Tissue and cell architecture are used to decide whether a growth is malignant.
- Pathology can distinguish between benign and malignant growths.
- Pathology defines the type of cancer.
- Pathology helps to determine prognosis and treatment.

Introduction

An understanding of pathology is essential to any description of cancer biology because it plays important roles in several clinical situations as well as helping to elucidate the steps in carcinogenesis. The steps in carcinogenesis were described in the previous chapter and so more general aspects of pathology will be dealt with here. Three types of pathology can be defined depending on whether intact tissues, individual cells, or chemical analysis of body fluids or tissues are involved (Table 3.1). Cancer is the growth of one or, occasionally, a few cell types at the expense of others and this differential growth disrupts the normal interrelationships between the different cell types and their extracellular matrix. These features can be visualised by microscopic examination of stained tissue sections (histopathology). Cytology on the other hand deals with single or small clumps of cells removed from a suspect site. Chemical pathology, which will be described more fully in Chapter 13, involves chemical analysis of tissue, blood or urine.

The term 'cancer' tends to be used differently in experimental and clinical settings; experimentalists adopt a more general usage than clinicians. Experimentalists use the term to include abnormal growth regardless of whether or not invasion and metastasis occurs. This is understandable as most chemically induced growths in animals tend not to metastasise and cultured cells have no opportunity to exhibit this property. Neoplasm (new growth) or tumour are terms that cover this broader definition of abnormal growth. Clinically, a cancer is more precisely defined as being invasive and able to metastasise (malignant) in contrast to benign growths, which remain localised. Use of the term 'cancer' should be confined to invasive growths. Other distinctions between benign and malignant growths are listed in Table 3.2 and further described below. Benign growths are sometimes, but not always precursors of malignant growths. Colon cancer and thyroid cancer are examples where benign growths turn malignant, whereas benign prostate and breast growths are not precursors of malignant growths.

Table 3.1 The objectives of pathology.

Pathology
Histopathology: tissues
Cytology: individual cells
Chemical pathology: analysis of tissue, blood and urine

Diagnosis
Is it cancer?
What type of cancer? Histogenesis
Has the surgeon removed it all?

Prognosis
What is the clinical outlook?

Identifying features
Cell and tissue architecture
Differentiation: degree it resembles normal
Cell structure: nucleus, mitoses, nuclear/cytoplasmic ratio
Localised or invasive (stroma, blood vessels)

Methods
Staining
Immunohistochemistry: protein
In situ hybridisation: mRNA
DNA characterisation

One role of pathology is to distinguish between benign and malignant cells, because benign cells are not usually life-threatening and therefore treatments of the two types of growth are different. A second function is to determine the cellular origin of a cancer (histogenesis), as a cancer in an organ can have several origins. Thus, in lung, smoking generates epithelial cancers whereas mesothelial cancers result from asbestos exposure. As treatments are different, the importance of determining histogenesis is clear. Likewise it is not axiomatic that a liver growth originated in that organ as it may have metastasised from elsewhere, and there are even tumours whose cellular origins cannot be determined (cancers of unknown origin).

Table 3.2 Comparison of benign and malignant growths.

Feature	Benign	Malignant
Edges	Encapsulated	Irregular
Metastasis	No	Yes
Invasion	No	Yes
Comparison to normal	Good	Variable, often none
Growth rate	Low	High
Nuclei	Normal	Variable, irregular
Life-threatening	Unusual	Usual

Carcinogenesis involves a series of changes that are reflected in an increasing departure from normal morphology. Pathology helps to define boundaries in this sequence of events, but as changes continue to occur after a cancer has formed, cell characterisation also has a role to play as a predictive (prognostic) tool to determine the likely course of the disease. Another function of pathology is in monitoring completeness of surgery. Because cancers have ill-defined margins, it is sometimes difficult for a surgeon to decide what should be removed; microscopic analysis of an excised lump can tell whether or not cancer cells occur at its edges and thereby provide evidence as to efficiency of removal.

Box 3.1　　**Classifying cancers**

Neoplasms are classified as being benign or malignant; malignant neoplasms are equivalent to cancer. Cancers are described according to their cell of origin and the tissue in which they arise (Table 3.3). Most common cancers

Table 3.3　Terminology.

General
Growth: a vague term that covers any collection of hyperproliferative cells
Neoplasm: general term used to identify a new growth without defining the characteristics of that growth
Tumour: general term used to describe any abnormal growth
Cancer: invasive growth with abnormal cellular and architectural features.

Epithelium (carcinoma)
Glandular, e.g. prostate: adenocarcinoma
Squamous, e.g. cervix: carcinoma

Mesenchyme (sarcoma)
Smooth muscle: leiomyosarcoma. Benign hyperproliferation is called a leiomyoma (fibroid)
Bone: osteosarcoma
Fat cells: liposarcoma. Benign hyperproliferation is called a lipoma

Nervous system
Eye: retinoblastoma
Astrocytes: astrocytoma

White blood cells (leukaemia)*
Myeloid cells: myelocytic leukaemia
Lymphocytes: lymphocytic leukaemia
Lymphoma: solid tumour derived from B or T lymphocytes

*Can be subdivided into chronic and acute forms.

arise in epithelial cells and they carry the suffix 'carcinoma' preceded by the name of the cell type involved. Frequently, the type of epithelium is additionally identified, so that a glandular epithelium generates an adenocarcinoma (e.g. prostatic adenocarcinoma) whereas a cancer of squamous epithelium would be a squamous cell carcinoma (e.g. cervical squamous cell carcinoma). Mesenchymal cells give rise to 'sarcomas' prefixed by the cell of origin, a format followed for other cancers. White blood cell cancers, leukaemias, are typical in this respect but are further defined according to the speed with which they develop. Thus, **a**cute **m**yelocytic **l**eukaemia (AML) and **c**hronic **m**yelocytic **l**eukaemia (CML) exhibit rapid and slow onset of symptoms respectively, and are different diseases with different causes. In contrast to leukaemic cells that circulate in the bloodstream, lymphomas of either B-cell or T-cell origin remain as solid cell aggregates. For historical reasons, some cancers are confusingly named after their discoverers: Burkitt's lymphoma is a B-lymphocyte cancer, Wilms' tumour is a renal carcinoma in young children and Kaposi's sarcoma arises from endothelial cells of blood vessels.

Histopathology

Histopathology is the routine method for characterising an excised lump. Diagnosis relies not only on the appearance of the cells but also on the tissue architecture, reflecting neoplastic cell relationships to the extracellular matrix and other cells (Figure 3.1). The main features that distinguish an epithelial cancer from its normal,

Figure 3.1

Glandular epithelium.

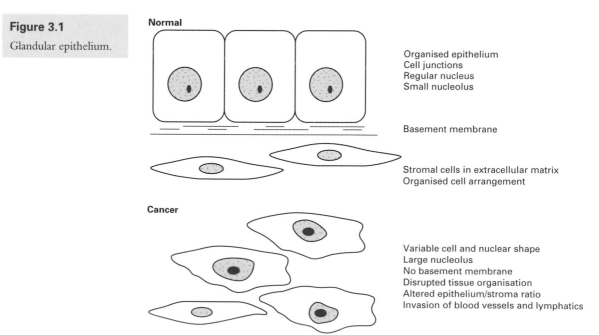

Normal

Organised epithelium
Cell junctions
Regular nucleus
Small nucleolus

Basement membrane

Stromal cells in extracellular matrix
Organised cell arrangement

Cancer

Variable cell and nuclear shape
Large nucleolus
No basement membrane
Disrupted tissue organisation
Altered epithelium/stroma ratio
Invasion of blood vessels and lymphatics

progenitor cells are shown in cartoon format in Figure 3.1 with a real example in Figure 3.2. The comparison of normal and cancerous colon in Figure 3.2 conveys the partial change in epithelial characteristics associated with a moderately differentiated cancer. The regular arrangement of crypt cells is retained in places but lost elsewhere in the section; invasive cancer cells are present in the stroma. The normal cells have regularly shaped nuclei in contrast to the heterogeneous sizes in the cancer; mitotic (proliferating) cells are evident in the cancer but not the normal colon. No secretory vacuoles are present in the cancer, indicating some loss of differentiated function. Such examples do not convey the remarkable heterogeneity of structures contained within a cancerous growth. Figure 3.3 is a section of a breast cancer that indicates this heterogeneity with normal ducts, *in situ* carcinoma, invasive carcinoma and infiltrating lymphocytes all present in one area of a cancer excised by surgery. This section provides a snapshot in time of what happens during carcinogenesis. The normal mammary epithelium surrounds a duct; during carcinogenesis the epithelium proliferates into and fills the duct but does not penetrate the basement membrane. The cells have the abnormalities represented in Figure 3.1 but they have not become invasive; this stage is known as *in situ*

Cellular stroma below a single layer of epithelial cells

Disorganised structure with few stromal cells.
Some residual crypt organisation

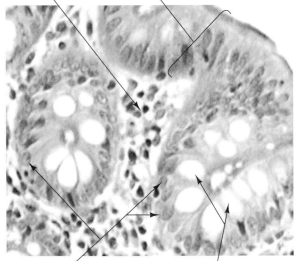

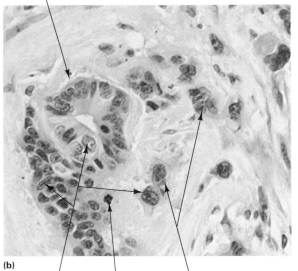

(a)

Regular shaped nuclei
No mitoses

Abundant secretion

Well-organised tissue with distinct glands and stroma

(b)

Irregular, large nuclei   No secretion

Mitotic figures   Cancer cells in the stroma

Figure 3.2

Colon epithelium:
(a) normal and
(b) a moderately
differentiated cancer.

carcinoma. Cancer cells that have become invasive are dispersed throughout the stroma (extracellular matrix proteins such as collagen plus mesenchymal cells). Blood vessels supplying nutrients and as potential routes for metastasis are also present in the stroma. This section has been immunohistochemically stained with an antibody against a heat shock protein (HSP27) to illustrate another aspect of heterogeneity within the cells that make up a cancer. Expression of specific proteins alters during

Figure 3.3

Histological sections of a breast cancer. NORMAL, mammary duct lined by epithelium. IN SITU, carcinoma that has not invaded the basement membrane (B). INVASIVE, carcinoma cells in the stroma; the stroma also contains infiltrating lymphocytes and blood vessels. The section has been stained with an antibody against a heat-shock protein (HSP27) to highlight differential expression of this protein in breast cells at different stages of cancer development.

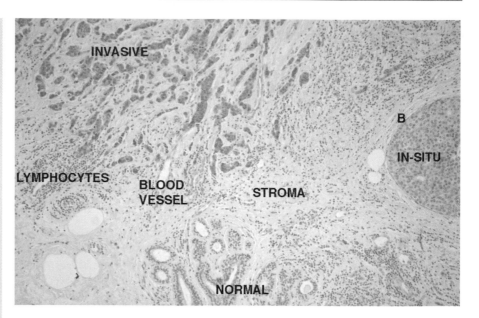

carcinogenesis and can be used for diagnostic purposes (Chapter 13). In this example, expression is low in normal epithelium, is slightly raised in *in situ* carcinoma but is greatly enhanced in the invasive cancer.

Benign growths, such as lipomas (fat cells) or leiomyomas (muscle cells) caused by overproliferation of specific cell types that resemble the cell of origin, are encapsulated and do not invade surrounding areas. Malignant lesions, on the other hand, can profoundly damage their surroundings. Epithelial cancers destroy the basement membrane and invade the stroma thus increasing the ratio of epithelial cells to stromal cells. Leukaemic cells take over the bone marrow and disrupt the balance of haemopoietic cells; sarcomas also disrupt normal architecture.

The cells themselves are also informative (Table 3.1). Benign cells closely resemble their normal antecedents and their nuclei have a regular shape with a small nucleolus. Malignant cells have a more aggressive appearance with convoluted cell membranes, irregularly shaped and large nuclei, pronounced nucleoli and little heterochromatin; the last two features reflect an active transcription machinery. If the cancer arose from cells with specialist functions, such as a glandular epithelium involved in production of a secretion, cytoplasmic changes are evident such as disorganisation of the endoplasmic reticulum and absence of secretions (Figure 3.2). This loss of differentiation (dedifferentiation) is a common accompaniment of carcinogenesis. Many cancers are graded on the above features to give an index of their degree of malignancy, which in turn can be used to predict subsequent behaviour of the cancer. Several grading systems exist (Chapter 13); some use all features of the cells and tissues, including number of mitotic figures, whilst others rely only on nuclear characteristics.

Cytology

This increasingly useful diagnostic technique relies on the characteristics of cells alone, but because it loses the benefit of tissue architecture, it provides less precise information than histopathology. It has the advantage over histopathology of requiring a less invasive procedure. Its most widespread use is in screening women for early signs of cervical cancer and with fine needle aspirates of suspicious breast lumps.

Immunohistochemistry

The use of antibodies to characterise antigen changes provides an additional way of defining abnormal cells. If a cellular antigen is gained, lost or altered in a cancer cell, that change can be used to characterise the cell. A good example is the repressor protein p53, which is mutated in many cancers (Chapter 6). Over half of such mutations result in a protein whose half-life is altered from minutes to hours; this longer-lived protein accumulates and can be detected. Thus, colon cancer cells are often p53 positive whereas benign (adenoma) or normal epithelial cells are not. As carcinogenesis involves progressive dedifferentiation and increased proliferation, markers of differentiation and proliferation are also useful (Chapter 13).

Molecular techniques

Techniques analogous to immunohistochemistry can also be used to monitor specific mRNAs (*in situ* hybridisation) or DNA (*in situ* PCR) in tissue sections, although they are mostly used for research rather than diagnostic purposes at the present time. The **p**olymerase **c**hain **r**eaction (PCR) is also used for detecting cancer cells in blood and lymph nodes (Chapter 13). Other molecular techniques, such as the detection of restriction length polymorphisms, are used to identify DNA mutations.

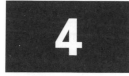

EPIDEMIOLOGY: IDENTIFYING CAUSES FOR HUMAN CANCERS

Key points

- Incidence of cancers in different populations provides clues about the causes.
- Risk factors can be identified that indicate causative events in cancer development.
- Geographical differences in cancer incidence indicate the importance of diet.
- The influence of diet on cancer is a complex one in which fat, vitamins, fibre and other agents are involved.
- Smoking, diet, sex hormones, increasing age and family history of cancer alter the risk of developing cancer.
- Most cancers could be prevented.
- Biochemical analyses provide additional information for epidemiological studies by identifying people at risk.
- Molecular epidemiology can be used to identify causative agents.

Introduction

Epidemiology, the study of disease distributions in human populations, is probably the single most important discipline that generates clues about factors that influence specific types of human cancers. Although laboratory experiments with animals and cell cultures can dissect molecular mechanisms and indicate the potential of chemicals or conditions to influence carcinogenesis, their applicability to real life can only be tested in humans. Epidemiological analysis is a major way of achieving that objective. This discipline involves comparisons of groups of people and its methodology has progressed markedly from the eighteenth-century observations that nuns get more breast cancer than other women and that scrotal cancer was common in chimneysweeps. The methods by which groups of people are compared are critical to decisions as to whether observed differences reflect a causal or artefactual link. Therefore those methods must be understood as well as the information generated therefrom.

Epidemiology is conveniently divided into two categories, descriptive and analytical, based on the type of data being used. A third category, molecular epidemiology, has entered the lexicon; here molecular analyses such as DNA or protein profiles are included as variables in the epidemiological studies.

Descriptive epidemiology

Descriptive epidemiology uses data from large populations; it draws general conclusions on which more specific analyses can be based. Figure 4.1 shows deaths from three cancers in the USA, indicating lung cancer to have been an increasing problem that has now reached a plateau, cancer of the stomach to be declining and colon/rectum cancer to be static. Such data indicate that a problem exists with lung cancer whereas something beneficial is happening for stomach cancer. However, the data tell us nothing about what causes those changes or what should be done to increase the benefits and decrease the adverse effects. Geographical distributions and influences of lifestyle, such as diet and environment, also provide important clues as to what might cause cancers.

Descriptive epidemiology is good at highlighting trends or differences, but more rigorous analytical epidemiology is needed to reveal aetiological relationships. Both methods are also useful for defining biological hypotheses that can be tested by other means.

Figure 4.1

Age-corrected male cancer deaths in the USA.

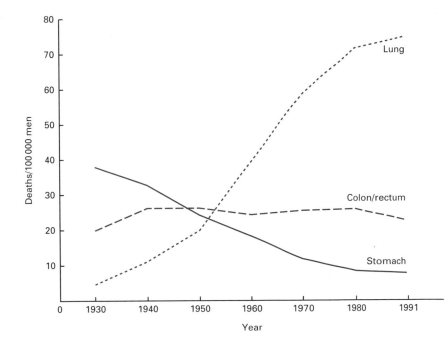

Box 4.1

Epidemiological methods and terminology

Descriptive epidemiology

Records of people's health and cause of death are used to correlate events such as the first detection of (*incidence*) or death from (*mortality*) a specific cancer with personal details like age, sex and race. Death certificates are an important source of information on mortality but incidence data is better obtained from population-based registries maintained by national and international organisations. From this data, *incidence rates* can be calculated like this:

$$\frac{\text{Number of people developing a cancer in a specific time period}}{\text{Total population at that time}}$$

A similar calculation is used to obtain *mortality rates*, but the number of people dying replaces those developing cancer. The time period can be one year or several years, and if the period is extended to encompass people of all ages throughout their life, it is called the *cumulative* or *lifetime rate*. This gives an index of the probability of getting (incidence) or dying from (mortality) a specific cancer sometime during a person's lifetime.

Population numbers are usually corrected per 100 000 people. According to Figure 4.1, the mortality rate from lung cancer in US men during the period 1989–91 was 75 per 100 000 population. The equivalent incidence rate for that population was 80 per 100 000 (not shown in Figure 4.1). US men born in 1940 have a 1 in 10 likelihood of getting lung cancer at some time in their life. These numbers are known as *crude incidence* or *mortality rates* because the data has not been corrected in any way. As many cancers occur in older people, it follows that an older population will have higher rates than a younger population, so uncorrected data can result in erroneous conclusions. For example, if one wishes to know how a Japanese lifestyle, based on a high-fish, low-fat diet, compares with a low-fish, high-fat Western diet, it is important not to let the different age profiles of the two populations confuse the results. This is remedied by correcting the crude data for age so that one can compare rates for populations of equivalent ages, a process that yields *age-corrected incidence* or *mortality rates*. *Prevalence* is analogous to incidence except that it represents *the number of cancer cases in a defined population at the time of data collection*, not just the new cases over a given period.

Age-corrected data are useful for comparing populations to get an idea of whether incidence of certain cancers is changing with time or whether a particular lifestyle correlates with specific cancers, but it gives little information on whether there is a cause-and-effect relationship. In the Japanese–Western comparison it turns out that stomach cancer is high in Japan whereas breast cancer shows the opposite pattern. But it would be wrong to immediately conclude that differences were due to diet, because breast cancer also correlates with number of typewriters! This highlights an important principle relevant to all epidemiological methods: any explanation for differences observed must be biologically plausible.

Analytical epidemiology

The essence of analytical work is the comparison of two or more groups of people with different characteristics. This generates a number called *relative risk* which indicates the risk associated with a given factor, e.g. smoking, as compared to an identical group not influenced by that factor. The term *odds ratio* approximates to the same thing. Because the range of values in a study can be large, it is important to obtain an estimate as to the limits within which the real risk lies. A commonly used method to achieve this is the *95% confidence limit*. This gives the range of values between which the real value has a 95% probability of lying. If the value exceeds 1.0 there is a strong probability that the exposure in question has a real effect.

There are two approaches for analytical analyses, case–control studies and cohort comparisons. In *case–control* studies, two groups of people are compared, one having cancer the other not. Because they rely on past events they are sometimes called *retrospective analyses*. In *cohort* studies, a healthy, well-defined population (a cohort) is followed for many years to identify the characteristics that distinguish people who subsequently get cancer from those who do not. Because they monitor events following the start of analysis, they are known as *prospective studies*. Cohort studies provide more reliable information than case–control studies but they are more complex and more expensive.

To avoid false conclusions, it is important that the groups being compared are in fact identical apart from the specific factor being analysed. This can be difficult to achieve and errors arise through *bias* and *confounding factors*. *Selection bias* occurs through inappropriate selection of people for comparison; *recall bias* occurs through inadequate measures of exposure. For example, in case–control studies it is common to ask both groups to recall past events. Compared to the controls, cancer patients have more reason to think about events that might have led to their disease, so the recall may be different in the two groups. In case–control studies, control groups are often selected from people attending hospital for non-cancerous conditions. This tends to underestimate real differences (selection bias).

Because several factors may be indices of the same underlying influence, if one wants to identify causative agents, it is important to identify the real agent rather than a *confounding factor*. For example, eating red meat is a risk factor for several cancers but this may be due to its fat content rather than the meat protein component. There are often difficulties in recruiting sufficient numbers of individuals for one study to provide the statistical power needed to detect small effects on risk. This problem can be overcome by using mathematical models to combine data from several different studies (*meta-analysis*).

Types of information obtained from descriptive data

Changes with time

If incidence or mortality change with time it indicates that something is happening for which an explanation must be sought. Figure 4.1 illustrates examples of male cancer deaths that are increasing (lung), decreasing (stomach) or showing little change (colon/rectum) over recent years. Analytical data (see below) indicate that the increase in lung cancer is due to smoking as the amount of tobacco smoked mirrors this increase and a decline in smoking lessens the rate of increase. Biological plausibility is provided by the identification of carcinogens in cigarette smoke. The decrease in stomach cancer is intriguing but conclusions about cause are elusive, although diet is a prime candidate.

Analytical epidemiological data have shown that high intake of fruit, vegetable, fibre, vitamins A and C and low intake of salted meat and fish all correlate with a low incidence of stomach cancer (see below). Laboratory data provide biological plausibility for such concepts. Highly salted foods contain nitrates capable of conversion to oxidising agents that damage cells; vitamins such as A (converted to retinoic acid) or C (ascorbic acid) are antioxidants that prevent these adverse effects.

Geography

There are enormous geographical differences in cancer incidence and their study has provided important insights into cancer causation. It has also given cause for optimism that a high proportion of common cancers may be preventable. These points are illustrated in Table 4.1, which compares incidence rates for selected cancers in high and low risk countries. Japan has high levels of stomach cancer but low numbers of melanomas, whereas China has low rates of prostate cancer but high rates of liver cancer.

From these types of data one can generate testable hypotheses as to what might be the causes of such large intercountry differences. Perhaps they could be explained by genetic differences between races, but according to studies of Chinese migrating to Hawaii or the USA (Figure 4.2), this does not seem to be the case. Both prostate and breast cancer incidence rates increase, although not to the levels in the

Table 4.1 Incidence of cancers in different countries.

Cancer	High	Low	Relative risk (high/low)	Cause?
Skin	Australia	Japan	155	Sunlight (UV)
Prostate	USA	China	70	?
Colon	USA	India	19	Diet
Stomach	Japan	Kuwait	22	Diet
Cervix	Brazil	Israel	28	Sexual practices
Liver	China	Canada	49	Virus/toxins

Figure 4.2

Cancer incidence for Chinese people living in three countries.

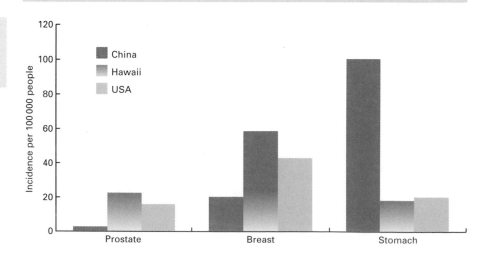

indigenous White population. Conversely, stomach cancer decreases in the migrating population. If the migrants maintain an Eastern diet, they retain an Eastern pattern of high stomach cancer and low rates of breast cancer; if they adopt a Western diet the incidence of these two cancers reverses to mimic that seen in the native US population. Analytical epidemiological studies indicate that fat is one culprit and laboratory studies are attempting to identify how this might work at a cellular level.

The large high:low cancer ratios illustrated in Table 4.1 plus the link between smoking and lung cancer indicate that many cancers are potentially preventable (see below). Identification of the reasons for the high:low risk ratios in various populations should facilitate corrective measures, although major problems exist for their implementation. The use of suntan creams containing UV-absorbing chemicals, coupled with decreased skin exposure, is effective in preventing skin cancer; but it is harder to persuade people to change their diet or sexual practices, perhaps to reduce transmission of papilloma virus.

Age

The older people get, the more likely they are to develop the common cancers. Carcinogenesis requires multiple cellular changes that take time to accumulate. Using data on cancer incidence at different ages, it is possible to obtain a minimal estimate of how many changes are required (Chapter 2).

Effects of treatment

Descriptive studies can also be used to generate information on effectiveness of treatment, although not as efficiently as with clinical trials. Alterations in five-year survival rates with time can provide clues as to whether or not changing clinical practices are beneficial (Figure 4.3). Success rates with ovarian cancer have changed

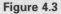

Figure 4.3

Five-year survival rates for consecutive three-year periods (US data).

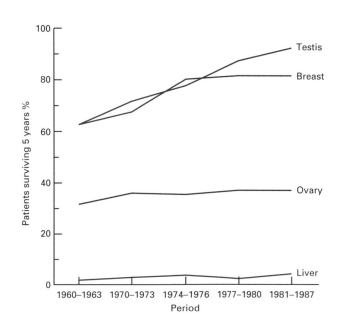

little whereas for testicular cancer the increased survival is such that one can begin to talk of a cure. Figure 4.3 also illustrates the markedly different life expectancies associated with various cancers, such that the majority of breast cancer patients survive 5 years whereas hepatoma patients do not. The latter reflects the essential functions performed by the liver, disruption of which has dire consequences.

Analytical epidemiology

Factors that influence the probability of getting cancer, such as where one lives or what one eats, are referred to as risk factors. They can be identified by comparing populations of people who have a given cancer with healthy people, or people exposed to a certain environment with people who are unexposed. An exposure example would be a comparison of lung cancers in smokers and non-smokers, which defines smoking as a bad risk factor; an example of the other kind would be relating the number of breast cancers in women who have had children (parous) with those who have not (nulliparous), which shows that having children reduces the risk. Thus the term 'risk factor' can be used in both positive and negative ways.

Analytical information is obtained from questionnaires on lifestyles and past events, but molecular data is increasingly being built into such analyses, a practice known as molecular epidemiology (see below).

Case–control studies

The method compares the characteristics of cases, either patients who have a cancer or healthy individuals with specific characteristics, with controls who do not have cancer or the characteristic in question. Details are compared to identify factors that are different between the two groups. Case–control studies have the advantage of providing quick answers because a relatively small number of people can be used and data is already available on both cases and controls. Major disadvantages are deciding on the appropriate controls and the fidelity of recall for past events. It is essential that the characteristics of cases and controls should be carefully matched so as not to confound the factors which do influence cancer.

A study designed to identify risk factors for cervical cancer (Table 4.2) illustrates the general features of a case–control study. In panel A of Table 4.2, all of the factors fall into this category except oral contraceptive use.

Women with cervical cancer were 16 times more likely than controls to be human papilloma virus (HPV) positive, with indices of sexual activity (number of partners, age at first intercourse) also indicating increased risk. If all women were included in the analysis, lack of schooling was a risk factor but oral contraceptive use was not. If the sexually transmitted virus HPV is a causative agent, then other indices of sexual activity that increase the likelihood of viral infection would also show up as risk factors. Lack of schooling would be an indirect index of promiscuity (a confounding factor) in Colombia for economic reasons or due to poor social

Table 4.2 Case–control analysis of cervical cancer in Colombia.

Factor	Relative risk	95% Confidence limits
A. All women		
HPV DNA positive	16	7–35*
>6 sexual partners	7	2–24*
First intercourse before 16	3	1–9*
Lack of schooling	3	1–8*
Oral contraceptive use	1.5	0.8–3
B. HPV-positive women only		
Oral contraceptive use	6	1.3–31*
Lack of schooling	3	0.6–12
>6 sexual partners	1	0.2–6
First intercourse before 16	2	0.5–6

* Statistically significant differences.
HPV = human papilloma virus.

environment. This is the case because if the analyses are undertaken only on HPV-positive women, schooling and indices of sexual activity are no longer risk factors (panel B). Interestingly, use of oral contraceptives becomes a risk factor in this subgroup, which indicates a synergism between the virus and hormones in the contraceptive.

Cohort studies

The principle is to start with a well-defined, healthy population (a cohort) and to compare those who get cancer in the ensuing years with those who do not. These prospective studies provide more reliable data by circumventing many of the defects of case–control studies. There are none of the problems of finding a control group, although confounding factors still occur. The reasons cohort studies are not used more widely are expense and time. Carcinogenesis is a long process, so cohorts must be followed for many years and they must contain large numbers of people to ensure enough cancers to analyse. There is also the problem of maintaining contact with those people over a long period. When the atom bombs were dropped on Japan in 1945, the radiation they released was a powerful carcinogen and people living at different distances from the epicentres were subjected to quantifiable levels of exposure. Those cohorts have been followed up with informative results. All age groups subsequently had increased likelihood of developing leukaemia but it occurred more rapidly in younger people than in older people (Figure 4.4). This was a common feature with all types of cancer induced by atomic radiation and it may reflect the increased sensitivity of cells to carcinogenic agents prior to reaching their fully differentiated state (Chapter 7).

Figure 4.4

Prospective cohort analysis of relative risks of developing leukaemia in people of the stated ages at the time of exposure to atomic radiation in Hiroshima/Nagasaki.

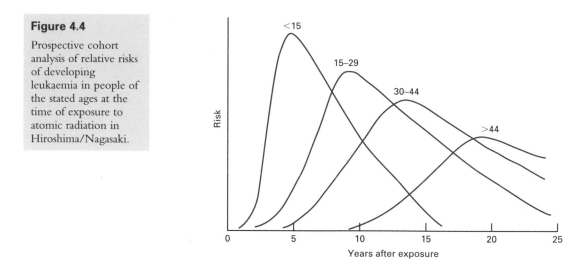

Criteria reqired to establish causality

With the exception of rare, genetically linked cancers, everything to do with human cancers concerns probabilities of events rather than black and white distinctions. This is also true for epidemiological conclusions about establishing causal links between risk factors and cancers. Conclusions can only be drawn from repeatable studies designed to minimise bias and identify confounding factors. There should be a dose–response relationship between 'factor' and cancer risk, the time course of events should be logical and a plausible biological link should be established.

Biomarkers

Inclusion of molecular data can greatly strengthen the power of epidemiological research. Recall bias is a problem in many studies in which exposure to an agent has to be quantitated: independent ways of assessing exposure help to determine that exposure. The HPV/cervical cancer study discussed above monitored viral infection by PCR methods. Another study on liver cancer in China used a urinary metabolite of the fungal hepatocarcinogen aflatoxin to indicate people who had been exposed. The results indicated a synergism between aflatoxin and hepatitis B virus such that a marginally increased risk with either agent alone was amplified fiftyfold when both agents were involved.

Biochemical markers are also useful when carcinogen exposure cannot otherwise be determined. Passive smoking is known to increase lung cancer risk in non-smokers. The extent of carcinogen exposure in this group is difficult to quantitate through questionnaires but plasma analysis of cotinine and polycyclic aromatic hydrocarbon–albumin adducts can be so used. Cotinine is a metabolite of nicotine whilst the albumin adduct of benzopyrene indicates exposure to this tobacco

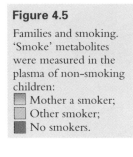

Figure 4.5

Families and smoking. 'Smoke' metabolites were measured in the plasma of non-smoking children:
- Mother a smoker;
- Other smoker;
- No smokers.

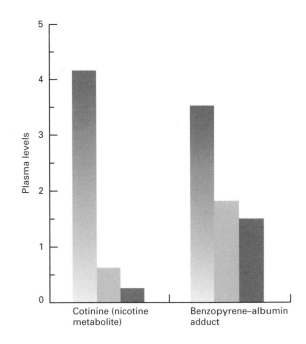

carcinogen. Figure 4.5 shows the levels of the two metabolites in plasma of children in three family categories: no smokers, mother a smoker and a member other than the mother who smokes. The children of smoking mothers are clearly exposed to elevated levels of noxious chemicals and the levels are related to the number of cigarettes smoked by the mother.

Molecular epidemiology

Molecular epidemiology combines epidemiological methods with molecular analysis to help determine carcinogenic events. The molecular dissection of colon carcinogenesis (Figure 2.11) was a forerunner of the approach but a better idea of the information obtainable involves p53 mutations. This repressor gene plays a pivotal role in the genesis of many cancers (Chapter 6) so changes in its structure are relevant to carcinogenesis. Over 2000 mutations have been identified, which has enabled correlations of mutation types with different cancers. This may point to causative agents (Figure 4.6). The Li–Fraumeni syndrome is due to a germline mutation in the p53 gene resulting in an inherited risk of breast, bone or brain cancers (Chapter 9). The pattern of p53 mutations is different in this syndrome to the pattern of somatic mutations in mouth and lung cancers, and variable patterns are seen in the various cancers generated by somatic cell mutations. This dissimilar mutational spectrum is even seen in comparisons of lung cancers from smokers and non-smokers. As different carcinogens generate different mutations (Chapter 7), molecular epidemiology may provide evidence as to the identity of causative agents independent of the evidence obtained by conventional epidemiology. Thus, the pattern of p53 mutations seen in lung cancers from smokers is consistent with

Figure 4.6

Types of p53 mutation in different cancers. Each segment represents the percentage of all mutations in the stated category.

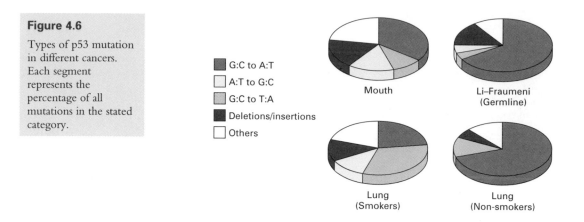

exposure to a spectrum of carcinogen types, each having a major influence, whereas the different pattern seen in non-smokers (Figure 4.6) suggests that one type of carcinogen is predominantly responsible. Another example of this approach is the spectrum of p53 mutations seen in liver cancers in China, Japan and Taiwan (Figure 4.7). Hepatitis B virus infection is a risk factor in all three countries but the Qidong province of China has an additional exposure to a fungal toxin, aflatoxin, from poorly stored peanuts. Most p53 mutations in liver cancers from that region are of one type $(G:C \rightarrow T:A)$ characteristic of an adduct between a guanine and a bulky carcinogen like aflatoxin. The other regions of Southeast Asia have more variable mutational spectra. Analysis of p53 mutational spectra to identify human carcinogens is discussed further in Chapter 7.

Figure 4.7

Liver cancers in Southeast Asia: p53 mutations.

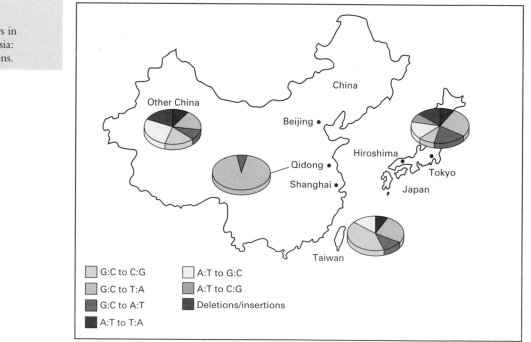

Factors that influence human carcinogenesis

If one looks at the five major cancers in men and women, four factors occur most frequently – smoking, diet, sex hormones and family history (Table 4.3) – each of which will be described separately.

Table 4.3 The incidence of the five main cancers in the USA and their risk factors.

Cancer	Percentage of all cancers	Risk factors	Possible mechanisms
Men			
Prostate	36	Sex hormones	Proliferation
		Diet	Hormones
Lung	13	Smoking	DNA damage
Colon/rectum	12	Diet	Antioxidants/toxic chemicals
		Family history	Gene defects
Urinary tract	9	Smoking	DNA damage
		Industrial*	DNA damage*
Leukaemia/lymphoma	7	?	?
Women			
Breast	33	Sex hormones	Proliferation
		Family history	Gene defects
		Diet	Hormones
Lung	13	Smoking	DNA damage
Colon/rectum	12	Family history	Gene defects
		Diet	Antioxidants/toxic chemicals
Leukaemia/lymphoma	6	?	?
Ovary	5	Ovulation	Tissue damage
		Family history	Gene defects

* No longer significant.

Smoking

The statistics related to smoking as a cause of premature death are frightening. In the USA 17% of deaths and 30% of all cancer deaths are due to smoking and the figures are similar in other countries. These figures translate into 3 million people worldwide each year dying uneccessarily (Table 4.4) and the outlook for people contracting lung cancer is poor, with less than 10% being alive 5 years after diagnosis. What is worse is that non-smokers (passive smokers) are also affected due to inhalation of tobacco-related products in the air. A non-smoker who lives with a smoker has a 30% higher risk of dying from lung cancer compared to their risk when living with a non-smoker.

Table 4.4 Some statistics associated with cigarette smoking in the USA.

	Annual number of smoking-related deaths
All deaths	400 000*
Lung cancer	150 000
Other cancers	30 000
Passive smoking	
All deaths	40 000
Lung	3 000

Smoking is responsible for 30% of all cancer deaths and 17% of all deaths

Less than 10% of lung cancer patients are alive 5 years after its first diagnosis

* Worldwide, this figure is estimated to be 3 million.

Table 4.5 Increased risk of cancers at different sites due to smoking.

Cancer	Relative risk smoker/non-smoker	Attributable to smoking (%)
Lung	22	90
Mouth	28	92
Bladder	3	47
Kidney	3	48

Although most attention is directed at lung cancer, there are also increases in mouth, pharynx, oesophagus, bladder and kidney cancer (Table 4.5). Smoking is the main cause of lung and mouth cancers and accounts for half of the bladder and kidney growths. Most of the affected sites are those that come into contact with the carcinogens in the smoke, but inhaled carcinogens enter the bloodstream through the lungs and are excreted via the kidneys and bladder. Both these sites are affected and it is interesting that inactivating mutations in the cancer repressor gene p53 are different in bladder and lung cancers (Chapter 7). This suggests that carcinogens in the smoke reaching the bladder are different from those acting on lung epithelium.

Causation has been established by all the criteria mentioned in the previous section. Over 40 potent carcinogens have been isolated from tobacco, including hydrocarbons such as benzopyrene and nitrosamines like dimethylnitrosamine. There is a dose–response relationship between the number of cigarettes smoked and the increased lung cancer risk (Figure 4.8). Maximal increased risk of contracting lung cancer occurs with more than 30 cigarettes per day but even under 10 cigarettes per day increases the risk twentyfold. There is a 20-year gap between increased tobacco consumption and lung cancer changes, and although stopping decreases the risk, it remains higher than in people who have never smoked for about the same period. There is a synergistic effect between smoking and alcohol consumption in mouth cancer, for example.

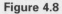

Figure 4.8

Lung cancer risk increases with the number of cigarettes smoked.

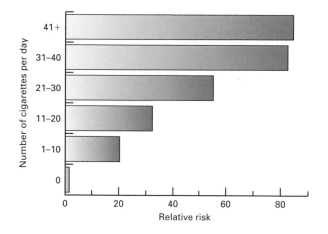

Diet

The evidence linking diet with several types of cancer is strong, but the basis of that link is obscure as both beneficial and detrimental components have been identified. Fruit and vegetables are protective against several types of cancer analysed whereas bad factors are more discriminating (Table 4.6). Not surprisingly, the biggest effects tend to be seen in the gastrointestinal tract but sites such as breast and lung, which do not come into direct contact with food, are also affected. Good factors identified in fruit and vegetables include fibre (non-starch polysaccharides), complex phenols and micronutrients such as carotenoids, and vitamins A, C and E.

The current conclusion about the influence of diet on carcinogenesis is that it is important, multifaceted, and confusing. Part of this confusion arises from the fact that altering diet changes several components so that it is difficult to decide whether a beneficial effect is due to addition of a 'good' factor or removal of a 'bad' one; both types exist. An Eastern diet, rich in plant products, contains many beneficial ingredients whereas fat-rich Western diets have the opposite effect. The so-called Mediterranean diet is thought to be beneficial because it has a high content of fruit and vegetable, red wine (phenols) and complex carbohydrate together with low saturated fat. The major dietary components that influence carcinogenesis will now be considered.

Table 4.6 Diet and major cancers.

| Site | Dietary factor | |
	Good	Bad
Lung	Fruit and vegetables	
Stomach	Fruit and vegetables	Salt, salt foods
Breast	Fruit and vegetables	Fat, alcohol
Prostate	Fruit and vegetables	–
Colon	Fruit and vegetables	Meat, alcohol
Mouth, pharynx, nasopharynx	Fruit and vegetables	Alcohol, salt fish

Fruit and vegetables

High fruit and vegetable consumption is associated with a decreased risk of many cancers and may have a general inhibitory effect (Table 4.6). This conclusion is based on epidemiological analysis of food consumption patterns in different communities at an international level (different countries) and within specific countries (vegetarian and non-vegetarian groups). Biologically plausible mechanisms exist to explain the beneficial effects via components such as antioxidants, vitamins, fibre and phytoestrogens (see below). However, in many cases the effect of these individual factors is less than is seen for the food as a whole; additional dietary components have yet to be identified. For simplicity, fruit and vegetables will be discussed as a single entity because common components are involved but beneficial effects have been noted with each on their own and with individual items within each group (green vegetables and lung cancer; citrus fruits and stomach cancer). The effect of vegetable intake on risk of lung cancer is shown in Figure 4.9. There is a 50% difference between the lowest and highest intake groups. A beneficial effect occurs in both smokers and non-smokers.

Fruit and vegetable consumption, linked with low fat intake (see below) goes a long way towards explaining geographical differences in incidence of cancers such as breast, prostate and colon (Table 4.1) but additional components have yet to be identified. Carotenoids are present in many plants; they are especially abundant in carrots. In theory they could have a twofold beneficial effect, as antioxidants and as precursors of vitamin A, which promotes cellular differentiation and blocks proliferation (Chapter 10). However, trials of β-carotene to prevent lung cancer in smokers have shown it to have a detrimental effect (Chapter 14). The plant-derived vitamins A (retinol), C (ascorbic acid) and E (tocopherol) have antioxidant properties that contribute to their protective effect. Reactive oxygen species such as superoxides or OH$^\bullet$ radicals are carcinogenic through their ability to damage DNA (Chapter 7); antioxidants counteract this effect. Two classes of plant phenols, lignans (metabolised by gut microflora to phenols) and isoflavones, have specific beneficial effects on cancers requiring sex hormones for their genesis. The phenols antagonise the mitogenic effects of the natural sex hormone oestradiol (Chapter 14).

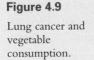

Figure 4.9

Lung cancer and vegetable consumption.

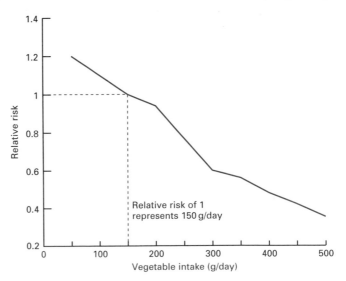

Dietary fibre such as cellulose from plant cell walls has little nutritional value and its mode of action in decreasing cancer risk is unclear. The major protective effects are seen in the gastrointestinal tract where the dietary agents are in close contact with the cells involved, although small effects are noted elsewhere. A protective effect of fibre was first suggested from the observation that elephants have bulky faeces because of the fibre they eat but they do not get colon cancer. It is unclear why fibre is protective but there are several suggestions. Fibre accelerates the rate of gut emptying and this might reduce the contact time between dietary carcinogens and nearby cells; fibre might help to bind or inactivate carcinogens in the gut; and fibre might alter the profile of microflora within the intestine. A high-fibre diet is often accompanied by low fat consumption but low fat consumption is unlikely to account for all its protective effect. Comparisons of groups with the same high fat intake but low (New York) or high (Finland) fibre indicate a lower incidence of colon cancers in the Finnish group. The same is true for breast cancer (Figure 4.10).

Fat and meat

A high meat consumption is linked with an elevated risk of colon cancers and possibly breast, prostate, pancreatic and kidney cancers. As meat is a major source of animal fat in Western diets (in the USA, one-third of saturated fat intake comes from red meat), meat will be assumed to be a surrogate measure of saturated fat intake. This may be an oversimplification of meat's true role, as high-temperature roasting may generate carcinogens from non-fat components.

Breast cancer incidence in different countries correlates with the total per capita fat consumption in that country (Figure 4.10). The same type of relationship exists if different ethnic groups within one country (Hawaii) are compared. A similar link exists between total fat intake and cancers of the colon, pancreas, prostate, kidney and endometrium. The potential importance of these data is illustrated by the theoretical calculation that, if total fat consumption in the USA was halved, the incidence of common cancers, such as those of the breast, endometrium and colon (women) or prostate and colon (men), would be reduced by up to two-thirds.

Figure 4.10

Deaths from breast cancer may be linked to fat consumption.

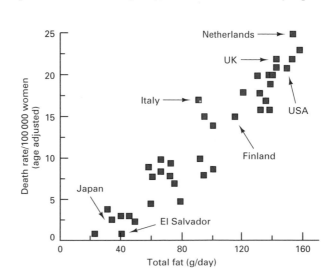

Unfortunately, this calculation is unrealistic because this degree of fat reduction is impossible to achieve and because we do not know why these international correlations between fat and cancer exist (the fat hypothesis). Sorting out the contribution of fat rather than the potential confounding factors has not been achieved for any cancer type. It is not clear whether reduced fat intake is beneficial because fat contributes a 'bad' factor or whether the switch to fruit and vegetables (see below) increases a 'good' factor. Both are probably important.

Animal feeding experiments support a causal relationship between fat intake and cancer production, but besides the international comparisons just mentioned, epidemiological studies in humans are equivocal. Retrospective, case–control analyses in which fat consumption by cancer patients was compared with fat consumption in controls, suggest a weak association; prospective cohort studies addressing the same question indicate little association (Chapter 14).

One factor that may help to clarify this confusion is the heterogeneous nature of the fat. There are animal and vegetable fats to consider, along with saturated and unsaturated fats, cholesterol and total calories provided by the fat. In the Western world, fat of mainly animal origin provides about one-third of the energy intake whereas fat consumption in developing countries primarily derives from plants and only constitutes about one-fifth of energy intake. There is also a qualitative difference between the two populations in that animal fat contains mainly saturated fatty acids whereas unsaturated fatty acids predominate in plants. The story is further complicated by the fact that the number and position of double bonds in unsaturated fatty acids influences their biological effects. Animal fat is also a rich source of cholesterol but plant fat does not contain this lipid. It is difficult to reach any firm conclusions about the relative contributions of individual components of fat except to say that a high total fat consumption, especially of animal origin, increases cancer risk at many sites (Table 4.7).

The uncertainty about the role of fat in carcinogenesis extends to ideas about its biological role in the process. Animal experiments indicate fat to be involved in promotion rather than initiation but, beyond that, ideas become speculative. High fat intake increases obesity; and obesity has been conclusively identified as a risk factor for breast and uterine cancers in women because of its effect on the production of female sex hormone (oestradiol). Fat cells can synthesise the mitogenic steroid oestradiol: increased fat equates to increased oestradiol and hyperproliferation (Table 11.5, Figure 13.12).

Table 4.7 Fat consumption and cancer.

---

1 These fats are correlated with an increased cancer risk:
   - Total fat: lung, colon, breast, prostate
   - Saturated/animal fat: lung, colon, breast, uterus, prostate
   - Cholesterol: lung, pancreas

2 Breast cancer shows no relationship to levels of cholesterol, monounsaturated fats and polyunsaturated fats.

3 Absence of other sites from the above indicates lack of data rather than no effect.

4 No protective effect of fat has been identified for any site.

Micronutrients

Micronutrients are constituents that are small in quantitative terms but not necessarily in terms of their biological effect. Vitamins and carotenoids were described above but minerals can also be important. A high salt (sodium nitrate) intake increases the risk of stomach cancer. The breast/fat data illustrated in Figure 4.10 can be mimicked by a graph of deaths from stomach cancer against the salt content of preserved soybeans in different rural prefectures in Japan. This practice of food preservation has now declined such that per capita intake has fallen in Japan by 16% and deaths from stomach cancer by 50% since 1970.

High selenium or calcium consumption may also be protective but the mechanism is obscure. Some proteins need these ions for their biological effect, e.g. glutathione peroxidase needs selenium to destroy mutagenic free radicals (Figure 7.8).

Alcohol

Alcohol is an important constituent of many diets, including students'! It has adverse effects on cancers of the breast, colon, liver and upper digestive tract (Table 4.6). For cancers of the oesophagus and larynx, the carcinogenic effect is seen in both smokers and non-smokers, but smoking and alcohol consumption have a synergistic effect rather than an additive effect. There is a twentyfold difference in relative risk between a daily consumption of 10 g alcohol or less (10 g is half a pint of beer) and a daily consumption of more than 160 g (8 pints of beer or 500 ml of spirits); see Figure 4.11

Figure 4.11

Oesophageal cancer and alcohol consumption.

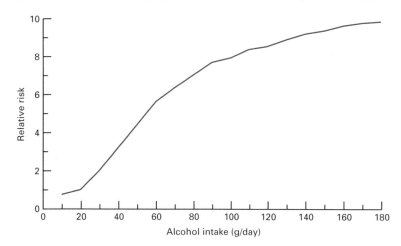

Sex hormones

Sex hormones are crucially involved in the most frequent non-smoking-related cancers in men (prostate) and women (breast) as well as others like those of the ovary and uterus (Table 4.3). The hormones are mainly produced in the testis (androgens, men) or ovary (oestrogens and progestins, women); people who have had these organs removed have a dramatically reduced incidence of the disease. Both male and female hormones influence proliferation of their respective target cells and this contributes to their promotional effects. Actions of these hormones are discussed elsewhere (Chapters

11 and 13) but note that they interrelate with other risk factors in a complex way. Diet influences both endogenous hormone levels and their bioavailability as well as providing plant compounds that antagonise the actions of endogenous hormones. Thus, a low-fat diet reduces androgen (testosterone) levels in men and is associated with a low prostate cancer risk, whilst obesity in women increases breast cancer incidence due to oestrogen synthesis in fat tissue. A woman's reproductive history (age at first birth, age at start and end of ovulation) are hormone-mediated features that influence the likelihood of breast cancer. Interestingly, the contraceptive pill, whose active ingredients are the two types of female sex steroid, oestrogen and progestin, has little influence on breast cancer although it can reduce the risk of both uterine and ovarian cancers by half. Ovarian cancer is listed in Table 4.3 as possibly being due to tissue damage resulting from ovulation, in which release of the egg requires disruption of the surrounding tissue. Hence there is decreased risk when ovulation is suppressed, as occurs with oral contraceptives containing oestrogen and progestin; but there is increased risk when ovulation is increased during fertility treatment.

Family history

Genetic association crops up with several of the major cancers but in none of these does it account for more than 10% of the cancers. This is not true for certain rare childhood tumours such as retinoblastoma (eye) or Wilms' tumour (kidney), where the majority of the children carrying the genetic trait are affected. Familial cancers are discussed in Chapter 9.

Other factors

Tables of carcinogenic agents are available; most agents relate to animal data but some have been proved to cause cancer in humans through epidemiological studies (Table 4.8). With improvements in occupational health regulations, many carcinogens have been eliminated, as in the case of bladder cancer. The original observations showed that people working in the rubber and dyestuff industries had a high incidence of bladder cancer; a metabolite of 2-naphthylamine, one of the culprits, forms adducts with DNA (Chapter 7).

Exposure still occurs to some forms of radiation that carry a degree of risk, mostly due to their DNA-damaging properties (Chapter 7). Ultraviolet (UV) light is a major determinant of skin cancer and debate continues over the nuclear industry's contribution to leukaemia. Build-up of radon-222 gas (α particles) in homes can increase lung cancers (Chapter 7).

What is interesting about lists of human carcinogenic agents is the paucity of viruses. Despite the enormous influence they have in animals and the information they have generated about molecular mechanisms of carcinogenesis, they make relatively minor contributions to human cancer. The four exceptions are human immunodeficiency virus (sarcomas), hepatitis B virus (liver), human T-cell lymphotropic virus (leukaemia) and human papilloma virus (cervix), of which only cervical cancer is a big contributor to cancer statistics outside China, Latin America and Africa.

Table 4.8 Agents known to cause human cancer.

Agent	Source	Cancer
Current		
Radon-222	Building materials	Lung
X-rays	Radiotherapy	Breast, thyroid, bone
Cytotoxic drugs	Chemotherapy	Leukaemia/lymphoma
Immunosuppression	Transplants	Leukaemia/lymphoma
Asbestos	Industry	Lung
Religion	Nuns	Breast/uterus
Aflatoxin	Diet	Liver
Human papilloma virus	Prostitutes	Cervix
Historical		
Soot	Chimneysweeps	Scrotum
2-Naphthylamine	Rubber, dye industry	Bladder
Chromium/nickel compound	Industry	Lung

Cancer prevention

Many of the risk factors identified by epidemiological means reflect elements of lifestyle that can be changed and therefore have the potential of altering cancer risk (Table 4.9). However, potential and reality do not equate, so although tobacco-related cancers could be prevented now by banning tobacco use, getting people to change their diets to include more fruit and vegetables and less fat is more problematic. This is even more true for reproductive factors such as when a woman has her first child or whether a barrier method of contraception is used to minimise HPV transmission.

Routes to preventing cancer formation in humans based on many of the factors described in this section are discussed in Chapter 14.

Table 4.9 Potential for cancer prevention.

Factor	Percentage of deaths that could be avoided	
	Potential	Achievable now
Diet	35	2
Tobacco	30	30
Reproductive factors	7	?
Alcohol	3	3
Food additives	<1	<1
Industrial products	<1	<1
Total	76	34

TUMOUR IMMUNOLOGY AND IMMUNOTHERAPY

Key points

- Patients with suppressed immune functions resulting from treatment (transplant patients) or viral infection (AIDS) are at increased risk of developing lymph gland tumours. Common epithelial cancers are not increased.
- Viral or chemically induced animal tumours generate immune responses; spontaneous tumours do not.
- Immunodeficient mice do not have a high incidence of spontaneous tumours.
- Immune surveillance can occur whereby host immune mechanisms can kill cancer cells. Their importance in preventing development of common cancers is questionable.
- Differences between normal and cancer cells in antigen expression are quantitative rather than qualitative. Viral cancers are an exception.
- Major histocompatibility antigens can be lost by cancer cells thereby decreasing their susceptibility to immune attack.
- Several mechanisms exist through which the immune system can attack and lyse tumour cells. Cell-mediated and antibody-mediated processes exist.
- Cytotoxic T-cells, natural killer cells and macrophages are important.
- Components of the immune system can be manipulated to provide forms of immunotherapy. Limited successes have been recorded.
- Monoclonal antibodies are useful diagnostic tools.

Introduction

Immunosuppressed patients, such as those receiving kidney transplants, are at increased risk of developing cancers of the lymph glands (lymphomas), so there is a clear link between decreased immune activity and cancer formation. However, it is not clear how important that link is for other types of cancer. Animal data also indicate that several components of the immune system can be manipulated to alter cancer growth but the relevance of this information to human cancers remains uncertain. The animal results are also difficult to interpret because demonstrable immune effects are limited to viral cancers and to cancers induced by high doses of chemical carcinogens; spontaneous cancers are little affected by immune manipulation.

The concept of immune surveillance, in which the immune system monitors the body for abnormal antigens/cells, is important in tumour biology as cancer cells can be considered to be abnormal. Immune surveillance therefore has the potential to prevent cancer formation by killing the abnormal cells. The core requirement for such surveillance is that the cancer cells activate the immune system whereas normal cells do not. The presence of tumour-specific antigens on the cancer cell but not on the normal cell would satisfy this requirement but such specificity rarely occurs and antigen differences are usually quantitative rather than qualitative.

Although there is debate about the overall importance of immune mechanisms in the development of cancers, there is no doubt about their role in the diagnosis and treatment of cancers. Antibodies are widely used as immunohistochemical or immunoassay reagents to characterise cancers, and labelled antibodies are given to patients to detect cancers *in vivo*. Trials are under way to use antibodies as a means of targeting drugs to specific sites, and other attempts are being made to manipulate the immune system in order to attack and kill established cancers. These two approaches are known as immunotherapy.

The immune system is complex and its potential impact on a complicated process like carcinogenesis can therefore be multifaceted. This chapter will only deal with features of the immune system that are directly relevant to cancer. The terminology used to describe immunological events can be daunting, so some of the more important terms will be introduced.

Box 5.1   Terms used in immunology

The characteristics of the main cells of the immune system that are related to tumour biology are given in Table 5.1; other terminologies are given in Table 5.2.

Table 5.1 Cells of the immune system relevant to cancer.*

Cells	Characteristics
Lymphocytes	General term for cells of the lymphoid lineage (T and B cells)
T-cells	Heterogeneous class of lymphocytes with specific surface receptors that recognise familial markers on other cells
Cytotoxic T-cells	Subset of T-cells capable of recognising and killing (cytotoxic) cancer cells to which they attach
Helper T-cells	Subset of T-cells that help B-cells to produce antibodies and enhance T-cell responses
Suppressor T-cells	Opposite of helper T-cells
B-cells	Heterogeneous class of lymphocytes. Mature B-cells (plasma cells) secrete antibodies
NK cells	Natural killer cells that are cytotoxic but which lack specificity and memory. Not T or B cells
K-cells	Functional description of killer cells that can kill by antibody-dependent cellular cytotoxicity
Phagocytes	Cells that phagocytose particles and proteins. Can be mononuclear or polymorphonuclear. Latter include neutrophils and eosinophils
Macrophages	Mononuclear phagocytes in tissues. Can be cytotoxic
Myeloid cells	General term for cells of the myeloid lineage (granulocytes, macrophages, platelets, erythrocytes)
Leukocytes	White blood cells
Dendritic cells	Bone marrow-derived cells that have efficient antigen-presenting properties

* For other definitions see Table 5.2.

Table 5.2 Definitions used in immunology.[*]

Term	Definition
Tumour antigen	Protein/glycoprotein on tumour cell
Epitope	Molecular sequence on antigen recognised by antibody
MHC	Major histocompatibility complex. In humans, called HLAs (human leucocyte antigens). Membrane protein receptors for processed antigen. Required for presentation of 'antigen' to T-cell receptor. Two classes: MHC-I on all nucleated cells and MHC-II on immune cells
T-cell receptor	Family of T-cell protein complexes that bind to processed antigen presented by MHCs on other cells
MHC restriction	T-cells subclassified with CD markers according to whether they interact with MHC-I or MHC-II
CD system	Classification (clusters of differentiation) of marker proteins that characterise specific types of lymphocytes. Not confined to lymphocytes and can have other names
CD4	Antigen on T-cells involved in MHC-II recognition
CD8	Antigen on T-cells involved in MHC-I recognition
Activation	Several immune system cells must be activated by contact with other cells/proteins
Complement	About 20 proteins involved in cascade of events that lead to phagocytosis and/or cell lysis and generation of molecules that are chemotactic for phagocytes in inflammation
Syngeneic animals	Animals of the same species with identical chromosomes
Allogeneic animals	Animals with dissimilar chromosomes
Cytokines	Proteins/polypeptides involved in signalling between cells of the immune system. Can also be growth factors (interferons, interleukins, colony stimulating factors, tumour necrosis factors)
Lymphokines	Cytokines produced by lymphocytes

[*] For cell definition see Table 5.1.

Immune surveillance and tumour development

There is clear evidence from animal and clinical studies that the host immune system can survey the body for the presence of abnormal cells and either destroy them or delay their development. The essential feature of this process is that immune cells recognise antigens on the cancer cells that facilitate attachment of the cells or proteins involved and this union results in death of the cancer cell. Normal cells should not be so monitored (Figure 5.1). Ideally, such a system requires that cancer cells have tumour-specific antigens capable of activating immune cells. It is now apparent that, with the exception of cancers induced by viruses or high doses of potent chemical carcinogens, antigen differences between normal and cancer cells are mostly quantitative rather than qualitative.

Animal data

Tumours can be transplanted from animal to animal provided the recipient is either syngeneic or has a defective immune system. Transplantation to other strains

Figure 5.1

Immune surveillance.

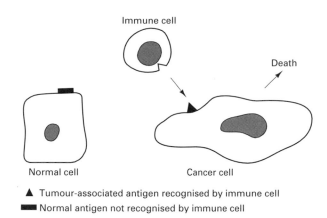

Immune cell

Death

Normal cell   Cancer cell

▲ Tumour-associated antigen recognised by immune cell

■■ Normal antigen not recognised by immune cell

(allogeneic) of the same species or to other species results in rejection. This simple observation provides powerful evidence that rejection mechanisms exist and also indicates how they might work. Syngeneic animals have been inbred so that their chromosomes are identical; allogeneic have not. The relevant difference between a syngeneic mouse in which a transplanted tumour will grow, and an allogeneic mouse, in which it will not grow, is in the genes coding for transplantation antigens, the **m**ajor **h**istocompatibility **c**omplex (MHC) antigens (see below). Mice with defective immune systems have been developed (Chapter 2) into which not only murine but human tumours can be successfully transplanted. Athymic, or nude, mice have no thymus gland in which T-cells can develop, so they are deficient in this cell type; this indicates a second component of the surveillance mechanism.

Virus-induced cancers express viral antigens on their surface that are recognised by the host as being foreign. These antigens generate host antibodies capable of killing the cancer. Thus, if SV40 virus-induced cancer is transplanted into a syngeneic mouse that has never encountered such a tumour, it will grow because the host immune system has not had time to develop its response (Figure 5.2). Removal of that tumour and reinjection of a smaller number of the same cells does not result in tumour growth. The host immune system responds to the first transplant to a degree that enables rejection of the second challenge. If a cancer induced by a different virus, such as polyoma, is used as the challenge, the transplant will grow because its viral-coded antigens are not the same as those of the first

Figure 5.2

Rejection of
transplanted tumour.

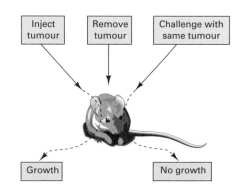

Inject tumour   Remove tumour   Challenge with same tumour

Growth   No growth

tumour. Similar results can be obtained with chemically induced cancers but spontaneous cancers will not elicit an immune response. The strong carcinogen causes major differences in antigen expression, whereas spontaneous cancers exhibit smaller changes that are not recognised as being abnormal.

The number of tumour cells is also important in determining whether or not a cancer is rejected. A small number of cells can be killed whereas larger numbers cannot. In part this reflects the inefficiency of the host immune system, but another problem is accessibility of antibodies or immune cells to cancer cells within a mass. The accessibility problem is also a major consideration with new methods of immunotherapy, which will often work with isolated cells but not solid tumour masses.

The immunodeficient mice provide evidence as to the likely importance of immune surveillance besides evidence obtained by injecting them with cancers. Nude mice have a deficiency in mature T-cells but do not have a higher than expected number of spontaneous tumours, so mature T-cells cannot play an overriding role in eliminating spontaneous tumours. Another strain, the beige mouse, has defective natural killer (NK) cells and does have a high incidence of spontaneous tumours.

In conclusion, animal studies indicate that host immune attack on cancer cells can occur in special cases but not in all situations. The relevance of animal studies to human cancers has been questioned on the grounds that human viral cancers are uncommon as are cancers induced by massive doses of carcinogen.

Clinical data

There is clear evidence in favour of immune attack mechanisms existing in humans but the picture is less clear as to the relevance of those mechanisms to cancer development other than in special situations. Kidney transplant patients receive immunosuppressant therapy, such as high-dose glucocorticoids or cyclosporin, to prevent transplant rejection. Such patients are at increased risk of developing lymphomas and, to a lesser extent, skin cancers. People who are immunosuppressed for other reasons such as infection with the human immunodeficiency virus (AIDS) are at increased risk of developing lymphoma about 2 years after the virus is first detected. Kaposi's sarcoma (blood vessel endothelial cell proliferation) is also increased in such patients whereas common epithelial cancers are not. These types of data indicate a role for immune surveillance in special cases but they do not suggest a major influence on the genesis of common cancers.

A second data set indicating the potential for immune surveillance relates to the presence of tumour-infiltrating lymphocytes (TILs) in tumours. These infiltrates are reminiscent of an inflammatory response to foreign antigens, consisting predominantly of macrophages and lymphocytes; lymphocyte subtypes are present. They can be isolated, activated in culture and used to treat patients (see below). Additionally, a high concentration of these cells in colon cancers indicates a good prognosis that could be explained by immune attack. The occurrence of large numbers of histiocytes (tissue macrophages) in lymph nodes of breast cancer patients is also a beneficial feature that could be used as evidence for a surveillance mechanism.

Mechanisms of immune surveillance

The components needed for immune surveillance are a tumour antigen capable of eliciting an immune response, immune cells that can interact with the tumour cell, and usually MHC antigens on the tumour cell to facilitate this interaction. Several mechanisms can be involved and not all of the components are required in each case. A successful outcome for immune attack is killing of the cancer cell; this cytotoxicity is achieved by lysing the cell and it can be either cell mediated or antibody–complement mediated. Both require tumour-associated antigens.

Tumour antigens

Tumour antigens were originally known as tumour-specific antigens; the term was changed to tumour-associated antigen when it became evident that differences between normal cells and cancer cells were mainly of a quantitative rather than qualitative nature. Tumour antigen is the preferred term as it makes no judgement about cell type specificity. The antigens are usually, but not necessarily, proteins; gangliosides and carbohydrates can be immunogenic. Four types of tumour antigen can be categorised (Table 5.3) according to whether (i) they have a tumour-specific expression, (ii) they are products of genes with point mutations, (iii) they are differentiation antigens or (iv) they are overexpressed in cancers. Note that the antigens described here are those identified by sophisticated techniques and which activate cytotoxic T-cells (see below). Cancers contain many other proteins that

Table 5.3 Tumour antigens (human) capable of eliciting an immune response.

Type of antigen	Cancer
Tumour-specific expression	
MART	Melanoma
MAGE	Melanoma, testis*
RAGE	Melanoma, kidney
gp100	Melanoma
Mucin	Breast, ovary
Products of genes with point mutations	
β-catenin	Melanoma
Cyclin-dependent kinase 4	Melanoma
Caspase 8	Head/neck
Differentiation antigens	
Tyrosinase	Melanoma
Prostate-specific antigen	Prostate
Carcinoembryonic antigen	Colon
Antigens overexpressed in cancers	
ErbB2	Ovary, breast
Common acute lymphoblastic leukaemia antigen (CD10)	Leukaemia

* Normal cells.

Table 5.4 Expression of tumour antigens on different cancers.

Cancer	Percentage of tumours expressing the antigen	
	MAGE-I	RAGE-I
Melanoma		
Primary	16	2
Metastasis	48	5
Kidney	0	2
Breast	18	1
Colon	2	0

would fall into one of these four categories but which do not elicit an immune response. Identification of such tumour antigens has opened up some new possibilities for therapeutic regimes. These regimes, plus the techniques involved, are discussed in Chapter 13. Melanomas predominate as the type of cancer expressing tumour antigens. In large part, this reflects the fact that melanoma cells have been the main experimental tool used to identify them. It does not mean that other cell types do not have tumour antigens.

Tumour-specific antigens The MAGE (**m**elanoma **a**nti**g**en **e**xpression) family of proteins are more frequently expressed in metastatic melanomas than in primary melanomas (Table 5.4). More modest numbers of other cancers express MAGE. The MAGE are also expressed by normal placental and testicular cells; this might lead one to question their categorisation as tumour-specific antigens. However, those two normal cells do not express MHC-I, required for antigen exposure to lymphocytes, so they are functionally tumour-specific. The RAGE (**r**enal **AGE**) family have a more limited expression (Table 5.4). The mucin mentioned in Table 5.3 has different characteristics in that the protein component in cancers is exposed due to its hypoglycosylation compared to the normal antigen. This antigen is also different in that it evokes an immune response by a non-MHC-I-mediated mechanism.

Point mutations For the technical reasons mentioned above, point mutations have mainly been identified in melanoma cells and are only those antigens that elicit a T-cell response. It is noteworthy that common cancer-related proteins like p53 or ras have not been so identified.

Differentiation antigens Tyrosinase is high in normal melanocytes as it is needed for the synthesis of the skin pigment melanin. **P**rostate-**s**pecific **a**ntigen (PSA) and **c**arcino**e**mbryonic **a**ntigen (CEA) are released into the bloodstream and can be used for diagnostic purposes (see below).

Antigens overexpressed in cancers The **c**ommon **a**cute **l**ymphoblastic **l**eukaemia **a**ntigen (CALLA) is readily detected in leukaemias but is difficult to find in normal blood lymphocytes. This is because CALLA is only found on B-cell precursors, which comprise <1% of normal bone marrow cells and which rarely escape into the bloodstream. Leukaemias result from clonal expansion of precursor cells, so larger numbers of these partially differentiated cells are present that enter the general circulation. CALLA can be detected because of this change in proportion of cell types in the blood. Growth factor receptors such as erbB2 are overexpressed in advanced cancers of the ovary, breast and cervix, a feature that is exploited to target antibodies to cancers (Chapter 13).

Major histocompatibility complex antigens

In normal cells, over 50 genes have been identified that determine recognition of foreign proteins by T-cells. These genes have been identified mainly through their role in coding for proteins involved in tissue transplantation, sometimes referred to as transplantation antigens. These cell membrane proteins, the MHC antigens, are classified into groups I and II. In humans these proteins have been defined through analysis of **h**uman **l**eukocyte **a**ntigens (HLAs) but the MHC terminology will be used here. Antibody production requires uptake and proteolytic cleavage of the antigen and these fragments must be presented to T-cells bound to receptors; MHC antigens act as those receptors. Each class of MHC gene is highly polymorphic so many different protein products exist. MHC class I (MHC-I) are found on all cell types whereas MHC class II (MHC-II) are confined to specific cells of the immune system. Hence, MHC-I on cancer cells are especially important for T-cell recognition, whereas MHC-II on macrophages are involved in the initial stages of antibody production. A third class of MHC antigens coding for cytokine-related proteins can also be defined.

MHC-I can be lost in cancers and therefore the cell interactions required for their lysis destroyed. The importance of MHC-I in immune surveillance has been demonstrated in animals in which MHC-I expression has either been increased or decreased. Mice reject transplanted tumours containing transfected MHC-I genes but they allow their untransfected counterparts to grow. Conversely, suppression of MHC-I expression by antisense olignucleotides promotes growth. In humans about half of breast and colon cancers have lost MHC-I expression, which may reduce the chances of immune attack.

Cytotoxicity

Cancer cells can be killed by immune mechanisms involving other cells, cell-mediated immunity, antibody-mediated immunity or complement-mediated immunity (Figure 5.3). Death of the cancer cell results from changes in membrane permeability that cause lysis or apoptosis.

Cell-mediated cytotoxicity

Antibody-independent mechanisms The T-cell receptor on the cytotoxic T-cell binds to MHC-I proteins on the tumour, provided that the peptide derived from the tumour antigen is bound to the MHC (Figure 5.4). The tumour antigen is digested to the peptide by proteasomes in the cancer cell and the peptide transferred

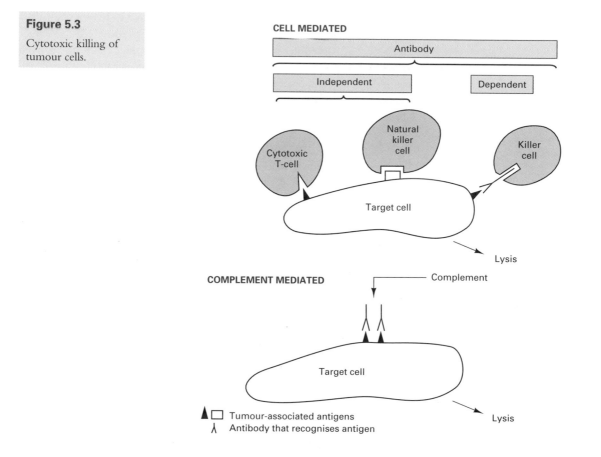

Figure 5.3

Cytotoxic killing of tumour cells.

to the extracellular face of MHC-I via the endoplasmic reticulum. In macrophages, the analogous process of peptide transfer to MHC-II is mediated by lysosomes. The peptide on the **a**ntigen **p**resenting **c**ell (APC) is 10–25 amino acids in length and is called the *immunodominant peptide*. An accessory protein of the **c**luster of **d**ifferentiation (CD) series on the T-cell determines whether they recognise antigen presented on MHC-I or MHC-II target cells. If CD8 is present, MHC-I is recognised, whereas CD4 dictates an MHC-II interaction. This is called an MHC-restricted process. As tumour cells express MHC-I, it is the CD8-positive cytotoxic T-cells that are most important in this type of tumour killing. Additional cell adhesion molecules stabilise interactions between the two cell types.

A second antibody-independent mechanism of cytotoxicity involves interaction between NK cells and tumour determinants (Figure 5.3). NK cells, derived from mononuclear granulocytic lymphocytes, are found in the bloodstream as large granular lymphocytes and in tumour infiltrates. They can kill isolated cancer cells in the bloodstream but they can also escape from capillaries into the surrounding tissue. NK cells can invade and kill clumps of metastatic cells without affecting normal cells. So tumour-specific recognition processes must exist. Two types of receptors have been identified that could mediate such recognition: one involving NK interaction with polysaccharides on the cancer cell, the other requiring

Figure 5.4

Interaction between cytotoxic T-cell and tumour cell. MHC-I is the major histocompatibility complex class I; LFA1, LFA3, ICAM, ICAM2, CD2 are adhesion proteins; CD8 is a protein that restricts recognition to MHC-1 positive cells.

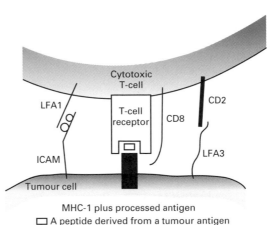

MHC-1 plus processed antigen

☐ A peptide derived from a tumour antigen

members of the KIR receptor family that recognise cancer-associated MHC-1 molecules. These NK receptors use a variety of adhesion and co-stimulatory molecules to mediate their entry into and attachment onto specific types of cancer. Macrophages and granulocytes such as neutrophils or eosinophils can also induce non-specific cell lysis.

Antibody-dependent mechanisms A category of leucocytes called K (killer) cells will lyse tumour cells provided the tumour cells have a tumour-associated antigen plus its bound antibody (Figure 5.3). As such antibodies are rarely present, this is not a major method of killing. This does not apply if the antibodies are supplied as a form of treatment (see below). K-cells are described by their killer function, not by their morphological characteristics, so both NK cells and some cytotoxic T-cells can exhibit K-cell activity.

Cell lysis

Interaction of the cytotoxic T-cell and cancer cell results in release of lymphocytic vesicles containing a monomeric protein, perforin. In the presence of Ca^{2+}, perforin polymerises in the target cell membrane to form a channel through which water and ions can travel and lyse the cell. The cytotoxic T-cell is not killed and can attack other cells.

Cytotoxic T-cells can also secrete tumour necrosis factor (TNF) or interferon (IFN), which bind to their respective receptors on the tumour and initiate intracellular signal transduction (Chapter 11). These cytokines can be used to treat patients (see below). Activated macrophages also kill by this pathway but can additionally generate toxic oxygen radicals or secrete proteases capable of destroying cells.

Escape from immune surveillance

Defects in any of the cytotoxic methods just described would enable a tumour to escape immune attack. Excluding the special cases of immune deficiency diseases, alterations in cells of the immune system do not occur, whereas loss of tumour cell MHC-I would facilitate escape. Two other features are important. Common tumours are poorly immunogenic because of the absence of tumour-specific antigens and the surveillance mechanisms are not activated. The second feature is a physical one in that antibodies and cytotoxic cells have difficulties accessing the surface of tumour cells within a mass.

Immunotherapy

Active immunotherapy

Active immunotherapy involves stimulation of the host immune system; the principle is illustrated in Figure 5.2 in which injected tumour is the stimulus. It works in animals with viral or chemically induced cancers but has not had success with human cancers. Living cancer cells could not be injected into humans so they are first inactivated, which might explain the lack of success. Antibodies are generated against the injected cells but few of those antibodies reach the cancer. However, a more likely explanation is that such tests have only been performed in patients with advanced cancers and poor outlook regardless of what treatment they receive. Such patients have cancers that are resistant to virtually any therapy.

An alternative approach has been to activate the host immune system with non-specific adjuvants such as BCG (bacillus Calmette–Guérin) or levamisole. BCG treatment of mice can result in rejection of nearly half of transplanted, chemically induced tumours but, worryingly, 10% of the transplants became larger. Clinical trials with melanoma and leukaemia have yielded unconvincing results although remission can be induced in bladder epithelium by direct application of BCG via a catheter. How this works is unclear as the requirement for local application rules out systemic activation of the immune system; activation of tissue macrophages is a possible mechanism. Transfecting BCG with genes for interleukins or tumour antigens enhances its adjuvant effect. The interleukin growth factors stimulate lymphocyte proliferation, and the tumour antigen increases the host immune response.

Passive immunotherapy

Antibody-based therapy

The principle is to provide immune effectors such as antibodies that will bind to tumour antigens (Figure 5.3). Availability of monoclonal antibodies against specific antigens present in high concentrations on tumour cells has facilitated the coating of these cells with such antibodies, which can activate either complement- or cell-mediated antibody-dependent lysis. These methods have been successfully used to clear circulating tumour cells from the blood of mice but have little effect on solid cancers, possibly because of difficulties in coating such cells with antibody.

An adaptation of this method may be more successful. Instead of relying on the cell-bound antibody alone to activate lysis, cytotoxic drugs, toxins or radioisotopes can be covalently attached to the antibody and the antibody can be used to target those drugs to specific cells. A subtype of lymphoma, non-Hodgkin's lymphoma (Appendix A), has been successfully treated by this approach. This cancer is radiosensitive and expresses a membrane protein, CD20, which can be targeted with a monoclonal antibody labelled with isotopes that emit β particles, e.g. iodine-131 or yttrium-90. The antibody is internalised and the free radicals generated from water by the β particles (Chapter 7) damage the DNA and kill the cell. Good response rates (over 75% of patients) of long duration have been obtained. An analogous approach with colon cancer using a different antibody (anti-TAG-72 protein) has achieved some responses but not as good as seen with lymphoma. A problem with this scheme is that most monoclonal antibodies are produced from mouse cells and mouse immunoglobulins are antigenic in humans. This results in their rapid clearance plus side effects due to the immune response against the mouse protein. Methods based on genetic engineering have been developed to circumvent this problem by making chimeric antibodies containing murine antigen-binding domains and human constant regions. Such antibodies are said to be 'humanised'. Examples of this approach are Vitaxin (anti-integrin $\alpha_v\beta_3$) and Herceptin (anti tyrosine kinase receptor, erbB2); see Chapter 13. ErbB2 (HER-2) expression is elevated in about one-third of breast and ovarian cancers, and appreciable tumour shrinkage (up to 50%) has been obtained with this antibody in 10% of women with advanced breast cancer; this response rate was increased by simultaneous use of cytotoxic chemotherapy.

Cell-mediated (adoptive) immunotherapy

Tumours contain lymphocytes such as cytotoxic T-cells and NK cells capable of specifically killing tumour cells. These TILs can be isolated, their numbers increased by culturing with cytokines such as interleukin-2, and returned to the host. An analogous approach can be used with peripheral blood lymphocytes rather than tumour-derived lymphocytes. Both methods generate **c**ytotoxic **T**-cell **l**ymphocytes (CTLs). Such methods will induce a limited number of responses in leukaemia patients but the remissions are of short duration with severe side effects because the CTLs also attack normal cells. The problem lies in part with the heterogeneous nature of the cells used. It has been calculated that only 1 in 2500 CTLs from a melanoma patient will recognise melanoma cells expressing a particular tumour antigen. This can be improved by better selection of CTLs and by improved characterisation of the immunodominant peptides mediating the T-cell–tumour interaction. More effective subpopulations of CTLs can be generated by cyclical activation with antigen-presenting cells in culture prior to reintroduction into the patient. Choice of tumour antigen and its immunodominant peptide can also enhance responses (Chapter 13) as can choice of the APC. The cancer cell itself is used for *in vitro* activation of cytotoxic T-cells but a subpopulation of cells with a characteristic dendritic morphology can be isolated with a high cytotoxic potential. A separate problem with currently available cell-mediated, adoptive immunotherapy is the poor survival and targeting of infused CTLs to the tumour. Potential ways of circumventing these defects include continual infusion of cytokines like interleukin-

2 to maintain CTL populations in the patient and attaching tumour-recognising antibodies to the CTLs to improve targeting. Culture of blood lymphocytes with interleukin-2 produces cells with an NK-like function except they are more active. These **l**ymphokine **a**ctivated **k**iller (LAK) cells can be returned to the host. Best results have been obtained with advanced CML patients but a limited number of kidney cancers also respond. Few of the LAK cells reach the cancer; inclusion of monoclonal antibodies against tumour antigens may improve targeting of the LAK cells.

Cytokines such as interleukins, interferons, colony-stimulating factors and TNF regulate various components of the immune response and are undergoing clinical trials as cytotoxic agents.

All these methods work to varying degrees in animal models and in cell culture but have had limited success thus far in humans. This may reflect poor information on how to use such reagents rather than their inherent ineffectiveness. Interferon-α can induce remissions in a rare form of leukaemia, hairy cell leukaemia, so there remains hope for a more general use of such approaches.

Diagnostic use of antibodies

The inherent specificity of monoclonal antibodies can be used to characterise cells either *in vivo* or on histological sections. Additionally, they are used to monitor tumour-related products in blood to see whether treatments are effective.

CEA is upregulated in colon cancers and is present in the cell membrane, where it can be recognised by monoclonal antibodies labelled with iodine-123 or iodine-131 that emit γ rays. These penetrative radiations can be detected by external monitors and thus localise the cancer without resorting to invasive methods. At the immunohistochemical level, monoclonal antibodies are in routine use as diagnostic tools. They can characterise a cancer but are also used to predict its subsequent behaviour and thus determine treatment. Antibodies against growth factor receptors, such as epidermal growth factor receptor, are particularly useful as high expression correlates with rapid growth and recurrence. High levels of such antigens indicate that additional treatments might be beneficial. Tumour-associated antigens like CEA and PSA are released into the bloodstream, where their presence can be used to monitor residual cancer after drug treatment (Chapter 13).

ONCOGENES, REPRESSOR GENES AND VIRUSES

Key points

- Oncogenes and repressor genes play major roles in carcinogenesis.
- Oncogenes are normal regulatory genes whose activity is increased as a consequence of genetic alteration. This gain of function can be due to qualitative or quantitative change in the protein product.
- Only one allele of an oncogene needs to be changed for a biological effect to occur. The effect is dominant.
- Oncogenes can be activated by mutation in a coding sequence that generates an altered product. Alternatively, chromosome rearrangement can result in increased production of a normal protein or a fusion protein with altered biological activity. Gene amplification commonly occurs during progression.
- The function of many metabolic pathways can be altered as a result of oncogene activation. These include membrane receptors, signal transduction and gene transcription.
- Repressor genes code for inhibitory proteins whose function is lost in cancers.
- Both gene copies of a diploid cell must usually be lost before a biological effect is seen. This type of repressor is recessive; p53 is an exception in that mutation in one allele generates an abnormal p53 that inactivates the normal product of the other allele. The first mutation is dominant-negative.
- Repressor proteins can be inactivated by protein phosphorylation, mutation or binding to other proteins.
- Some carcinogenic RNA viruses carry an oncogene. Others cause cancers by influencing host genes through viral regulatory sequences (insertional mutagenesis).
- Carcinogenic DNA viruses code for repressor-binding proteins or may act by indirect methods.
- Many pathways are influenced by repressors including those regulating cell proliferation and death.
- Inactivating mutations can occur at many loci within a repressor gene.
- Oncogenes and repressors cooperate in the genesis of cancers.

Introduction

These two categories of genes, and the proteins for which they code, describe the functional features that drive carcinogenesis at a molecular level. The names of the two terms have historical origins. Oncogene, or cancer gene, was so named to account for the properties of a viral gene that caused cancers in animal cells. Repressor genes were identified later when it became clear that normal cells contained inhibitory functions (repressors) whose loss resulted in uncontrolled growth. Repressors are sometimes referred to as anti-oncogenes, which is not a good term as it erroneously implies that they always act by counteracting the function of oncogenes. In fact, the two functions synergise in carcinogenesis. Oncogenes can be described as genes whose protein products gain a function as a result of mutation, whereas repressors lose a function.

This chapter will mainly be concerned with molecular changes in the genes and their products; the biological consequences of these changes are discussed in Chapters 9 to 12. Terminology and molecular detail can create problems for those not immersed in the topic, so some general points are explained in Box 6.1.

Box 6.1   Molecular terms relevant to genes and their regulation

Abbreviations

Oncogenes are described by a three-letter code usually derived from their first discovery. Thus, the ras oncogene refers to a gene originally identified in **rat** **s**arcomas and abl derives from its first discovery in the **Abl**eson virus. Sometimes, the three-letter code is followed by a letter or number. This became necessary when a function allocated to one 'gene' was subsequently found to have multiple activities. The erb gene, identified in the **er**ythro**b**lastosis virus is now divided into erbA and erbB categories. The functions of the genes were originally unknown but, even when rectified, the original nomenclature is retained. Thus, erbA is the viral homologue of the thyroid hormone receptor and erbB is homologous to the epidermal growth factor receptor. Allocation of a number conveys the fact that many of these genes are members of closely related families. The number refers to its place in the family.

Repressor genes have a more varied terminology; two- and three-letter codes are used in some situations and the size of the protein product is used in others. Thus, Rb refers to the **r**etino**b**lastoma gene and Bcl2 describes a gene first identified in a **B-c**ell lymphoma. The **2** was added to distinguish it from another gene in the same tumour type. The p53 gene is so named because the protein synthesised from its coding sequence has a molecular mass of 53 000 daltons (53 kDa). It is also known as TP53 (**t**umour su**pp**ressor).

The protein products from these genes are named using the molecular mass in kDa, preceded by a '**p**' or by the same code as the gene. Thus, the ras gene produces the ras protein or p21. Little can be done about these multiple nomenclatures and common sense has to be used in deciding whether a term refers to a gene or its protein product. The confusion is confounded by the fact that different genes can produce proteins of the same size. The ras p21

GTP-binding protein (Chapter 11) has different functions to the p21 cyclin-dependent kinase inhibitor (Chapter 10); once again, all that can be done is to translate the abbreviations in the context of their use.

Genetic terminology

Most cancers arise in somatic rather than germ cells and somatic *mutations* are therefore said to underlie most types of cancer. As somatic cells are diploid, they carry two copies (alleles) of each autosomal gene and, as both alleles can be transcribed, it follows that a mutation in one allele will only influence cell activity if the change results in a gain of function that is *dominant* over that of the unaffected allele (Table 6.1). This gain of function is characteristic of oncogene mutations such as ras that generate a constitutively active protein. Where a mutation in one allele has no effect, that mutation is said to be *recessive* and biological consequences only result when the second normal or **w**ild-**t**ype (wt) allele is lost. When the second allele is lost, the cell changes from being *heterozygous* to *homozygous* (loss of heterozygosity, LOH), which is characteristic of repressors such as Rb whose normal function is inhibitory. Functional loss of each of the two alleles can be via different mechanisms. Thus, inactivation of the first p53 allele is often by a point mutation whereas a deletion/insertion destroys the second allele. However, the function of one repressor, p53, is altered after a single allelic mutation. This protein is a transcription factor and two p53 molecules must interact (homodimer) as part of the activation process. If mutant p53 is formed from one allele, the normal and mutant products form an inactive dimer (heterodimer). Oligomer is the general term used for these protein interactions. The single mutation in the first allele is *dominant but negative*.

Table 6.1 Terminology used to describe effects of gene changes.

Diploid alleles

Normal: both alleles active

Dominant: gain of function in one allele overrides activity of the normal allele

Dominant-negative: mutation results in loss of usual function but will block normal activity

Recessive: loss of function of one allele has no effect. Must change both alleles to generate change

Loss of heterozygosity (LOH): Change from heterozygous to homozygous state due to mutations in second normal allele

Oncogenes and repressor genes produce key regulatory proteins, so there is a tendency for homologies, at both nucleic acid and protein levels, to be conserved throughout evolution, such that similarities are seen in genes from yeast, fruit flies, frogs and humans. This has helped elucidate functions, as information is available from lower organisms that has relevance to humans. But it has confused the terminology as non-mammalian names become adopted for functions of human cells.

DNA structure   In mammalian nuclei, DNA exists as two strands twisted into a double helix. This forms part of a higher structure, the chromosome, described in Box 9.1. Each DNA strand has a backbone of deoxyribose units joined to each other by phosphate groups. One end of the chain has free 3′-hydroxyl group, known as the *3′ end*, and there is a terminal 5′-hydroxyl at the other end, the *5′ end*. This polarity is such that the two chains of the double helix are of opposing polarity (Figure 6.1). The polarity determines the direction in which the genetic code is read because the enzyme RNA polymerase, which reads (transcribes) the code into messenger RNA (mRNA) will only do so in a 5′ to 3′ direction. Local regions within the helix have to be separated (melted) so that the code can be read into mRNA; the strand being read is called the *sense strand* in contrast to the complementary *antisense strand*. The genetic code is formed by the sequence of four bases attached to the deoxyribose phosphate backbone. The two pyrimidine bases, thymine (T) and cytosine (C), and the two purines, adenine (A) and guanine (G), can pair with complementary bases on the other strand of the DNA double helix in the format G:C and A:T (Figure 6.1). The cytosines can sometimes be methylated (Figure 8.2). Each amino acid is coded by three bases (a codon) specific to that amino acid.

Gene regulation

The DNA bases code for the sequence of amino acids in a protein, with each amino acid being specified by a three-base sequence known as a *codon* (Figure 6.1). Mutations in the bases can result in their being misread so that a different base is inserted at the next round of DNA synthesis. In colon cancers, the middle base of –GGC– (codon 12) in the ras oncogene is often mutated to an adenine, which results in aspartate rather than glycine being incorporated into the protein. Other types of mutation result in complete loss of protein, a truncated protein or fusion proteins derived from two genes; these are described in Box 9.1.

A gene is composed of a *coding sequence* that codes for a protein and *regulatory regions*. The regulatory regions can occur at several places within a gene but they are usually depicted at each end (Figure 6.1). The 5′ end contains base sequences that are recognised by DNA-binding proteins. These include RNA polymerase (R), which transcribes the DNA sequence into messenger RNA (mRNA), and *transcription factors* that regulate transcription. Several types of transcription factor are required but some features are

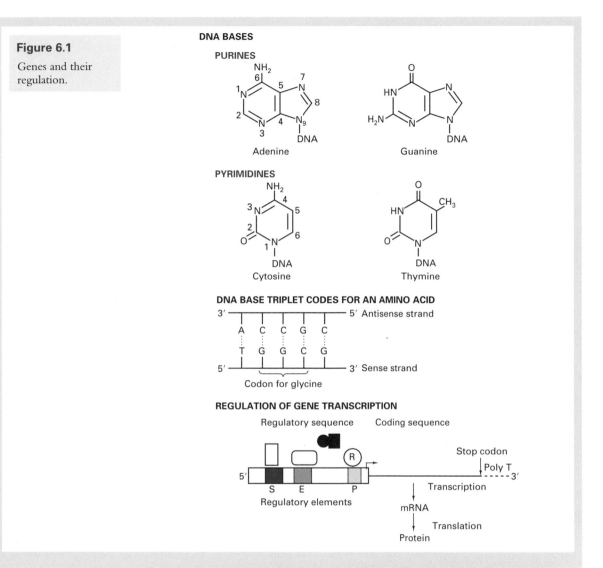

Figure 6.1

Genes and their regulation.

DNA BASES

PURINES

Adenine

Guanine

PYRIMIDINES

Cytosine

Thymine

DNA BASE TRIPLET CODES FOR AN AMINO ACID

3′ ——————————————— 5′ Antisense strand

A C C G C

T G G C G

5′ ——————————————— 3′ Sense strand

Codon for glycine

REGULATION OF GENE TRANSCRIPTION

Regulatory sequence   Coding sequence

R

Stop codon

Poly T

5′   3′

S   E   P   Transcription

Regulatory elements

mRNA

Translation

Protein

especially relevant to carcinogenesis. Many of the metabolic pathways by which the cancer cell responds to extracellular signals are focused into altering the function of transcription factors that either enhance (E) or silence (S) gene transcription. Both these functions are mediated by proteins called *enhancers* or *silencers* binding to DNA base sequences (regulatory elements). Proteins that act in this way have the ability to recognise specific DNA bases and other proteins that must be recruited into the transcription complex (*coactivators*). Many DNA-binding proteins of this type do not bind as single molecules but as dimers. Dimers can consist of two similar proteins (homodimer) or two dissimilar proteins (heterodimer).

At the 3′ end of the gene are triplet bases that stop transcription, often followed by polythymine tails. The coding sequence is transcribed into RNA but some of them are removed (spliced out) to give mature mRNA that will be translated into protein. The DNA sequences that are eventually transcribed and translated into protein are called *exons*; those that are transcribed and then spliced out are called *introns*.

Protein structure   The first amino acid translated from the 5′ end of the mRNA has a free amino group (N-terminus) whereas the last amino acid has a free carboxyl group (C-terminus). Regulatory proteins are composed of different regions (domains), each with a specific function. Thus, the DNA-binding transcription factors have a DNA-binding domain and a transactivation domain. The transactivation domain is responsible for binding other proteins, thereby forming the transcription complex. Other proteins are described later with domains responsible for ligand binding (e.g. hormones, growth factors), GTP binding (e.g. ras) and tyrosine kinase activity (e.g. growth factor receptors). There can be complex interactions between domains, so the function of the full protein does not simply reflect the sum of the individual domains. The domain function of regulatory proteins is often altered by phosphorylation of protein hydroxyl groups. One class of protein kinase phosphorylates serine and threonine residues whilst another group phosphorylates tyrosines.

Proteins are destroyed by proteolysis either in lysosomes or by macromolecular complexes called *proteasomes*. The lysosomal pathway is relatively non-specific whereas proteasomes can selectively inactivate proteins. They do this by attaching the polypeptide ubiquitin to the protein; this marks the protein for proteolysis within the proteasome. As proteolysis destroys function, it represents an off-switch for biochemical reactions.

Oncogenes

Oncogenes are genes that gain oncogenic or transforming potential as a result of genetic changes in either their coding region or regulatory sequences. The gene present in normal cells is called a *proto-oncogene* to distinguish it from the altered gene in the cancer cell. The term 'proto-oncogene' can be misleading as it implies a latency in normal cells that is unwarranted since the normal genes have important functions. The normal gene is sometimes referred to as a cellular oncogene (c-onc) to distinguish it from its viral homologues (v-onc). This arose for historical reasons as the original oncogene, v-src, was first identified as a viral gene responsible for the sarcoma-producing properties of the Rous sarcoma virus; a cellular homologue, c-src, was subsequently identified in normal cells. Virus-induced cancers are not as important in humans as in animals, so the term v-onc has minimal application to humans. The term 'proto-oncogene' can be synonymous with c-onc, which becomes an oncogene after its expression is altered. However, additional clarification is necessary about the use of the term c-onc. Figure 6.2 depicts the

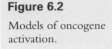

Figure 6.2

Models of oncogene activation.

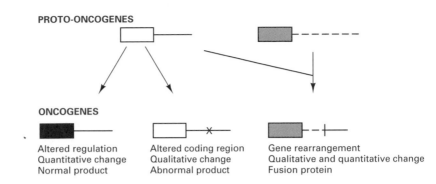

oncogene model of carcinogenesis in which gene modification results in either qualitative or quantitative changes in gene expression. Altered regulation can bring about quantitative change in a normal product. As shown in Figure 6.2, the $5'$ upstream regulatory sequences are changed, thereby altering transcription. However, post-transcriptional effects can occur, as in the fos gene where mutations in the $3'$ non-coding region increase the half-life of fos mRNA. Overproduction of a normal product is also achieved by gene amplification, as in the case of the growth factor receptor erbB2.

Qualitative changes due to the generation of an abnormal product can occur either by mutation in the coding region or by gene rearrangement resulting in production of a fusion protein made up of parts of each participating gene. In the latter case there may be confusion as to which of the two genes is the proto-oncogene. The confusion is circumvented if one considers the gene to include both coding and regulatory sequences.

Examples of each type of change are described later.

Viral carcinogenesis

Analysis of mechanisms whereby viruses cause cancer was fundamental to the understanding of molecular carcinogenesis, the original concept being that the virus carried a gene capable of disrupting cell regulation. This has since been modified to include viruses that do not carry such genes but which alter cell function in other ways. Table 6.2 gives examples of viruses that contribute to carcinogenesis and it is evident that they influence many different host functions. The RNA viruses shown all relate to animal cancers and have little impact on human carcinogenesis except for human immunodeficiency virus (HIV, sarcomas) and human T-cell lymphotropic virus (HTLV, leukaemia). This is less true of the DNA viruses mentioned in Table 6.2, as only adenovirus and simian virus 40 (SV40) are not human related.

RNA viruses

RNA viruses infect competent cells and, by reverse transcription, their RNA is converted into DNA and incorporated into the host genome, hence their classification

Table 6.2 Viral carcinogenesis.

Virus	Gene	Function	Compartment
RNA			
Rous sarcoma	$pp60^{src}$	Tyrosine kinase	Cytoplasm, membranes
Rat sarcoma	ras	GTPase	Cytoplasm, membranes
Erythroblastosis	erbA	Thyroid hormone receptor	Nucleus
Feline osteosarcoma	fos	Transcription factor	Nucleus
Simian sarcoma	sis	Platelet-derived growth factor	Secreted
Mouse mammary tumour	None	Insertional mutagenesis	–
DNA			
Human papilloma	E6, E7	Bind repressors (p53, Rb)	Nucleus
Adenovirus	E1A, E1B	Bind repressors (p53, Rb)	Nucleus
Simian virus 40	Large T antigen	Binds repressors (p53, Rb)	Nucleus
Epstein–Barr	BZLFI, EBNA5	Binds p53; rearranges myc genes?	Nucleus
Hepatitis B	HBX	Binds p53	Nucleus

as retroviruses. The DNA generated from the virus is called the provirus. Carcinogenesis is influenced in one of two general ways (Figure 6.3): by provision of an oncogene, or insertional mutagenesis in which regulatory viral sequences alter host gene activity. The former, acutely transforming group has a short latent period, as oncogene insertion does not have to be at a specific locus. The latter group shows a prolonged induction period because of the low probability of being inserted in the right place next to a relevant host gene. In humans, insertional mutagenesis is unknown although it is a common cause of animal cancers.

Provision of an oncogene Many oncogenic RNA viruses contain an oncogene additional to the sequences needed for viral replication (Figure 6.3). The case

Figure 6.3

RNA viral carcinogenesis.

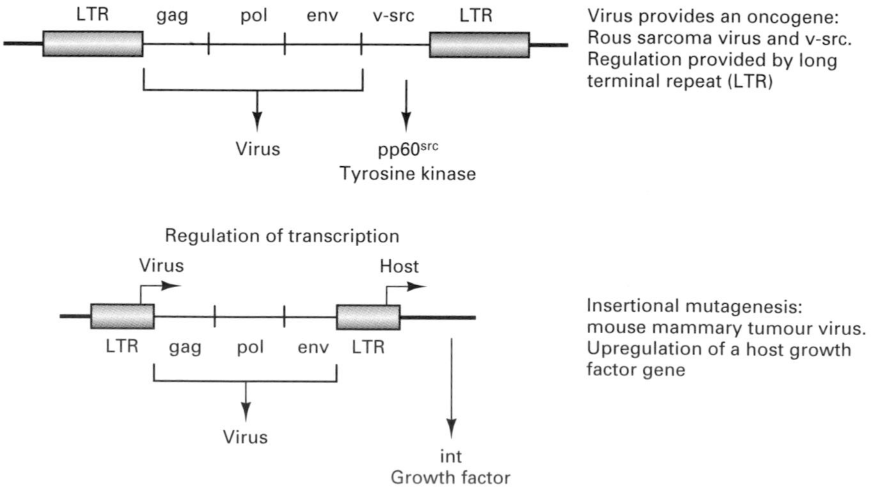
LTR
gag
pol
env
v-src
LTR
Virus
pp60src
Tyrosine kinase
Virus provides an oncogene: Rous sarcoma virus and v-src. Regulation provided by long terminal repeat (LTR)
Regulation of transcription
Virus
Host
LTR
gag
pol
env
LTR
Virus
int
Growth factor
Insertional mutagenesis: mouse mammary tumour virus. Upregulation of a host growth factor gene

illustrated is Rous sarcoma virus in which the oncogene v-src codes for a 60 kDa phosphoprotein (pp60^{src}) that has tyrosine kinase activity. In its active form, it is bound to the inner face of the cell membrane but it can also be found in the cytoplasm and other membranes. It is attached to the membrane by a 14-carbon side chain, myristic acid. Viral oncogenes differ from cellular oncogenes in both specific and general ways: c-oncs are typical eukaryotic genes in possessing both introns and exons, the introns being spliced out in the mRNA; v-oncs have lost their introns during the evolutionary time since the virus acquired the gene from the host cell. In the src example, specific differences include a longer C-terminal region in c-src and the last 12 codons of v-src differ from their c-src counterparts.

Insertional mutagenesis **M**ouse **m**ammary **t**umour **v**irus (MMTV) does not contain a v-onc but its regulatory sequences can stimulate adjacent host genes (Figure 6.3). The regulatory sequences are repeated at each end of the viral genome (**l**ong **t**erminal **r**epeats, LTRs) and so either end of the virus has the potential to influence host genes. LTRs contain enhancer sequences capable of increasing transcription from nearby genes. The DNA base sequences that make up the enhancer are effective in either 5′–3′ or 3′–5′ orientations so the orientation of the virus relative to host genes does not matter. Mapping MMTV in mouse mammary tumours indicated that, although the insert locus could vary, it was always near a gene (int) that codes for a fibroblast growth factor (Figure 6.3).

The modes of action of the two human retroviruses HIV and HTLV are indirect but obscure. Neither carries an oncogene and no meaningful pattern of tumour insertions has been identified. HIV may work by suppressing immune attack on early cancers but this is not a complete answer. HTLV can code for transcription factors that regulate host genes such as fos but the link with carcinogenesis is tenuous.

DNA viruses

DNA viruses can act directly by virtue of their v-onc protein product binding to and inactivating host proteins (Table 6.2). The repressor protein p53 was first identified by its interaction with large T-antigen of the SV40 virus, whereas E7 of **h**uman **p**apilloma **v**irus (HPV) binds to and inactivates the Rb repressor protein. The consequence of either of these interactions is altered cell proliferation. Note that there is frequently viral production of proteins capable of binding p53 and Rb repressors; this may represent a common pathway for the carcinogenic effects of directly acting DNA viruses. In some cases (HPV, adenovirus) the virus codes for two separate proteins, one inactivating p53 the other Rb; by contrast SV40 codes for a single protein, large T (tumour) antigen with separate domains for recognising p53 and Rb.

DNA viruses are important in several human cancers: cervix (HPV), liver (hepatitis B virus), nasopharynx and Burkitt's lymphoma (Epstein–Barr virus). There are many members of the HPV family involved with different pathologies. Thus, HPV 16 and 18 are involved with cervical cancers whereas HPVs 6, 10 and 11 are associated with epithelial warts, which are not cancers. The varying cellular responses to the different types of HPV are related to the E6 and E7 proteins produced therefrom. These proteins from high-risk forms of HPV can transform cultured cells, whereas those from low-risk viruses cannot. The synergy of actions of these two proteins is helped by the fact that both genes are transcribed as a single (*polycistronic*) mRNA regulated by one promoter; the individual E6 and E7 mRNAs are generated by cleavage of the larger RNA.

In HPV the viral DNA initially exists as individual elements (episomes) within the host cell nucleus (Figure 6.4), but as part of the carcinogenic process, specific segments become inserted in a random way into host chromosomes. For cervical cancer to occur, the viral E6 and E7 sequences have to be present. Given the randomness in the choice of viral segments and their positions of insertion in the host DNA, it is not surprising that increasing the viral exposure of cervical epithelium raises the risk of developing cancer. This is not a single-hit process as transient HPV infections are not carcinogenic; prolonged exposure is required. This may be related to the fact that carcinogenesis is a time-dependent, multistage process (Chapter 2); inactivation of Rb and p53 by viral E7 and E6 proteins, respectively, is required at several stages.

Viral DNA can have indirect effects that are difficult to define. Most people have been infected with Epstein–Barr virus whereas Burkitt's lymphoma is only common in certain regions such as Central Africa, so other factors must be required for carcinogenesis; infection with the malarial parasite may be one such cofactor. With this B-cell lymphoma one result of viral infection is a translocation that places the c-myc gene (chromosome 8) adjacent to an immunoglobulin promoter (chromosome 14) so that myc is constitutively expressed. This mechanism is sometimes referred to as promoter insertion (see below). The mechanism for this remains obscure but the virus may increase the likelihood of this specific chromosome translocation early in B-cell differentiation. EBV stimulates the proliferation of B-cells that could contribute to the elevated chromosome damage. Inactivation of p53 by viral proteins (Table 6.2) could be a mechanism by which increased proliferation and chromosome translocation occur (Chapter 10).

Figure 6.4

Cervical cancer and human papilloma virus (HPV). See Chapter 10 for consequences of E6 and E7 production.

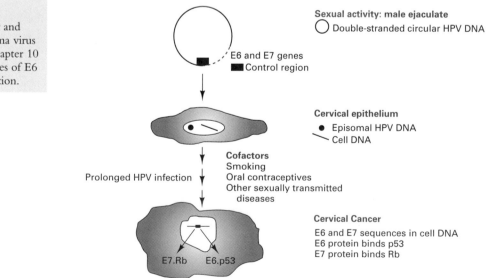

Sexual activity: male ejaculate
○ Double-stranded circular HPV DNA

E6 and E7 genes
■ Control region

Cervical epithelium
● Episomal HPV DNA
Cell DNA

Prolonged HPV infection

Cofactors
Smoking
Oral contraceptives
Other sexually transmitted
  diseases

Cervical Cancer
E6 and E7 sequences in cell DNA
E6 protein binds p53
E7 protein binds Rb

E7.Rb   E6.p53

Table 6.3 Characteristics of eurkaryotic oncogenes.

Oncogene product	Chromosome	Function
Extracellular		
sis	22	Platelet-derived growth factor
Membrane		
ras	11	GTPase
erbB2	7	Growth factor receptor
fms	5	Growth factor receptor
*Cytoplasm**		
src	20	Tyrosine kinase
raf	3	Serine/threonine kinase
Nucleus		
myc	8	Transcription factor
fos	14	Transcription factor

* Can be transferred to membranes.

With cervical cancer, cofactors that synergise with HPV in increasing risk include smoking and use of oral contraceptives (Figure 6.4). Genotoxic carcinogens (Chapter 7) in tobacco smoke can explain the smoking effect but the role of oral contraceptive actions is more problematic. A possible mechanism involves the active hormonal ingredient of the contraceptive. Commonly used forms contain progestins which, in combination with receptor proteins (Chapter 11), can bind and activate HPV promoter sequences.

Specific examples of oncogene changes

More than 60 oncogenes have been identified; an oncogene is contained in each of the diverse regulatory pathways that govern cell behaviour. Selected examples are shown in Table 6.3 and are referred to in later chapters dealing with biological functions. This section presents specific examples from human tumours to illustrate the main features of oncogene involvement in carcinogenesis.

Increased normal product

Increased normal product is achieved by either amplifying the gene or altering its regulation. Amplification is common in advanced cancers but is infrequently a causative event in early stages of carcinogenesis. Altered regulation is encountered at both early and late stages of tumour development.

Altered regulation In some cancers, chromosome rearrangement results in the coding sequence of an oncogene coming under the influence of the strong

Figure 6.5

Increase in a normal protein: c-Myc and Burkitt's lymphoma translocation between chromosomes 8 and 14.

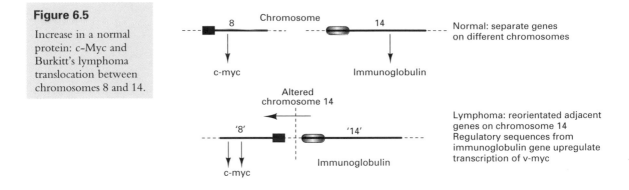

regulatory (promoter) sequences of another gene (promoter insertion). Little is known about mutations in regulatory regions of oncogenes in the absence of chromosome rearrangements.

Increased c-myc due to promoter insertion is found in Burkitt's lymphoma, a B-cell cancer common in Africa where malaria and Epstein–Barr virus infection are cofactors of unknown function (Appendix A). In the majority of such tumours, the c-myc gene on chromosome 8 is translocated next to an immunoglobulin (Ig) gene on chromosome 14 (Figure 6.5). The Ig remains silent, so the body's defence mechanisms are not compromised, but normal c-myc is overproduced because the strong Ig promoter can upregulate the adjacent myc gene. The c-myc protein heterodimerises with another protein, Max, to generate a transcription factor that regulates genes involved in both proliferation and apoptosis (Chapter 10).

Different lymphomas have different chromosome breakpoints and the orientation of the two genes can be head-to-head (5′ of c-myc to 5′ of Ig) or head-to-tail (5′ of c-myc to 3′ of Ig) although head-to-head is more common. As depicted in Figure 6.5, the c-myc promoter is unaffected by the translocation but this is not always the case. Whatever happens to the myc promoter, the coding region is always retained and is upregulated by the strong Ig promoter.

Gene amplification This common feature of advanced cancers often accompanies the acquisition of increased aggressiveness, a good example being the c-erbB2 oncogene. This is a transmembrane growth factor receptor whose cytoplasmic domain has tyrosine kinase activity capable of upregulating growth-promoting signal transduction pathways (Chapter 11). Cancers of the breast and cervix overexpress normal protein due to gene amplification. The chromosome instability associated with cancer progression is accompanied by multiple duplications of specific regions of DNA due to defective start signals at DNA replication forks (Chapter 8). In rat neuroblastomas, the erbB homologue neu has a T → A mutation that changes a glutamate to a valine in the transmembrane region. This may facilitate ligand-independent dimerisation of the receptor and therefore it is constitutively active. Hence increased receptor activity is achieved by increased normal protein in humans and an abnormal, constitutively active product in rats.

Altered product

Two commonly used ways of achieving this result are mutation and production of a fusion protein made up of incomplete parts of two separate genes.

Normal-sized product with altered activity   The ras oncogene is commonly mutated in tumours such as colon and pancreas. The term ras is a generic one covering different members of a family that includes H-ras, K-ras and N-ras, the prefixes referring to the condition in which they were first identified: H and K refer to **H**arvey and **K**iersten murine sarcoma virus and N indicates **n**euroblastoma. The proto-oncogene codes for a key intermediary in signal transduction between cell membrane and nucleus (Chapter 11) – it is a GTP-binding protein with latent GTPase activity, active when bound to GTP and inactive when the GTP is hydrolysed to GDP (Figure 6.6). The 21 kDa ras protein (p21) has intrinsic GTPase activity that is regulated by other proteins (Chapter 11).

The GTP-binding region (domain) is diffuse, involving five codons between 12 and 69 and four between 116 and 147 (Table 6.4), although all the carcinogenic mutations occur in the first group. Ras is bound to the cytoplasmic face of the cell membrane via a 15-carbon isoprenyl (farnesyl) group linked to a C-terminal cysteine. Experimentally engineered loss of this isoprenylation site inactivates the protein.

Ras protein is a focal point in the signal transduction pathways for several input signals and it relays those signals to a number of effector pathways. This requires ras

Figure 6.6

Functional change in oncogene product. Ras: mutation in a coding sequence.

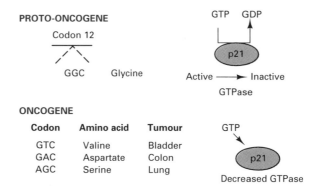

Table 6.4   Domain functions of the ras oncogene.

Functions	Codons
GTP phosphates	12, 13, 59–69
GTP guanine	116–119, 147
Bind other proteins	32–40
Prenylation of CAAX motif (cysteine.alanine.alanine.any amino acid)	C-terminal end
Carcinogenesis; decreased GTPase	12 (frequent) 13, 1 (infrequent)

to interact with other proteins (Chapter 10). The codons responsible for these interactions are located between positions 32 and 40.

Point mutations in ras have been identified in several codons, notably 12, 13 and 61, the first being most commonly affected but, whatever the codon, the result is decreased GTPase activity resulting in constitutive ras activity. This heterogeneity in affected codons is also seen when individual base changes within codon 12 are identified; different tumours exhibit different point mutations such that the glycine in the proto-oncogene can be substituted with either valine, aspartate or serine (Figure 6.6). In the human we know neither the mechanism behind these mutations nor the carcinogens involved but more complete information is available in the rat. Chemically induced tumours have codon 12 mutations due to covalent interaction between the carcinogen (N-methylnitrosourea) and the O-6 of guanine (Chapter 7).

Abnormal-sized product: retinoic acid receptor α/acute promyelocytic leukaemia   **A**cute **p**romyelocytic **l**eukaemia (APL) is a form of leukaemia in which differentiation is blocked at the promyeloid cell stage (Appendix A). It is characterised by a reciprocal chromosome translocation such that the **r**etinoic **a**cid **r**eceptor **α** (RARA) gene from chromosome 17 is translocated next to the **p**romyelocytic **l**eukaemia gene (PML) on chromosome 15 (Figure 6.7). The altered chromosome 15 is said to be 15+ and the altered chromosome 17 is referred to as 17−; the translocation is designated t(15;17) (Box 9.1). There are two classes of breakpoints that result in the production of two different PMLRARA fusion proteins (Figure 6.7). Both have a common RARA segment that has lost the N-terminal region including part of the transactivation domain (Figure 11.21) but the PML contribution differs in the two sets of patients. A subtype of acute promyelocytic leukaemia is characterised by a different t(11;17) chromosome translocation; the RARA gene is involved but the fusion protein (PLZFRARA) has a different N-terminal sequence. The presenting symptoms of the two types of APL patient are similar; this suggests that those symptoms are a consequence of the altered RARA gene but it does not rule out a contribution from the other partner of the fusion protein, as treatment responses differ between the two types of patient.

In normal cells, RARA is a transcription factor whose DNA-binding activity relies on the presence of the ligand, *trans*-retinoic acid. The RARA receptor plus the *trans*-retinoic acid form a functional transcription factor by heterodimerising with the **r**etinoic acid **X** **r**eceptor (RXR) plus its ligand, *cis*-retinoic acid. RXR also heterodimerises with receptors for vitamin D and thyroid hormone; heterodimerisation is essential for the biological function of all these ligands (Chapter 11). Hence anything that disrupts RXR availability interferes with the actions of these other agents. Both retinoic acid isomers, vitamin D and thyroid hormone promote cell differentiation so their blockade inhibits differentiation; this is a hallmark of leukaemias (Chapters 2 and 15). The normal function of PML is less clear but it is expressed in the nuclei of most cells and the protein is a component of the nuclear matrix, possibly involved in regulating gene function. Its predicted structure indicates the presence of DNA-binding and dimerisation domains characteristic of some transcription factors. PML protein can form homodimers with itself and heterodimers with another member of the RARA family, RXR.

Figure 6.7

An abnormal fusion protein. Acute promyelocytic leukaemia: translocation between chromosomes 15 and 17.

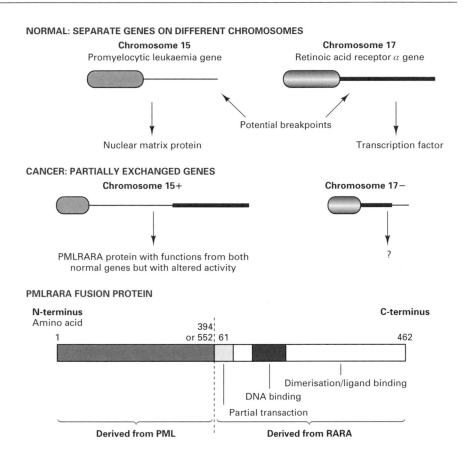

NORMAL: SEPARATE GENES ON DIFFERENT CHROMOSOMES

Chromosome 15
Promyelocytic leukaemia gene

Chromosome 17
Retinoic acid receptor α gene

Potential breakpoints

Nuclear matrix protein

Transcription factor

CANCER: PARTIALLY EXCHANGED GENES

Chromosome 15+

Chromosome 17−

PMLRARA protein with functions from both normal genes but with altered activity

?

PMLRARA FUSION PROTEIN

N-terminus
Amino acid

C-terminus

1   394 or 552 61   462

Dimerisation/ligand binding
DNA binding
Partial transaction

Derived from PML

Derived from RARA

The protein produced from the chromosome rearrangement is a fusion of partial products from each participating gene (Figure 6.7). The PMLRARA fusion protein contains most of the functional domains of both PML and RARA but the RARA is the major contributor to the genesis of leukaemia. Nevertheless, RNA transcripts from the 17− fusion gene are detected in some APL cases and so additional effects may derive from this product. The PMLRARA product is under the regulation of the PML promoter and the fusion protein made therefrom is mainly cytoplasmic. The RARA part of the fusion protein retains its DNA-binding, dimerisation and ligand-binding domains but it has lost part of the transactivating mechanism. The protein can bind *trans*-retinoic acid, dimerise and interact with DNA but it inefficiently recruits other transcription factors. At least two features of this fusion protein contribute to blocked promyelocyte differentiation and their resultant accumulation in the blood. PMLRARA fusion protein will heterodimerise with RXR and interfere with RXR function. This also has the potential to disrupt vitamin D and thyroid hormone effects on differentiation; vitamin D can induce promyelocyte differentiation. Secondly, loss of part of the RARA transactivation domain interferes with *trans*-retinoic acid function. Nevertheless, high concentrations of *trans*-retinoic acid induce remission in most APL patients, so some elements of normal RARA function are retained. Whatever the mechanisms involved, they are lost in the t(11;17) type of APL as these patients are unresponsive to *trans*-retinoic acid.

In this example and others, such as chronic myeloid leukaemia (Chapters 2 and 11), components from both the normal genes contribute to the oncogenic potential of the fusion protein, so the terminology becomes problematic about whether one or both of the normal genes are proto-oncogenes.

Repressor genes

Repressor genes have proved to be of critical importance in human carcinogenesis and their limited number indicates a more general role than the more diverse oncogenes. The basis of their importance is that in normal cells growth and other functions are restricted by inhibitory (repressor) proteins that must be reversibly inactivated for growth to occur.

The relevance of such repressor proteins and their genes to human cancer is apparent from two data sets, one clinical and the other experimental. Familial retinoblastoma is caused by loss of both alleles of a gene, Rb, encoding a repressor protein; loss of functional protein results in uncontrolled growth (Chapter 9). The experimental data come from studies in which normal and cancer cells are fused, the hybrids having a normal phenotype. The normal cells express repressor proteins that inhibit the cancerous properties (Chapter 2).

The involvement of a repressor gene is advertised by the requirement for inactivation of both alleles so that neither can make an inhibitor. However, the converse is not always true: biological change resulting from inactivation of only one allele does not exclude a repressor mechanism. This is exemplified by p53, which can act in a dominant-negative manner. When first identified, p53 was described as an oncogene on the basis of its ability to transform cultured cells. When the original p53 was shown to be mutant and not the wild-type product, it was reclassified as a repressor. The original experiment worked because the mutation was dominant-negative so that heterocomplexes with wild-type protein from the other allele produced an inactive complex. Hence the presence of one mutant allele was sufficient in this situation to generate an inactive product.

Repressor inactivation

Repressor proteins inhibit cell functions by complexing with other effector proteins and blocking their action. Inactivation of the repressor gene product and therefore the lifting of its blocking effect is achieved by preventing its binding to the effector protein, a process that can be achieved in several ways (Figure 6.8). In quiescent normal cells, proliferation is blocked because Rb protein binds and inactivates a transcription factor. Serine/threonine phosphorylation of Rb protein disrupts this interaction thereby releasing the cell cycle block characteristic of this protein. Mutation resulting in altered product or loss of product is another way of escaping

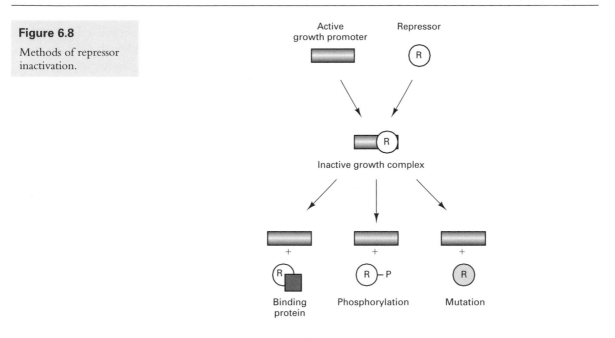

Figure 6.8

Methods of repressor inactivation.

Table 6.5 Repressor genes.

Name	Chromosome	Location	Function
Rb	13	Nucleus	Cell cycle
p53	17	Nucleus	DNA repair, apoptosis
Bcl2	18	Mitochondria	Apoptosis
nm23	17	Mitochondria	Metastasis
BRCA2	17	Nucleus	DNA repair
APC	5	Cytoskeleton	Cell–cell recognition

from this inhibition. Alternatively, a repressor gene need not be changed but the normal product can be inactivated by other proteins. Rb and p53 adopt both mechanisms depending on the cancer concerned (see below).

Examples of repressor genes inactivated in human cancers are given in Table 6.5; many more are known by virtue of their loss of heterozygosity in various tumours but their functions are unknown. Repressors are found in various cell compartments and influence varied functions. Because Rb and p53 have such a wide and interrelated involvement in carcinogenesis, molecular aspects of their actions will be considered here; biological implications are discussed in Chapters 9 to 12. Biological features of the other repressors listed in Table 6.5 can be found in Chapters 2 (APC), 9 (BRCA2), 10 (Bcl2) and 12 (nm23).

Retinoblastoma

The retinoblastoma gene codes for a 110 kDa nuclear protein of the same name, first identified because its loss of function is a causal event in retinoblastoma development

(Chapter 9), but loss has also been noted in a proportion of common cancers such as those of lung, prostate and breast. Rb is a big gene (300 kb), although most mutations are in the 3 kb coding region and mostly involve gross chromosomal changes. However, about one-third of the cases are point mutations. Several retinoblastomas can arise in one eye, each with a different Rb mutation. This illustrates both the clonal origin of these tumours and the varied ways in which one gene can be inactivated. The gene is crucial for normal development, so homozygous Rb $-/-$ mice die as embryos whilst heterozygous animals develop pituitary and thyroid cancers. The normal protein inhibits proliferation. In these events it synergises with p53, so that in many tumours there is loss of both repressors (Chapter 10).

The Rb protein has more than 10 phosphorylation (ser/thr) sites mainly in the C and N terminal regions. Conversion from hypo- to hyperphosphorylated states alters the ability of Rb to interact with other proteins. Over 25 Rb-binding proteins have been identified with functions relating to nucleosome structure (Brm), tyrosine phosphorylation (abl), protein dephosphorylation (phosphatases, pp-1a2), oncogenes (Mdm2) and transcription (E2F, DP) of genes involved in proliferation. Thus, Rb can influence many cell functions but most attention has been directed at its influence on gene transcription. Hypophosphorylated Rb binds and inactivates the transcription factor E2F, whereas the hyperphosphorylated (se/thr) form will not (Figure 6.9). The proliferation cycle of the cell, the cell cycle, is regulated by a series of protein kinases that are activated by another set of proteins, the cyclins. These **c**yclin-**d**ependent **k**inases (CDKs) phosphorylate and inactivate Rb thereby relieving the cycle block (Chapter 10). Little is known about dephosphorylation mechanisms except that they involve a protein phosphatase. The released E2F stimulates transcription of genes that regulate growth such as cdc2, myc and DNA polymerase α. The active transcription complex is a heterodimer of E2F with DP protein. Rb also inhibits transcription from ribosomal and transfer RNA genes by binding with transcription factors UBF (**u**pstream **b**inding **f**actor) and TF-IIIB (**t**ranscription **f**actor **IIIB**) respectively (Figure 6.10 and Chapter 10). Rb thus influences the mass of a cell (protein content) as well as its replicative ability.

Figure 6.9

Actions of the retinoblastoma repressor protein (Rb).

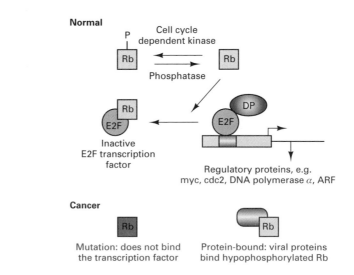

Figure 6.10

Rb inhibits several types of RNA synthesis by binding to different proteins.

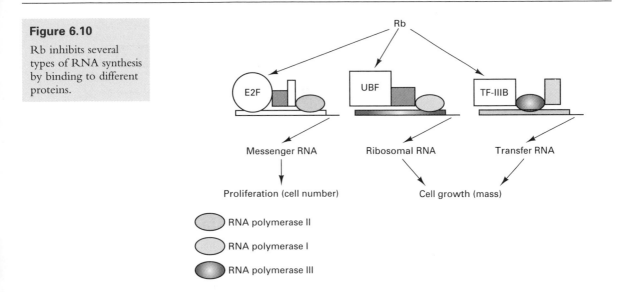

Relief of Rb repression occurs normally by hyperphosphorylation and abnormally by Rb mutation or binding to other proteins. Binding occurs with hypophosphorylated Rb and human papilloma virus E7 or adenovirus E1B proteins (Figure 6.9). Thus, Rb is inactivated by mutation in retinoblastoma, by E7 protein in cervical cancer and by phosphorylation in the normal cell cycle.

p53

The p53 gene, which produces the p53 repressor protein, is the gene most frequently altered in human cancers. If one had to nominate one protein to illustrate the multiplicity of molecular mechanisms involved in carcinogenesis, p53 would be that protein. There are other members of the p53 family (p41, p51, p73) but information on their functions is sparse. In normal cells it has been well described as the 'guardian of the genome' because it protects DNA from insults as varied as radiation and drugs. It achieves this protection by coordinately blocking cell proliferation, stimulating DNA repair and promoting apoptotic cell death (Chapters 9 and 10). Given the importance of p53 in cell function, it is surprising that mice in which both alleles have been deleted or humans who have a germline mutation in one allele (Li–Fraumeni syndrome) develop at all, although they do have a propensity to develop multiple tumours in adulthood. This suggests that knocking out p53 destabilises the genome in a general way so that deleterious agents such as mutagens are more likely to be effective and errors are more likely to accumulate.

The p53 gene can be inactivated by mutation or the normal p53 protein rendered non-functional by binding to other proteins.

Normal p53   Over 2000 inactivating p53 mutations have been identified in human tumours; to understand how such diverse and numerous changes achieve the same end result, it is essential to understand the domain structure of p53 (Figure 6.11). It has four functional domains involved in regulation of transcription (*transactivation*),

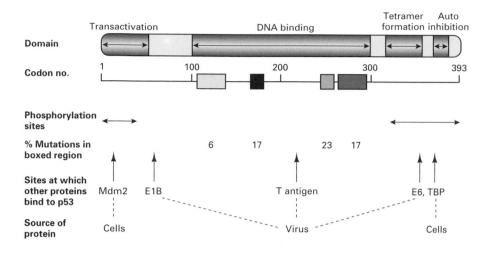

Figure 6.11

Domain structure of p53 protein and how its function may be altered.

binding to specific DNA sequences, reacting with other p53 molecules (*oligomerisation*), and a C-terminal, 30 amino acid tail capable of inhibiting functions relating to DNA binding (autoinhibitory domain). The transactivation domain stimulates transcription indirectly by binding other nuclear proteins and recruiting them into the transcription complex. Normal cells can produce a protein, Mdm2, capable of inactivating wild-type p53 by binding to the transactivating domain as well as increasing p53 degradation. The functional p53 unit that interacts with DNA is a tetramer made up of two dimers; the oligomerisation domain is the determinant for this process. The autoinhibitory domain contains many basic (positively charged) amino acids and is thought to block the DNA-binding domain as agents that bind to or alter the charge (phosphorylation) of the inhibitory region activate DNA binding. These agents include synthetic peptides, antibodies, non-specific DNA and protein kinases. Other proteins that regulate p53 function bind to each of these domains (see below). p53 can be phosphorylated (ser/thr) at several sites in both the C and N terminal regions. Kinases such as protein kinase C, cycle-dependent kinases and mitogen-activated protein (MAP) kinases can catalyse C-terminal phosphorylations whereas DNA-dependent protein kinase and the ATM kinase coded by the ataxia telangiectasia gene (Chapter 9) phosphorylate the N-terminal end (see below). Other proteins that regulate p53 function bind to each of the domains (see below).

The three-dimensional structure of the DNA-binding domain indicates a core scaffold region from which three loops extend (Figure 6.12). The first loop, composed of two separate regions of the DNA-binding domain (Figure 6.11), contacts the major groove of the DNA, the second loop contacts the minor groove and the third loop stabilises the second one via a zinc atom coordinated to cysteine residues in the loop.

Numerous genes are influenced by p53, mostly but not entirely mediated via the cell's transcription machinery (Figure 6.13). Genes whose transcription is increased by p53 have a response element that specifically binds a p53 tetramer via the tetramer's DNA binding domain. The N-terminal domain recruits additional transcription factors (proteins) required for mRNA synthesis. BAX, p21, insulin-like

Figure 6.12

Regions of the DNA-binding domain of p53 that interact with DNA. The loop symbols compare directly with those in Figure 6.9 to indicate the regions in which most inactivating mutations occur.

Figure 6.13

Actions of p53 that depend on transcription.

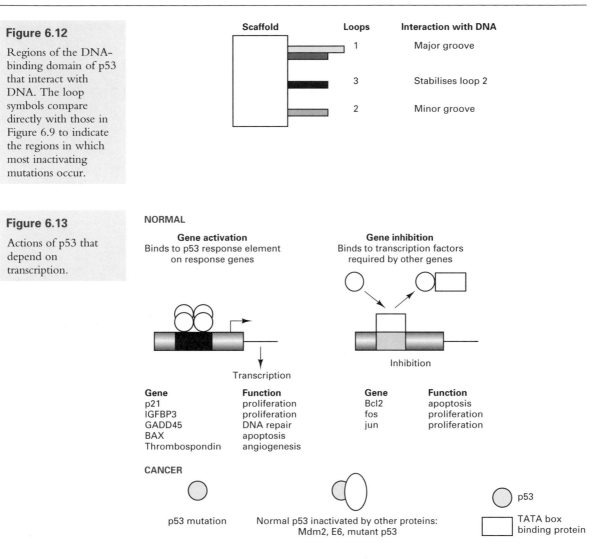

growth factor binding protein 3 (IGFB3), GADD45 and thrombospondin are all increased by this mechanism. Expression of genes such as Bcl2, fos and jun can be inhibited by p53. Such genes do not have a p53 response element but they do need a transcription factor, the **TATA-box binding protein** (TBP) for gene transcription. p53 will bind and inactivate TBP via the C-terminal domain of p53 and thus inhibit transcription from those genes. However, not all inhibitory functions of p53 are mediated by this mechanism. p53 can bind to and influence serine (casein kinase) and tyrosine kinases (abl oncogene), calcium-binding proteins (S100b) and excision repair proteins (XPD, XPB). These non-transcriptional effects could influence functions that are important in carcinogenesis.

Normal cells contain latent p53; the amount and function are influenced by phosphorylation and interaction with other proteins. In such cells the half-life is low (< 2 min) and the p53 is bound to Mdm2 protein (Figure 6.14). This interaction

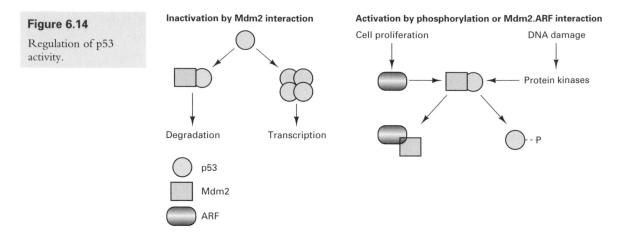

Figure 6.14

Regulation of p53 activity.

serves two functions: prevention of transcription activity and acceleration of p53 degradation via ubiquitin-mediated proteolysis. The Mdm2–p53 interaction is regulated either by p53 phosphorylation or sequestration of the Mdm2 protein by the ARF protein. Thus, increasing ARF or using p53 phosphorylation are two independent ways of increasing p53 availability without requiring protein synthesis (post-transcriptional regulation). DNA damage activates serine protein kinases which rapidly phosphorylate p53 and release it from Mdm2, thus increasing cellular levels of functional p53 (up to a hundredfold). This feeds through to decreased proliferation and increased apoptosis (Chapter 10). *In vivo*, mitogen-stimulated proliferation is followed by a smaller wave of apoptosis. Mitogen-induced phosphorylation of Rb results in E2F-activated transcription of the **a**lternate **r**eading **f**rame (ARF) gene as well as those that stimulate proliferation (Figure 6.9). The mitogen-activated apoptosis could be a consequence of ARF releasing p53 from Mdm2.

Four cellular responses are influenced by p53-sensitive genes: cell proliferation, apoptotic death, DNA repair and angiogenesis (Figure 6.13). The important question of how p53 inhibits proliferation without stopping DNA repair in some situations but promotes cell death in others is only partially resolved. One key may be the gene that codes for a **c**ycle-dependent **k**inase **i**nhibitor (CKI), p21, which inactivates the cyclin–cycle-dependent kinase complex essential for DNA synthesis (Figure 10.5); p21 also binds to a protein, PCNA (**p**roliferating **c**ell **n**uclear **a**ntigen), needed for both DNA synthesis and repair. PCNA forms part of the DNA polymerase complex and PCNA interaction with p21 blocks the synthesis but not repair function of this complex. Hence p53 might inhibit DNA synthesis while allowing repair to continue. Note that this p21 is different to the similarly named product of the ras gene. GADD45 interacts with PCNA whereas IGFB3 binds and inactivates the growth factors IGF1 and IGF2, so both these p53-induced gene products contribute to the inhibition of proliferation.

Apoptosis can be blocked by the products of two other p53-sensitive genes, Bcl2 and BAX (Chapter 10). Inhibition of Bcl2 and stimulation of BAX expression (Figure 6.13) disrupts this block and apoptosis can proceed.

The thrombospondin gene codes for a protein that inhibits angiogenesis and is therefore important in the metastatic process (Chapter 12).

DNA damage activates p53 function by post-transcriptional and cell-type specific mechanisms. One pathway is by activating protein kinases that phosphorylate p53 (see above and Chapter 8). Binding of short stretches of single-stranded DNA to the autoinhibitory domain is an alternative that relieves the inhibition of the DNA-binding domain and is a possible route whereby damage blocks proliferation and facilitates repair. Whatever the mechanisms, they are very sensitive as they can be triggered by a single double-strand break in the DNA.

p53 effects on growth suppression and cell transformation (Chapter 10) can be divorced because experimental mutants lacking C-terminal sequences are capable of suppressing transformation, whereas growth inhibition requires the presence of both C- and N-terminal regions.

Mutations   These are mostly missense mutations. All the tumour-related mutations are in the DNA-binding domain, albeit widely dispersed between codons 112 and 286 (Figure 6.11). Importantly, they all disrupt DNA binding, either directly by preventing interaction with DNA bases or indirectly by destabilising the loop structures needed for this interaction (Figure 6.12). Mutations are sometimes described as conformational if they are in the scaffold region or as contact if they are present in the loops that directly interact with DNA bases. The most frequent mutation is in codon 248, coding for an arginine that directly reacts with the DNA. This codon is affected not only in somatic cells but also inherited germline mutations as in Li–Fraumeni syndrome patients who get multiple cancers (Chapter 9). Mutation in the adjacent codon 249, as seen in aflatoxin-induced hepatic tumours, only disrupts DNA binding in an indirect way, indicating how small differences can alter biochemical mechanisms.

The codon and type of p53 mutation varies according to cancer type and even geographical distribution. Mutational hot spots occur at codon 273 in ovarian and pancreatic tumours but additional ones at codons 157, 248 and 249 are seen in lung cancer. Codon 249 mutations are high in liver cancers in China but not the USA, which correlates with aflatoxin exposure in China but not the USA. Likewise, tobacco carcinogenesis generates different patterns of p53 mutation in lung and bladder. All these features are further discussed in Chapter 7.

The DNA domain mutations have minimal influence on dimerisation so that mutant and wild-type p53 can heterodimerise but will not bind to the DNA consensus sequence. This is the molecular basis of the dominant-negative effect of a p53 mutation in only one allele. The autoinhibitory effect of the C-terminal region on the DNA binding domain (see above) can be exploited to reactivate some mutant forms of p53. Small peptides corresponding to this domain disrupt the autoinhibitory effect, and in culture they can restore p53-mediated apoptosis to cells containing mutant p53. The concept of reactivating mutant repressors has potential therapeutic benefits.

In normal cells, p53 protein has a very short half-life (minutes) but this can be increased either by mutation or by interaction with other proteins and it thus accumulates within the cell. This feature is exploited clinically to identify cancers with p53 mutations, but not all mutations are so detected. Wild-type p53 is rapidly destroyed by Mdm2/ubiquitin-mediated proteolysis whereas mutant forms are not. Heterodimers of wild-type and mutant p53, as occur in Li–Fraumeni cells (Chapter 9) also have extended half-lives.

Inactivation of normal p53 by protein binding   Adenovirus codes for a protein, E1B, that binds to the transactivation domain of normal p53 and blocks its transcriptional activity; some human sarcomas have Mdm2 gene amplifications that have the same end result. The human papilloma virus encodes a protein, E6, that binds to the oligomerisation domain and prevents dimerisation, whilst the HBX protein of hepatitis B virus binds and inactivates p53. Normal p53 alleles are polymorphic in that the codon for amino acid 72 can code for either a proline or an arginine, depending on which allele is present. This has no obvious effect on any of its normal functions but it does influence the p53 half-life when complexed with the E6 protein from the HPV virus. The p53arg.E6 complex is degraded faster than the p53prol.E6 oligomer. Women with two copies of the arginine gene have a sevenfold greater risk of getting HPV-associated cervical cancer as compared to those homozygous for the proline form. Presumably the increased risk is linked to the faster degradation of p53.

p53 is a nuclear protein in normal and most cancer cells, but in neuroblastomas and some breast cancer cells it is cytoplasmic. Wild-type p53 is present in neuroblastomas, so presumably something is blocking nuclear retention and thus preventing p53 function.

Oncogenes and repressors cooperate

Although some oncogenes can generate cancers on their own, the more usual situation is for synergism between cooperating oncogenes. Thus, transgenic mice containing the neu oncogene (homologue of the human erbB2 gene) have a high incidence of breast tumours, whereas either ras or myc alone are poorly carcinogenic in such mice and a combination of ras plus myc results in breast tumours in most of the test mice (Figure 2.4). At a general level, the commonest type of cooperation seen in experimental systems is between an oncogene that will immortalise a cell and an oncogene that changes additional aspects of cell function. Frequently, but not always, this shows up as a complementation between a nuclear and a non-nuclear oncogene (Table 6.6).

Most cooperations between oncogenes have been identified in cell culture as changes in behaviour like density regulation and anchorage independence (transformation); see Chapter 2. They should not be considered in too rigid a manner although the concept of cooperation has clear relevance to the multiple changes required for human carcinogenesis. Loss of a repressor gene, as in

Table 6.6 Cooperation between genes.	
Immortalising (nuclear)	Transforming (non-nuclear)
myc	ras
fos	src
p53	erbB2
Rb	abl

retinoblastoma, is a frequent event in human cancers, although cooperation between different repressors or between an oncogene and a repressor is often observed. The ras and p53 mutations in colon cancer are examples of cooperation between different repressors; p53 and Rb synergisms occur in several cancers. DNA viral carcinogenesis frequently involves production of proteins that inactivate both p53 and Rb. Rb and p53 mediated functions also intercommunicate in non-viral situations. One such example is phosphorylation of Rb followed by induction of ARF and subsequent activation of p53 (see above). These p53 and Rb examples illustrate the point about not treating the nuclear/non-nuclear cooperation too rigidly as they are both nuclear proteins.

CHEMICAL AND RADIATION CARCINOGENESIS

Key points

- Chemicals and radiation can both cause cancers.
- Chemical carcinogens can act by damaging DNA (genotoxic) or by other means (non-genotoxic).
- Genotoxic carcinogens can damage DNA by direct interaction or after metabolic activation.
- Activation commonly requires cytochrome P450-dependent oxygenases.
- A carcinogen is converted to a proximate and then ultimate carcinogen; the ultimate carcinogen forms covalent adducts with purine and pyrimidine bases of DNA.
- Guanine is a frequent target of carcinogenic attack.
- Adduct formation requires electrophilic groups on the carcinogen and nucleophilic centres on DNA.
- Many genotoxic carcinogens have been identified that humans may encounter. They include polycyclic aromatic hydrocarbons, aromatic amines, nitrosamines and alkylating agents.
- Reactive oxygen species, generated naturally or from artificial sources, damage DNA and alter signal transduction.
- Antioxidants such as dietary vitamins can protect against cancer formation.
- Non-genotoxic carcinogens are important for major human cancers. Their mode of action is unclear.
- Laboratory tests that identify putative carcinogens are widely used but not foolproof.
- Ionising radiation from atomic particles, γ-rays and X-rays generates single- and double-stranded breaks in DNA.
- Several sources of natural and synthetic radiation can cause cancers.
- Ultraviolet light causes skin cancers.
- Partial predictions can be made about which agents are involved in human carcinogenesis from the type of DNA damage seen in different cancers. This is called mutational spectrum analysis.

Introduction

A working definition of a carcinogen is 'any agent that can induce cancer'. An enormous range and number of carcinogenic agents have been identified since the original eighteenth-century observation that soot causes scrotal cancer in chimney sweeps. To this list of chemicals has been added atomic radiation, ultraviolet and X-radiation. A feature common to most, but not all of these agents is that they damage DNA and generate changes that result in a growth advantage for the affected cell. Agents that damage DNA, either directly or indirectly through metabolic activation, are classified as genotoxic carcinogens; agents that exert their carcinogenic effects in other ways are non-genotoxic carcinogens.

This chapter will deal separately with carcinogenesis mediated by chemicals and by the various forms of radiation. It will then discuss the consequences of changes to DNA structure generated by such agents.

Chemical carcinogenesis

Carcinogenic chemicals range from the simple, such as arsenic and chromium, to the complex, like aflatoxin from a fungus. As living organisms such as viruses and bacteria are chemical, albeit a complex mixture thereof, they also fall within the definition given at the start of this chapter. Viral carcinogenesis is discussed in Chapter 6, whilst bacterial involvement is limited to the ancillary role of *Helicobacter pylori* as a cofactor in human gastric cancer. Diet is also a major determinant of human carcinogenesis that also reflects the effects of complex chemical mixtures. The general effects of diet on human cancers are discussed in Chapter 4 but more specific points about antioxidant mechanisms of dietary compounds such as vitamins will be included here.

During the 1930s, identification of carcinogenic chemicals and the chemical features that confer carcinogenicity on a compound were a major emphasis of cancer research and resulted in the identification and elimination from use of many industrial carcinogens. Bladder cancer was common in workers in the dyestuff and rubber industries, the cause being 2-naphthylamine (β-naphthylamine) whilst lung cancer was linked with the chromium industry. These beneficial findings generated a feeling that many human cancers could be eliminated if the causative chemical could be identified. Attention was directed at chemicals in manufactured items such as food, drink, medicines and plastics, and tests were devised to determine the carcinogenic potency of compounds. Such tests became mandatory before a product could be used by humans. This approach ensured that many potentially dangerous products were either not marketed or withdrawn from use. However, as evidence accumulated about causes of cancer, it became clear that industrial products and food additives accounted for less than 2% of such cancers and that it might not be possible to eliminate cancer by such a route. This 2% value does not include the large number of tobacco-related cancers (lung, bladder, mouth) for which data are available but about which little is done (Table 4.4).

Although data obtained thus far have had only a minor impact on reducing the major human cancers, chemical carcinogenesis is an important topic because its study has defined pathways by which different classes of chemical can generate inheritable changes in cell function. With this knowledge it is becoming possible to invert some of the concepts. Instead of defining which chemicals cause DNA base changes, mutations can be identified from which it may be possible to characterise the chemical nature of the causative agents. This approach of mutational spectrum analysis using molecular techniques is being applied to the p53 repressor gene and may provide clues as to causative events in major cancers whose aetiology is unclear.

Genotoxic carcinogens

Four major classes of compounds exert their effects by forming covalent adducts with bases of DNA: the polycyclic aromatic hydrocarbons, the aromatic amines, nitrosamines and alkylating agents. A feature common to all these compounds is that they have electrophilic groups (electron deficient) or groups that can be metabolically converted to such. These groups form covalent bonds with nucleophiles (electron rich) such as amino, sulphydryl and hydroxyl groups on other molecules. Nucleophiles are present in proteins, RNA and DNA; although carcinogen interactions with each of these macromolecules have been identified, DNA adducts are the ones most closely linked to carcinogenesis.

In non-proliferating cells, the two strands of DNA form a double helix that limits the accessibility of a carcinogen to individual bases. During DNA synthesis the two strands separate and this is a period when the DNA is especially vulnerable to carcinogenic attack.

Adduct formation distorts the DNA structure such that DNA replication is disrupted. Normally this can be repaired but if not, an inappropriate base is introduced into the new strand (a mutation). Different carcinogens form different adducts which in turn generate different mutations. It implies that all mutagens are carcinogens, but this is only approximately true. Some mutagens are so toxic that the cell is killed rather than surviving with a growth advantage over its neighbours (Figure 7.1).

Many genotoxic chemicals must first be activated by the introduction of epoxide or hydroxyl groups catalysed by **cy**tochrome **P**450-dependent enzymes (CYP). The general reaction sequence and terminologies involved are shown in Figure 7.1. Where activation is required, the administered carcinogen is converted first to a proximate and then to the ultimate carcinogen; the ultimate carcinogen reacts with the DNA.

Figure 7.1

Conversion of a carcinogen into a DNA adduct and the consequences.

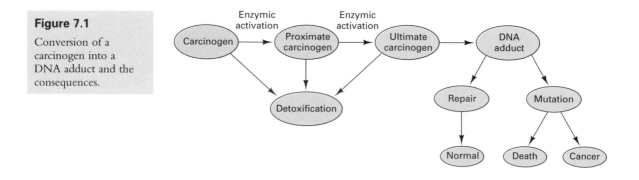

Environmental carcinogens taken up by the body are eventually excreted, mainly in the urine. As urine is stored in the bladder, any carcinogens present may be in prolonged contact with bladder epithelium, so it is not surprising that bladder cancer commonly results from carcinogen exposure.

Detoxification of carcinogens can also occur by CYP-dependent hydroxylations as well as by sulphation and glucuronide formation. The genes for some of these enzymes vary from individual to individual and can be detected as restriction length polymorphisms. Some of these polymorphisms indicate altered enzyme activity and could therefore influence carcinogenesis. One such polymorphism in CYP2D6 has been implicated in lung carcinogenesis. This hydroxylase was first detected by its ability to metabolise the drug debrisoquine. People with polymorphisms resulting in slower metabolism might not activate carcinogens in tobacco smoke and they would be less likely to develop lung cancer. Epidemiological evidence supports this concept but the beneficial polymorphism is rare so it has little impact in the general population.

Polycyclic aromatic hydrocarbons (PAHs)

Many PAHs have been identified in the environment and this class of compound has been widely used in experimental carcinogenesis models. They were originally characterised as pyrolysis products of oils and biological materials but they are also generated in tobacco, whisky, grilled meat and by incomplete combustion of fossil fuels such as coal and petrol. These few examples illustrate the potential impact of PAHs on human carcinogenesis.

The fused rings that make up PAHs come in many configurations but some basic chemical features have been defined that determine whether or not a compound is carcinogenic. The parent compound is phenanthrene (Figure 7.2), composed of three fused aromatic (benzene) rings. Additional rings and substituents can be added to the inactive phenanthrene structure to convert it into a carcinogen. The minimum requirement for carcinogenicity is (i) three fused aromatic rings in the phenanthrene configuration; (ii) additional fused rings; and/or (iii) a methyl group in the bay region.

The additional fused ring is only effective when joined at specific regions of phenanthrene. Thus, the extra ring in benzanthracene (Figure 7.2) yields a very weak or inactive product, whereas dibenzanthracene is a somewhat stronger carcinogen. Addition of two rings in the benzopyrene configuration results in a very potent carcinogen. Addition of one methyl group in the bay region of benzanthracene (12-methylbenzanthracene) generates a moderate carcinogen, whilst a second methyl group (7,12-dimethylbenzanthracene, DMBA) generates one of the most potent carcinogens known. Much interest centred on the K-region (Figure 7.2) as being important, but this is now known not to be the case as it can be modified without destroying potency.

There are two naturally occurring derivatives of phenanthrene: the steroid hormones and cholesterol plus its bile acid derivatives. Cholesterol has not been linked with human carcinogenesis but steroid hormones are involved in the genesis of major cancers such as those of breast, endometrium and prostate. This has led to many attempts to show analogies between PAHs and steroids, none of which have been productive. In fact, they have very different actions as steroids are non-genotoxic carcinogens (see below).

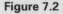

Figure 7.2

Carcinogenic potency of polycyclic aromatic hydrocarbons. Figure 7.3 shows the numbering system.

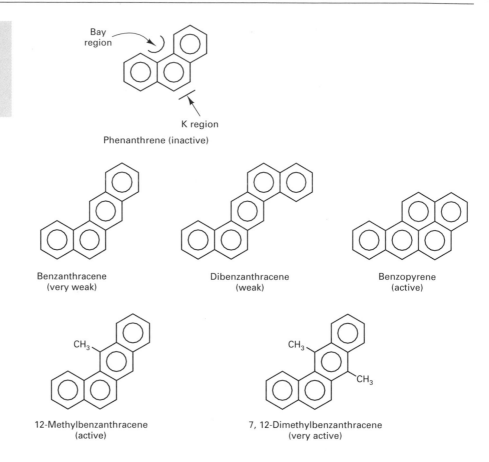

Phenanthrene (inactive)

Benzanthracene (very weak)

Dibenzanthracene (weak)

Benzopyrene (active)

12-Methylbenzanthracene (active)

7, 12-Dimethylbenzanthracene (very active)

PAHs form adducts with purine bases, especially guanine, but only after enzymic activation via proximate and ultimate carcinogens. The example shown in Figure 7.3 is benzopyrene but analogous reactions occur with other PAHs. CYP monooxygenases generate an epoxide that is converted to a diol by an epoxide hydrolase. A second epoxide is then formed, often in the bay region and this covalently attaches to DNA. This can be to the 2-amino of guanine or the 6-amino of adenine.

Aromatic amines

Aromatic amines, also known as arylamines, were identified as being hazardous through their use in the dyestuff and rubber industries. An example is 2-naphthylamine (Figure 7.4), which has been banned because it caused bladder cancer in the workers who handled it. Another compound dimethylaminobenzene, butter yellow, was so named because it was used to colour margarine in the 1930s. It was withdrawn from use when shown to cause liver and bladder cancers in animals.

The carcinogenic action of aromatic amines has been best analysed with 2-acetylaminofluorene (AAF, Figure 7.5), which causes multiple cancers in animals, such as bladder, liver, ear, intestine, thyroid and breast. It was originally used as an insecticide and related compounds can be detected in cooked meat. This illustrates one of the unresolved problems with carcinogen identification through animal

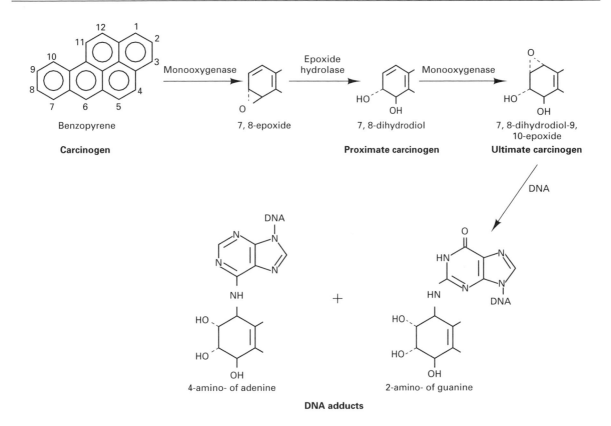

Figure 7.3

Activation of benzopyrene and the formation of DNA adducts.

studies and their relevance to humans. Milligram quantities of AAF are needed to generate cancers in rats of body weight about 0.2 kg whereas a millionth of that level has been detected in cooked meat to be eaten by much bigger humans (70 kg). Given the differences in both quantities and body volumes through which the carcinogen will be distributed, is it appropriate to say, as some do, that meat eating may cause cancer (Chapter 2)?

AAF is only carcinogenic after metabolic activation through a CYP-mediated N-hydroxylase and sulphotransferase (Figure 7.5). The first metabolite, N-hydroxy-AAF (proximate carcinogen) will not form DNA adducts but sulphation or acetylation (not shown) of the N-hydroxyl group generates the ultimate carcinogen that reacts with guanine bases in DNA. There are large variations in the susceptibility of different species to AAF and this is correlated with the activity of hepatic sulphotransferase and N-hydroxylase in those species. The sulphate and acetyl esters are unstable and undergo a spontaneous reaction to form a nitrenium ion, which generates a qualitatively major adduct via the C-8 and a minor one via

Figure 7.4

Carcinogenic aromatic arylamines.

2-Naphthylamine

Dimethylaminoazobenzene
(butter yellow)

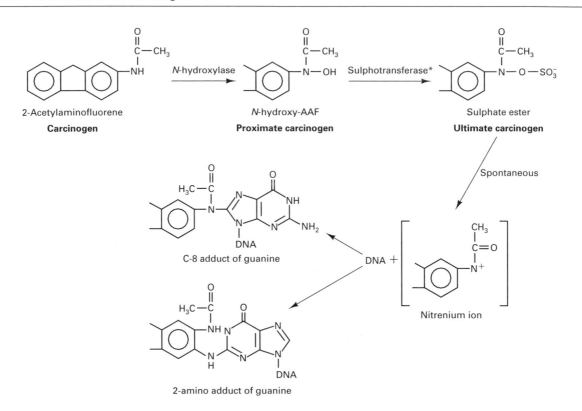

the 2-amino group of guanine. However, the minor occurrence of the 2-amino adduct is counterbalanced by its longer period of attachment to DNA before being removed. Both adducts are probably important.

Other aromatic amines are activated by analogous mechanisms through hydroxylation and ester formation at their amino group.

Nitrosamines

Humans can be exposed to nitrosamines in a number of ways. They are formed in smoked meats and fish by interaction of natural amines with nitrites added as preservatives but their most significant presence is in tobacco and its products. Nitrosamines in tobacco and its smoke contribute to lung and bladder cancers, whilst their presence in snuff and chewing-tobacco cause nasal and oral cancers respectively.

Enzymic activation is required to form ultimate carcinogens that methylate guanines of DNA (Figure 7.6). N^7-Methylguanine is the major product but its formation does not correlate with carcinogenicity whereas the minor O^6-methylated product does. Hence formation of the latter product reflects the major carcinogenic event. The O-2 of thymine is also a site of adduct formation.

N-Methylnitrosourea (Figure 7.6) is a nitrosamine widely used to generate cancers in experimental systems, its advantage being that it spontaneously forms the methyldiazonium ion without requiring enzymic activation. It is therefore classified as a direct-acting carcinogen, with no metabolic activation being required.

Figure 7.6

N–nitrosodimethyl-amine and *N*–methyl-nitrosourea: activation and DNA adducts.

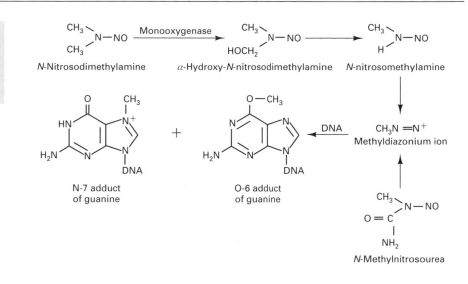

Other alkylating agents

Mustard gas (dichlorodiethylsulphide, Figure 7.7) was used during the 1914–18 war; affected soldiers subsequently developed a higher than expected incidence of cancers at exposed sites such as nose, bronchus and larynx. Mustard gas is a bifunctional compound, having two chlorine groups capable of reacting directly with nucleophilic amino or hydroxyl groups, as with the nitrosamines; it can therefore form intrachain and interchain cross-links with adjacent bases. It can also form single adducts. It is a direct-acting carcinogen as the chlorine groups are sufficiently electrophilic that metabolic activation is not required.

Monofunctional alkylating agents can also be carcinogenic due to adduct formation. An example is vinyl chloride (Figure 7.7), used in the plastic industry as **p**oly**v**inyl **c**hloride (PVC) for products such as food wrappers.

The ability of bifunctional alkylating agents to damage DNA has been turned to beneficial effect in developing drugs for killing cancers. Cyclophosphamide (Figure 7.7), a derivative of dichlorodiethylsulphide in which the S is replaced with N, is widely used for this purpose (Chapter 13). It can, however, cause second cancers (leukaemia, bladder) in a small proportion of patients about 5 years after being treated with the drug (Appendix A). This side effect is considered minor relative to preventing death from the first cancer.

Figure 7.7

Carcinogenic alkylating agents.

Bifunctional agents

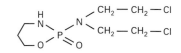

2, 2-Dichlorodiethylsulphide   Cyclophosphamide

Monofunctional agents

$CH_2 = CH - Cl$

Vinyl chloride

Oxidation as a cause of cancer

A considerable number of reactive free radicals or chemicals capable of being converted thereto are generated in cells by normal metabolic pathways. They can oxidise nucleic acids, proteins and lipids, and they have many of the characteristics of carcinogens. They generate structural alterations in DNA, decrease DNA repair by damaging essential proteins and activate signal transduction pathways. It has been suggested that cells are under 'oxidative siege' and it follows that antioxidant mechanisms will correct that siege. The oxidation status of a cell is sometimes known as its redox (**red**uction/**ox**idation) state. By analysis of urinary metabolites of purine and pyrimidine bases, it has been calculated that, under normal circumstances, DNA in each cell receives 10^4 oxidative hits per day. This substantial number of base changes are mostly repaired but any that escape the process might alter cell functions and contribute to carcinogenesis. The main source of damaging agents is **r**eactive **o**xygen **s**pecies (ROS) but additional contributions are made by **r**eactive **n**itrogen **s**pecies (RNS).

Reactive oxygen species   Several types of ROS exist that are mainly formed as by-products of mitochondrial electron transport or exposure to ionising radiation, but they can also be produced from other sources such as phagocytic cells and lipid peroxidation. Endogenously produced ROS are important contributors to the natural mutation rate (Chapter 8). The term 'spontaneous mutation' is often used inappropriately given that something has to generate the base change.

Oxidative phosphorylation, in which mitochondrial electron transport converts energy into ATP, is the major source of ROS. About 10^{12} oxygen molecules are processed per cell per day, about 1% of which are incompletely used and result in ROS formation. Hence the 10^{10} potential ROS are more than adequate to explain the 10^4 DNA hits mentioned above. However, superoxide and hydroxyl free radicals only travel short distances ($<0.1\,\mu$m) before being destroyed. Given a cell diameter of about $10\,\mu$m, it follows that direct interaction of mitochondrial ROS with nuclear DNA is unlikely. Perhaps chain reactions can be initiated by ROS that could transfer effects over longer distances, or ROS may be generated within the nucleus (see the section on DNA damage).

The main ROS are superoxide and hydroxyl radicals and hydrogen peroxide produced by electron capture, as shown in Figure 7.8. Hydrogen peroxide, a

Figure 7.8

Production and destruction of reactive oxygen species.

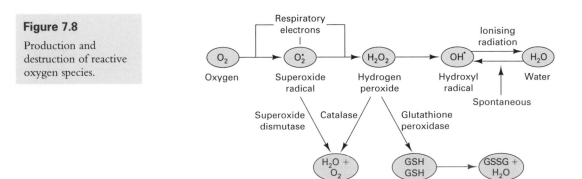

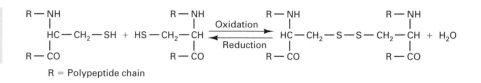

Figure 7.9

Oxidation of cysteine residues in proteins.

R = Polypeptide chain

component of the production pathway, is not a free radical but it is a precursor. Furthermore, it can have direct oxidative effects of its own on other proteins such as the transcription factor NFkB. The hydroxyl radical is the most reactive ROS and therefore the most damaging. Given concerns about destruction of the protective ozone layer in the atmosphere and increased risk of skin cancer, it should be noted that ozone (O_3) is converted to oxygen by free radicals. This has the deleterious effect of reducing the amount of atmospheric ozone available to protect the planet from harmful radiation. The protective effect of the ozone is also achieved by a free radical mechanism. Superoxide dismutase catalyses the conversion of superoxide to hydrogen peroxide; Fe^{2+} and Cu^+ accelerate hydroxyl radical formation from hydrogen peroxide. Hydroxyl radicals can also be produced from water by radiation (see below). ROS are also generated as products of reactions catalysed by cyclooxygenases, lipoxygenases and NADPH oxidase. Oxidising agents in tobacco smoke, such as nitric oxide, could also contribute to carcinogenesis via ROS formation.

The cell contains proteins and other molecules such as glutathione (Figure 7.8) and vitamins A, C and E, all of them capable of inactivating ROS. Enzymic proteins include catalase and glutathione peroxidase, which convert hydrogen peroxide to water. The other product of catalase is oxygen and, for glutathione peroxidase, oxidised glutathione. Glutathione peroxidase requires selenium, and this might account for selenium's beneficial effects (Chapter 4). Thioredoxin is a protein with adjacent cysteine residues that can be reversibly oxidised to cystine (Figure 7.9). It can thus act as a sink for ROS and it is noteworthy that thioredoxin is involved in the NFkB signal transduction pathway (see below). The protein metallothionine chelates divalent metal ions such as Fe^{2+} and Cu^{2+}, so it can destroy their role in hydroxyl radical formation.

Reactive nitrogen species These include nitric oxide (NO•), nitrogen peroxide (NOO•) and peroxynitrite (ONOO•) radicals; the nitric oxide radical is not as reactive as the other two. All three can be formed endogenously but their main interest is as carcinogenic products of the oxides of nitrogen in tobacco smoke.

Antioxidants as protective agents Antioxidants that destroy ROS without damaging cell function are protective. Natural products that fall into this category are ascorbic acid (vitamin C), tocopherol (vitamin E), carotene (precursor of vitamin A) and glutathione. Each of these compounds will protect animals against the effects of carcinogens, whilst dietary supplementation trials with carotene are looking optimistic as a means of preventing some cancers in humans. Fruit and vegetables are important sources of antioxidant vitamins and polyphenols, which may account for the protective effect of these foods against colon and stomach cancer in humans (Chapters 4 and 14).

Figure 7.10

Types of DNA damage caused by reactive oxygen species.

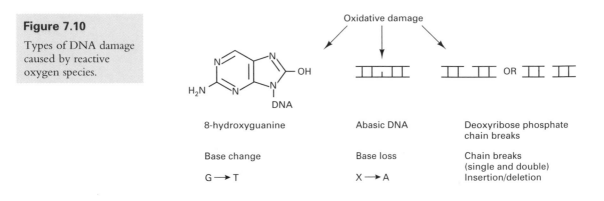

8-hydroxyguanine   Abasic DNA   Deoxyribose phosphate chain breaks

Base change   Base loss   Chain breaks (single and double)

G → T   X → A   Insertion/deletion

DNA damage Hydroxyl radicals can oxidise guanine to 8-hydroxyguanine, and generate abasic sites or strand breaks in DNA (Figure 7.10); 8-hydroxyguanine is misread as a thymine and therefore paired with an adenine during DNA replication. If the C-1 of deoxyribose is oxidised, the DNA chain remains intact but the base is lost with the generation of an abasic site. This is preferentially replaced with an adenine during repair. Oxidation at C-4 of deoxyribose breaks the DNA strand and a single-strand break is formed. Double-strand breaks can also be produced.

Oxidations thus generate various types of change, such as G → T point mutations, deletions and insertions; they are described more fully in Chapter 8.

Hydroxyl radicals are so reactive that they do not diffuse far from their site of formation. Their highest concentration is in mitochondria so the high concentration of 8-hydroxyguanine in mitochondrial DNA is to be expected, but mitochondrial genes primarily code for respiratory chain proteins in contrast to the much broader spectrum of cell functions coded for by nuclear genes. Although mutations in mitochondrial genes do occur and may increase with age, it is unlikely that they contribute directly to carcinogenesis; inherited defects in mitochondrial DNA exist but none are linked with an increased cancer risk. The sources of oxidative mutations in nuclear DNA cannot be identified with certainty but they undoubtedly exist as 8-hydroxyguanine is present in nuclear DNA, albeit at much lower levels than in mitochondria. Potential sources of nuclear hydroxyl radicals include precursors formed within the nucleus or extranuclear products like mitochondrial hydrogen peroxide which, being less reactive, can diffuse within the cell.

Protein oxidations and signal transduction The cysteine–cystine interconversion (Figure 7.9) was mentioned earlier in relation to thioredoxin function, but other proteins require cysteines for their normal function; oxidation to cystine alters those functions. When cells are exposed to mitogenic growth factors such as EGF and PDGF, there are two consequences: DNA damage and increased signalling to the nucleus. Several signalling components can be activated (i) at the level of transduction between cell membrane and nucleus via protein phosphorylation/dephosphorylations and (ii) within the nucleus (Table 7.1). Activation of **n**uclear **f**actor **kB** (NFkB) is indirect in that ROS activate phosphorylation/ubiquitin-dependent proteolysis of the **i**nhibitory factor IkB, which thus releases its cytoplasmic bound NFkB for translocation to the nucleus. ROS can thus act as

Table 7.1 Signal transduction proteins whose activities are altered by ROS.

Protein	Activity	Effect of oxidation
Tyrosine phosphatase	inhibited	Increased effectiveness of mitogenic tyrosine kinases
Mitogen-activated protein kinase	activated	Increased effectiveness of extracellular, mitogenic signals
Nuclear factor kB	activated	Increased transcription
AP1 transcription complex for jun/fos sensitive genes	activated	The Ref-1 transcription factor reduces cystines and increases transcription

second messengers in signal transduction pathways and this effect is achieved at lower concentrations than required to generate mutations in DNA. Another difference between this effect and cysteine oxidation in proteins is that different ROS may be involved; hydrogen peroxide can directly alter the function of proteins such as NFkB but without damaging DNA.

Hypoxia and signal transduction Inadequate oxygen supply (hypoxia) can also influence cell function (Chapter 12), some features of which are analogous to those just described for ROS; the term 'oxidative stress' is sometimes used to cover both circumstances. The biological consequences of hypoxia are mediated by **h**ypoxia-**i**nduced transcription **f**actors (HIFs) and are most relevant during metastasis (induces angiogenesis) and in response to chemotherapy (less effective). These processes are described in Chapters 12 and 13 respectively.

Non-genotoxic carcinogens

The aetiological chemicals of major cancers such as those of breast, prostate and endometrium are hormonal steroids, which do not damage DNA. Hormones are classified as tumour promotors in contrast to initiators, which do react with DNA; this is discussed in Chapter 2. These hormones are mitogens, increasing cell proliferation by binding to intracellular receptors, which are transcription factors. The tumour promotor phorbol ester also binds to its receptor, protein kinase C, thereby activating mitogenic pathways, but remember that the ester is not a naturally occurring agent (Chapter 11). Proliferation is a risk factor for carcinogenesis and its role in mutation accumulation is discussed in Chapter 2. Another factor linking proliferation with increased cancer risk is that bases in single-stranded DNA are more susceptible to attack by genotoxic carcinogens than when paired with other bases in double-stranded DNA. As regions of single-stranded DNA occur during DNA synthesis, it follows that increased proliferation increases the probability of DNA damage. If that damage is to the DNA repair processes, an autocatalytic effect would be generated.

Asbestos is a chemically inert silicate that causes a special type of lung cancer (mesothelioma) in exposed workers. How it does this is not clear but cells can phagocytose the asbestos fibres, which physically damage DNA. Another possibility is that the asbestos may carry bound PAHs. Thus, although asbestos is classified as non-genotoxic because it does not alter DNA bases, that classification may be suspect.

Tests for carcinogens

With so many chemicals having the potential to cause cancer, methods for testing environmental, industrial and nutritional components are important in the drive to lower human exposure to carcinogens. Such tests are impossible with humans so surrogate models have been devised. These models fall into three categories (Table 7.2): ability to cause cancers or damage DNA in animals, ability to damage DNA in cultured mammalian cells and ability to generate mutations in microorganisms. Each category has its own advantages and disadvantages so that reliance is not placed on data from a single type of test. The overriding principle behind the application of test results is that it is better to err on the side of caution rather than be wise after the event, even if this means misclassifying some compounds as being carcinogens when they may not be.

Animal tests

Government agencies that license compounds for human use have testing criteria that must be satisfied. These criteria vary in different countries but long-term testing for cancer production in animals is the most important criterion common to all agencies.

Varying doses of test compound are given to animals that are then monitored for cancer development. This most closely resembles the human situation in that it makes no prejudgement as to mechanisms by which carcinogens act: both genotoxic and non-genotoxic agents can be detected. The main criticism concerns the relevance of animal studies to humans. Several features contribute to that concern some of which are listed in Table 7.3.

Dose schedules   The highest dose tested is the maximal tolerated dose, usually determined by lack of gross signs of toxicity with less than 10% weight loss. Such doses are often orders of magnitude higher than those to which humans are exposed. Thus, aflatoxin causes liver cancers in rats at 10^{-6} g/kg body weight, whereas 10^{-10} g/kg is hepatocarcinogenic in humans. This problem is minimised by constructing dose–

Table 7.2   Methods for testing carcinogenic potential of compounds.

Animals	Tumour appearance
	Abnormal chromosomes in bone marrow
Cell culture	DNA damage
Microorganisms	Reversal of a mutation

Table 7.3 Problems in interpreting animal carcinogenesis tests.

Doses used: very high compared to human exposure

Timescale: short compared to human

Species: relevance of animal studies to humans

Metabolism: activation/deactivation variable in different species

response curves; however, the minimum effective dose is often greater than the potential human exposure and so the animal curve must be extrapolated downwards in order to assess effects of human doses. It is unclear whether the extrapolation should be as a straight or curved line or whether there is a threshold dose below which no effect is seen. This question has been most closely analysed with ionising radiation. Survivors of the atom bombs in Japan have provided good dose–response data for several cancers but even the lowest exposure levels were higher than those likely to be encountered around an atomic power station. The majority of bomb-induced cancers require more than 1 Gy exposure whereas the areas adjacent to nuclear power stations have a small fraction of this (<0.001%) at any one time. This is discussed more fully in the section below on radiation carcinogenesis but the best estimate is that for leukaemias, but not solid tumours, the risk is less than predicted from a linear downward extrapolation of the dose–response curve.

The other criticism related to dosage concerns duration of exposure. Animal tests involve giving a single or limited number of treatments whereas human carcinogenesis, such as by dietary factors or smoking, involves prolonged exposure.

Test species   Compounds can be classified as carcinogens or not depending on the species in which they are tested. The carcinogenicity of aflatoxin in humans and rats is such an example. Aflatoxin produces liver cancers in rats at μg/kg body weight levels but is ineffective at a thousand times that level in mice. Even different strains of the same species vary in their sensitivity to carcinogens. Dimethylbenzanthracene will produce breast cancers in Sprague–Dawley rats but not in Wistar rats. In part this variability reflects different levels of enzymes that activate or deactivate the putative carcinogen. An example of wider importance is the sex steroid medroxyprogesterone acetate. This had great potential as a contraceptive agent and as a treatment for hormone-sensitive cancers, but because it caused breast cancers in dogs, it was not granted a licence. This judgement was subsequently shown to be wrong, because hormone influences on dog breast are very different to those in humans.

Best practice is that more than one species should be used.

Cytogenetic tests   Animals dosed with test compounds can also provide cells that can be monitored for DNA damage. Bone marrow cells are often used and damage assessed by staining chromosome spreads. The presence of micronuclei or abnormal chromosomes is indicative of a potential carcinogen. These tests generate quick answers but are subject to the same criticisms as those based on cancer formation in animals.

Cultured cells

Test compounds are added to cultured cells and they are monitored for effects on cell functions relevant to carcinogenesis. Human cells can be used, which minimises species variation but metabolic activation of the test compound may not occur in the cultures. A source of activating enzymes (rat liver microsomes plus NADPH) is added to cultures to overcome this defect. In practice it is usual to monitor features of DNA damage such as the appearance of abnormal chromosomes or unscheduled DNA synthesis. Unscheduled DNA synthesis refers to the incorporation of labelled nucleotide triphosphates during DNA repair (Chapter 8) occurring at abnormal times in the cell cycle.

Ability to cause mutations in specific genes is another endpoint of such tests. A commonly used gene codes for hypoxanthine–guanine phosphoribosyl transferase, mutations in which can readily be detected by altered sensitivity of the cells to antiproliferative drugs such as 8-azaguanine. This is incorporated into DNA and blocks DNA synthesis. The enzyme is necessary to convert the drug into the nucleoside monophosphate, essential for its incorporation into DNA. If mutant (inactive) enzyme is present, 8-azaguanine is not incorporated and the cells proliferate whereas non-mutagenised cells are killed.

The advantage of this type of test is that a result is obtained quickly; the disadvantage is that the test does not detect non-genotoxic carcinogens.

Microorganisms

This widely used type of test relies on the ability of a mutagen to change the function of a growth-related enzyme. The microorganism most frequently used is the bacterium, *Salmonella typhimurium*, engineered so that it cannot synthesise the amino acid histidine. Chemically induced mutations are detected as a reversal of the engineered mutation so that the bacteria will grow in histidine-deficient medium. To minimise complications due to the fact that bacteria do not have the CYP enzymes needed to activate many carcinogens, a source of these enzymes (rat liver microsomes plus a supply of NADPH) is included in the growth medium. The test will only detect point mutations. This reverse mutation test is named after its originator, Ames.

The Ames test is simple and can handle large numbers of test compounds or biological fluids in a short time but only detects genotoxic agents. It gives a number of false positive and negative results, typically identifying 50–70% of known carcinogens, but about one-quarter of non-carcinogens can be misclassified. Despite the high error rate and the fact that it does not detect non-genotoxic carcinogens, the Ames test is used justifiably as a screening test for putative carcinogens prior to animal testing.

Radiation carcinogenesis

Humans encounter many types of radiation, several of which cause cancers. Radon, a radioactive gas produced by uranium, caused lung cancers in miners involved in producing the ore from which radium was extracted, whilst bone cancers also

Table 7.4 Types of radiation that cause cancers in humans.

Agent	Source	Cancer
Ultraviolet light	Sunlight	Skin
X-rays	Medical treatment	Leukaemia, thyroid
Atomic radiation	War	All types
Radon	Mining, building materials	Lung

increased because of radioactive deposition in bone. The atom bombs dropped on Japan in 1945 provided tragic proof of the carcinogenicity of atomic radiation as has the Chernobyl nuclear power station disaster. Other types of radiation such as X-rays and ultraviolet light are also carcinogenic (Table 7.4).

Radiation is energy whose power depends on its source and type. There is overlap of energy spectra between the different radiation types but, in descending order of energy release, the sequence is atomic particles > X-rays > ultraviolet (UV) light > visible light > infrared, microwaves and electrical waves. Only the first three have been shown to be carcinogenic. Atomic particles encompass energy sources of different types, such as β particles (electrons), α particles (2 protons + 2 neutrons), neutrons and γ radiation.

Each of the carcinogenic forms of radiation, except UV light, can generate ions in the media through which they travel and are termed ionising radiations. As ionising and UV radiations are carcinogenic by different mechanisms, they will be considered separately.

Ionising radiation

The types of cancer generated by such energy sources were described in the previous section and all involve DNA damage. Ionising radiations contain energies much greater than that in chemical bonds, so chemical bonds can therefore be broken by radiation. Whilst many molecules are so affected, water and DNA are the principal compounds involved as far as cancer formation is concerned. The energy released by the radiation as it passes through water produces electrons, which in turn generate reactive radicals in much the same sequence of reactions as those in the mitochondrial electron transport chain (Figure 7.8). This physical stage of radiation carcinogenesis occurs within a fraction of a second, followed by the chemical stage in which DNA bonds are broken. The consequences of the chemical changes become apparent in the final cell and tissue stage, and this can take years to appear.

Ionising radiations produce single- and double-strand breaks in the DNA, resulting in chromosome damage involving mainly deletions and rearrangements rather than the point mutations generated by chemical carcinogens and UV light. Another difference between the types of carcinogen is that cells are most sensitive to ionising radiations during the G_2/M phases of the cell cycle whereas early S phase is the sensitive period for chemical agents and UV light.

Table 7.5 Biological effects of 1 Gy on cultured cells.

- 2×10^5 ionisations per cell
- 100 DNA strand breaks per cell
- Start to see chromosome changes
- High LET radiation: 1% cells survive
  30 transformations per million cells (0.003%)
- Low LET radiation: 90% cells survive
  3 transformations per million cells (0.0003%)

LET = linear energy transfer.

The unit used to define energy release is the **gray** (Gy); 1 Gy is the release of 1 J/ kg tissue. The gray replaced the rad, an older unit equivalent to 0.01 Gy. As different forms of radiation release their energy at different rates, the concept of **linear energy transfer** (LET) is used to define the energy released per unit path length. A given amount of energy released in a short distance does more damage than the same amount over a longer distance. To convert from gray units to low LET values there is no multiplying factor. But to convert from gray units to high LET values there is a multiplying factor of up to 10; this is to account for high LET effects. When a Gy unit has been multiplied by this quality factor, the unit becomes a **sievert** (Sv). It is usual to refer to high and low LET radiation; high LET radiation is more dangerous than low LET radiation.

Some approximate indications of the effect of 1 Gy on cultured mammalian cells are given in Table 7.5. The large number of ionisations are more than sufficient to generate the strand breaks observed, which in turn account for the gross chromosome abnormalities that start to appear at this exposure. High LET radiations, as produced by α particles or neutrons, generate so much DNA damage that the cells die; whereas low LET radiation (X-rays and γ-rays) is much less cytotoxic. Anchorage-independent growth is a reasonable cell biological marker of carcinogenesis (Chapter 2) and the number of cells acquiring this property (transformants) also increases with LET, although only a small proportion are so affected. To put these values into the context of human exposure, the total lifetime exposure of an average individual is only 0.1 Gy and the majority of cancers in Japanese survivors of the atom bombs occurred in people exposed to more than 1 Gy.

Background radiation

Human beings are exposed daily to radiation, which can be categorised as either natural or synthetic. Natural radiation is the so-called background radiation and mainly derives from radon gas released by building materials (Table 7.6 and see below). The two other contributors are cosmic radiation reaching the earth from space and terrestrial radiation emitted by rocks and soils. Additional artificial sources of ionising radiation, such as medical X-rays and treatment with radioactive products, make up the components that an average person might encounter.

How much these types of radiation contribute to human cancers is a subject of

Table 7.6 Human lifetime exposure to ionising radiations.

Source	Percentage of total*
Natural	
Radon gas	55
Cosmic radiation	8
Terrestrial radiation	8
Synthetic	
Medical X-rays	11
Nuclear medicine	4
Consumer products	3
Other	<1

* Total lifetime exposure = 0.1 Gy.

debate. Individual sources of radiation such as radon and the atomic power industry are considered below; however, part of the debate centres on uncertainty about the biological effects of low levels of radiation. There are good dose–response data for levels greater than 1 Gy to indicate that atomic radiation increases all types of cancer, with leukaemia being the most sensitive. However, these dose–response curves have to be extrapolated back to zero to get the low radiation values encountered in everyday life and it is not clear what type of extrapolation is valid. Fewer leukaemias seem to occur than predicted from a linear extrapolation but that may not be true for solid cancers.

Radon

The radon-222 isotope is released as a gas together with an α particle from uranium-238 occurring naturally in building materials. Radon-222 also releases an α particle to generate polonium, another radioactive element. It is therefore a particularly dangerous natural agent because it degrades to another radioactive product but also because the radon gas can accumulate in poorly ventilated rooms and be inhaled. There are large local variations in radon levels but, taking an average, it has been calculated to cause about 1500 lung cancers per year in the UK and about 10 times that number in the USA. Important as these figures are, they should be seen in the context that they represent a fraction of 1% of the smoking-related cancers. The different patterns of p53 mutation in lung cancers of smokers and non-smokers (Figure 4.6) are informative as the non-smokers have a high proportion of guanine to thymine mutations, which is compatible with radon-induced oxidation of guanine (Figure 7.10).

X-rays

A number of medical conditions such as ankylosing spondylitis require high-dose (1–10 Gy) X-ray treatment; follow-up data from such patients suggest a threefold increased risk of leukaemia and a 30% increased risk of other cancers such as those of lung and colon. Modern X-ray machines used for diagnostic purposes generate

Table 7.7 Predicted carcinogenic effect of the Chernobyl nuclear accident.

Group	Exposure (Gy)	Percentage increase in lifetime cancer risk
Local inhabitants	10^{-1}	2
Europe (except former USSR)	10^{-2}	0.1
USA	10^{-5}	0.0001

much lower doses than those used in treatments and, provided they are not used too frequently, they are not a health risk.

Nuclear fuels

Debate continues about the health effects of the nuclear power industry. The concern originated from the increases in cancer demonstrated with atom bomb survivors but was kindled by the occurrence of a higher than expected incidence of childhood leukaemias in 'hot spots' around the nuclear processing plant at Sellafield. Two possible explanations, direct contact with radioactive material and chromosome damage to a father's sperm, have been discounted on scientific evidence. The estimated dose of radiation in the vicinity of Sellafield is about one-fifth of that received from natural sources, plus the types of leukaemia are not inherited and would require an implausible mutation rate if radiation were a cause. The cause of these leukaemias remains unclear.

Less contentious is the safety concern after the Chernobyl nuclear power plant disaster. Based on the atom bomb experience, predictions have been made as to the likely increase in cancers in different regions affected by the radioactivity released into the atmosphere (Table 7.7). Whilst the increase is significant, especially for those people in the immediate vicinity of the explosion, the global effect is fortunately much smaller.

Ultraviolet light

UV light has limited penetration, so the tissue it affects is skin, especially in areas such as the head that are exposed to sunlight. As a consequence of the cosmetic desirability of skin exposure to sunlight the incidence of skin cancer is increasing at a faster rate than any other cancer. The energy spectrum of UV light is divided into three regions according to its wavelength, UVA (>320 nm), UVB (290–320 nm) and UVC (200–290 nm); UVB is the most important fraction for skin carcinogenesis. Most UVB is filtered from solar radiation by the ozone layer, so ozone depletion is bad news for skin cancer.

Skin creams that minimise UV access to the skin are widely available and are based on UV-absorbing organic chemicals such as cinnamates or inorganic pigments containing zinc or titanium oxides.

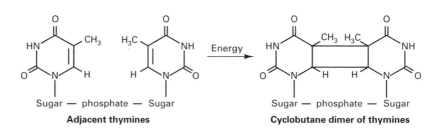

Figure 7.11

UV-induced formation of pyrimidine dimers.

In contrast to ionising radiations, DNA is most sensitive to UV light during early S phase of the cell cycle, because the pyrimidine bases that are altered by UV are more exposed during this period and therefore subject to attack.

UV radiation has lower energy than ionising radiations and therefore has less potential for breaking chemical bonds. However, it does excite other molecules, making them more reactive. As far as DNA is concerned, this involves the formation of covalent links between adjacent pyrimidines. Thymine–thymine, cytosine–cytosine and cytosine–thymine dimers can be formed. An example of a thymine–thymine dimer is illustrated in Figure 7.11. Cyclobutane dimers are read as thymines, so mutations only result if cytosine is a component of the dimer. This can result in a C → T transition (Tables 7.8–7.10) sometimes as unique double tandem mutations. Other photoproducts are formed with only a single bond linking the two pyrimidines, (6–4) photoproduct and its isomer. All the photoproducts are mutagenic but the cyclobutane dimer is probably most important in skin carcinogenesis as the other products are repaired more quickly.

Other forms of radiation

It has been suggested that microwaves from ovens and electromagnetic radiation from power lines and transformers might cause leukaemias but no substantive data exists to indicate that this low-energy radiation can do so. However, low-energy forms of radiation can influence rates of chemical reactions without breaking covalent bonds, so adverse effects remain theoretically possible.

UV-induced dimers activate melanin formation (tanning), which is the natural defence mechanism against overexposure to sunlight. The DNA damage also activates repair but this is a delayed response. Intermittent UV exposure is more deleterious than prolonged exposure as the delayed repair results in the accumulation of DNA damage.

Consequences of DNA damage

The three consequences are (i) repair and return to normality; (ii) extensive damage leading to cell death; and (iii) misreading of modified bases at the next round of DNA synthesis. DNA synthesis generates mutations whose types depend on the nature of the damage (Table 7.8). The commonest result of chemical damage or

Table 7.8 Mutations caused by DNA-damaging agents.*

Modifying agent	Example	Recognised as	Base pairing Old	Base pairing New
Small adduct	G → Me.G	A	G:C	A:T
Large adduct	G → G.BP	T	G:C	T:A
Ultraviolet light	Cytosine dimers	T	G:C	A:T
Oxidations	G → 8-OH.G	T	G:C	T:A
Oxidations	Strand breaks		deletions	
Ionising radiations	Strand breaks		deletions	
Spontaneous	C/MeC deamination	T	G:C	A:T

* These are the major mutations; others occur with each agent.
A, G, C, T, DNA bases; Me, methyl; BP, benzopyrene

UV light is a point mutation in which one base is replaced by another. Depending on the base involved and its location within a given region of DNA, such a point mutation can result in no effect (redundant DNA), replacement of one amino acid by another (altered codon), truncated protein (generation of nonsense or stop codon), altered regulation (regulatory sequences) or abnormal-sized protein (altered intron:exon boundaries, chromosome rearrangements). Specific examples of each type of change are given in Chapter 8.

Ionising radiations generate a wider spectrum of alterations with deletions being frequent and point mutations less common.

Base transitions and transversions

Small adducts, such as the O-methylguanine generated by N-methylnitrosourea, are treated as an adenine and become paired with a thymine rather than the normal cytosine at the next round of DNA synthesis. Subsequent divisions generate A:T pairs instead of the original G:C pairs. This G → A mutation is referred to as a transition, a term used when a purine is substituted by a different purine or a pyrimidine with a pyrimidine. Oxidative damage commonly produces a G → T mutation as does the presence of a bulky adduct such as benzopyrene or aflatoxin on guanine. This change from purine to pyrimidine is called a transversion. The changes listed in Table 7.8 are those most frequently, but not exclusively, associated with the carcinogens mentioned.

Relevance of model changes to real genes

Given that only a small fraction of the bases in DNA have a coding or regulatory role, it follows that the majority of mutations are silent and have no functional effect.

Table 7.9 Mutations in adenosyl phosphoribosyl transferase gene generated in cultured cells.

Agent	Most frequent change	Percentage of all mutations
Spontaneous	G → A	71
Benzopyrene diol epoxide (large adduct)	G → T	62
Nitrosamines	G → A	63
Ultraviolet light	C → T	61
Ionising radiation	deletions	31
	G → A	19
	A → C	19

Therefore, it is important to show that the adducts and base changes determined by experimental interaction of carcinogens with DNA have relevance to functional DNA in whole cells. To do this, cultured human cells have been exposed to different carcinogens and a housekeeping gene, adenosyl phosphoribosyl transferase, has been sequenced to see what mutations have occurred. The results (Table 7.9) fit the predictions from model experiments with non-specific DNA (Table 7.8), but in the gene analysis there were 30–40% of mutations besides those which had been predicted. Thus, the G → T transversion predicted for benzopyrene accounts for 62% of mutations with G → C transversions accounting for another 14%. More information is required to identify the molecular basis of those other mutations.

Deletions predominate with ionising radiations but some point mutations are also observed. Agreement also occurs if an oncogene rather than a housekeeping gene is analysed. In rat N-methylnitrosourea-induced bladder cancers, H-ras is activated by a G → A transition, as predicted for the formation of a small alkyl guanine (Table 7.8). A carcinogen such as 3-methylcholanthrene forms a bulky adduct with the consequential G → T transversion at codon 12 of H-ras. Mutations in the repressor gene p53 are discussed in the next section.

Predicting the type of carcinogen by mutational spectrum analysis

As types of mutation can be predicted by knowing the carcinogen, the logic should be reversible, i.e. the type of carcinogen can be identified from mutations detected in cancers. This approach is being used with some success, even though certain problems have still to be resolved. Epidemiological methods have been the main approach in identifying carcinogenic risks in humans, so molecular epidemiology is the name given to molecular methods such as gene sequencing that are used for epidemiological purposes (Chapter 4).

The approach is to select a gene known to be involved in many cancers and then analyse the types of mutation (mutation spectrum) in those cancers. The gene coding for the repressor protein p53 has generated most information because the majority of human cancers contain aberrant p53 and more than 2000 mutations have been identified. These can be looked at in a general way by determining the proportion of transversions and transitions in different cancers, and in a more specific way through the actual bases involved.

Transversions and Transitions in p53

The pattern of change is different in each of colon, lung, breast and liver cancers (Figure 7.12), suggesting that different carcinogenic events are involved in each case. Transversions predominate in lung cancers and their number increases with number of cigarettes smoked. Liver cancer follows a similar pattern to lung cancer, but transitions are the dominant feature in colon cancer. The mixed pattern seen in breast cancers suggests a complex aetiology. Non-genotoxic female sex steroids are the major known factor for breast carcinogenesis. It is not clear why these steroids are carcinogenic but increased proliferation and generation of genetic instability is a possibility (see above). Such general mechanisms might be expected to generate diverse mutational changes.

Specific base changes in p53

The data just described indicate that different pathways of carcinogenesis are operative in the relevant cancers. Identifying the specific base changes involved can provide clues as to what might be causing those changes in the p53 gene (Table 7.10). Lung cancers caused by smoking have a high transversion of G → T, compatible with both bulky adduct formation and oxidations. Potential adducts like benzopyrene and oxidants such as nitric oxide have been identified in tobacco smoke. Smoking also increases bladder cancer, and G → T transversions of the lung type are present, but there is also a high frequency of G → C mutations. This suggests that other carcinogens are carried by body fluids to the bladder. The high

Figure 7.12

p53 in human cancers: transitions and transversions.

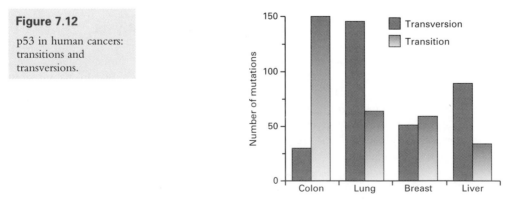

Table 7.10 p53 mutations in human cancers.

Cancer	Most frequent Mutation	Codon	Predicted agent
Lung	$G \rightarrow T$	273	Benzopyrene, oxidations
Colon	$G \rightarrow A$	175, others	Small adduct
Liver	$G \rightarrow T$	249	Aflatoxin
Skin	$C \rightarrow T$	–	Ultraviolet light
	(plus tandem double mutations)		

$G \rightarrow T$ transversion rate in liver cancers (Table 7.10) is compatible with bulky adduct formation such as from aflatoxin in foodstuffs (Figure 4.7). The high $G \rightarrow A$ transition pattern in colon cancer might indicate involvement of carcinogens generating a small DNA adduct. Skin cancers exhibit the anticipated $C \rightarrow T$ transition expected from pyrimidine dimer formation, and there are some double transitions in adjacent cytosines. Such double mutations have only been observed in cancers induced by UV light.

Not only do certain types of base change occur in different cancers but the affected codon within the p53 gene can vary (Table 7.10). This could be due to differential access of carcinogens to specific bases in various cancers. With the ras oncogene, another situation arises in that the same codon (codon 12) is affected in lung and bladder cancer but different bases within that codon are altered. In bladder cancers, $G \rightarrow T$ transversions predominate, whereas $G \rightarrow A$ transitions are more common in lung cancers, again pointing to different tobacco-related carcinogens being involved at the two sites. Interestingly, not all the p53 mutation hotspots identified in model systems *in vitro* coincide with those reported for human tumours *in vivo*. This may be due to faster repair *in vivo* at some sites than others, masking some of the hotspots detected *in vitro*.

Conclusions

These examples of mutational spectrum analysis indicate the potential of the approach but refinements are required to make the predictions more accurate for identifying human carcinogens. Both large adducts and oxidative damage generate $G \rightarrow T$ transversions and so at present it would not be possible to distinguish between these two sources of mutation. However, they can be distinguished from small adducts. A $G \rightarrow A$ transition characteristic of this type of carcinogen also occurs with UV light (secondary to the causative $C \rightarrow T$ mutation) but this is characterised by dual tandem mutations because of its cross-linking effect.

8 MUTATIONS, DNA REPAIR AND GENETIC INSTABILITY

Key points

- DNA is continually exposed to endogenous and exogenous damaging agents. It is efficiently repaired in normal cells so that errors (mutations) are not inherited by daughter cells.
- Cancer cells acquire defects in the repair process that accelerate the mutation rate.
- Genetic instability is a consequence of defective repair.
- The damaged region of DNA is detected and excised, together with adjacent nucleotides, then the correct nucleotides are inserted. Several mechanisms exist for doing this with different abilities to handle specific types of damage.
- Repair processes can be strand specific or strand independent.
- Strand-specific mechanisms can repair errors caused by the introduction of bases into the newly synthesised strand that do not pair with bases on the template strand. This is termed mismatch repair.
- Instability of microsatellite DNA is a common feature of cancers. It is an index of genetic instability due to inefficient mismatch repair.
- Strand-independent mechanisms such as nucleotide excision repair, which are less specific about the type of damage, can cope with damage caused by carcinogens, ionising radiations and UV light.
- There are strand-independent mechanisms to remove oxidised or methylated guanines; this is called base excision repair.
- DNA damage activates p53, which then inhibits proliferation and promotes DNA repair and apoptosis.
- Several clinical conditions are due to an inherited defect in DNA repair; patients with the conditions have an increased risk of developing specific types of cancer.
- Lynch's syndrome is due to an inherited defect in one allele of genes required for mismatch repair. Cancer results from loss of the second allele.
- Patients with Li–Fraumeni syndrome develop cancers at several sites caused by an inherited mutation in the p53 gene.
- Patients with xeroderma pigmentosum have an inherited defect in nucleotide excision repair that results in increased risk of skin cancer.

Introduction

Cancer results from changes in DNA sequence called mutations. The mutations are reflected in proteins which have an altered amino acid sequence, and these altered proteins ultimately change the cell function. DNA changes are generated by normal intracellular metabolic events and by external factors such as diet, lifestyle and solar radiation. It is therefore important to identify the mechanisms whereby cells minimise adverse effects of mutations. The preceding chapters have discussed the various agents capable of causing and propagating mutations; this chapter will deal with mechanisms used to repair altered DNA sequences. Repair of damaged DNA is an important defence mechanism that prevents most people developing cancers. The original clues came from bacteria in which repair defects increased the appearance of mutations. This link between repair and mutations also became evident from observations that patients with rare inherited diseases such as Bloom's syndrome, ataxia telangiectasia and xeroderma pigmentosum, which have the common feature of deficient DNA repair, have an increased risk of developing certain cancers (Chapter 9). The importance of DNA repair defects has now widened to include cancers such as those of colon and breast.

Decreased efficiency of repair is now viewed as being an important event in the succession of changes required for cancer formation, because such defects accelerate the rate of genetic change. This opinion developed from several data sets. Spontaneous mutation rates were too small to explain the speed with which multiple changes occurred that resulted in a cancer. The concept of a 'mutator phenotype' arose, in which cells with a faster mutation rate gained a survival advantage over their neighbours. Defective DNA repair could be the molecular engine for such a process because the inability to normalise damaged DNA would accelerate the accumulation of errors in DNA bases (mutations). If the defect was in the repair process itself, an autocatalytic process would be generated. Such defects have been identified in a subtype of inherited colon cancer, hereditary non-polyposis coli cancer (HNPCC, Chapter 2), and shown to be present in a number of spontaneous cancers. However, there is debate as to whether the accelerated accumulation of mutations is solely a characteristic of cancer cells. Mutation rates also increase with age in normal cells and it may be a normal phenomenon, with carcinogenesis being a normal consequence of the ageing human life cycle. Regardless of whether the mutator phenotype reflects normal or abnormal events, there must be causative agents. There has been an emphasis on external agents as the most important but they may be supplemented by spontaneous events generated through normal cell metabolism. The human data are supplemented by animal information such as the observation that mice develop cancers much more readily than humans, they have a higher spontaneous mutation rate and they have a less active DNA repair system.

The elucidation of DNA repair mechanisms is a good illustration of the multidisciplinary contributions to cancer biology. Many of the molecular characteristics of the repair processes were first elucidated in microorganisms and subsequently shown to have relevance to human cells. Characterisation of the cellular defects in patients with xeroderma pigmentosum required the expertise of clinicians, geneticists and molecular biologists, as did investigations on the patients with HNPCC. Cell biologists contributed by isolating cultured cells possessing the molecular characteristics of the parent tissues, thereby facilitating analysis of the cellular defects.

Although a decreased ability to repair DNA is an important factor in carcinogenesis, many cancers do not have defects in the repair processes themselves but in ancillary pathways concerned with regulation of repair and/or the transfer and accumulations of DNA defects to daughter cells. Cell proliferation is the prime determinant of the accumulation, and over time the number of mutations accumulated per cell is proliferation dependent. For this reason, proliferation has been defined as a risk factor for cancer. For similar reasons, cell death is also part of the equation that determines whether sufficient mutations accumulate to generate a cancer.

Cells have several repair pathways capable of dealing with various types of abnormal base sequence which are described below. Additionally, a special type of DNA repair is used to correct changes to telomeric ends of chromosomes (Chapter 10).

Mutations

Changes in DNA base sequence advertise themselves in several ways; single or multiple bases can be changed, deleted or inserted. Sophisticated molecular techniques may be required to detect such changes, but they can sometimes appear as gross changes in DNA content per nucleus (ploidy), as chromosome rearrangements or as gene amplifications. Data are sparse on mutation rates in normal human cells but three factors are clearly important in determining that rate: age, cell type and DNA characteristics (Table 8.1). The higher frequency in kidney epithelium relative to that in blood lymphocytes is important because it might account for the high frequency of cancers in epithelial cells. Little is known as to why some somatic cells have higher mutation rates than others, but rates are

Table 8.1 Mutation frequencies in normal human cells.

	Mutations per million cells*	
Cell type and age of individual		
Kidney epithelium	40 (young)	250 (old)
Lymphocytes	3 (young)	8 (old)
DNA type		
Microsatellite	10 000	
Hypoxanthine phosphoribosyl transferase gene	10	
Other factors		
Potent carcinogen	100-fold increase	
Theoretical value to account for age–incidence data	1000-fold increase	

* Approximations from a wide range of values.

probably set during embryonic development. Efficiency of DNA repair is one factor that influences mutation rates but additional components related to a cell's redox state may also be involved. A cell with a high free radical production may be more vulnerable than a cell with minimal production of these DNA-damaging agents. Answers to these points might solve the question of why cancers are more common at some sites than others. The increase in mutation rate with age is analogous to the age-dependent incidence of common cancers (Chapter 2), and this comparison between mutation rate and cancer incidence has another similarity in that both increase in an exponential manner rather than a linear manner.

Mutations are more likely to occur in stretches of DNA containing repeat sequences because of misalignment of multiple repeats on the template and daughter strands than in a gene with few such repeats. This accounts for the higher number of mutations in microsatellite DNA, which consists of these sequences, than in the hypoxanthine phosphoribosyl transferase gene.

From the figures for normal epithelial cells in Table 8.1, it is possible to calculate theoretical mutation rates for a repressor the size of the crucial colon cancer gene, APC (Chapter 2). The spontaneous mutation frequency for one allele would be 1 per 1000 cells per generation, and for both alleles the figure would be 1 per million cells. This is not a large number of cells, being the equivalent of a sphere about a millimetre in diameter. A similar number emerges from a different data set – normal urinary excretion of metabolites of purine and pyrimidine bases – suggests that about 10 000 bases are destroyed per cell per day. If DNA repair of this damage is 99% efficient, 100 mutations per cell per day would result. Such calculations are subject to major errors and should not be overinterpreted, but they do indicate that spontaneous mutations could generate initial carcinogenic changes in normal cells.

Genetic instability

In cell culture, potent carcinogens such as N-methylnitrosourea increase mutation rates between tenfold and a hundredfold (Table 8.1) but sufficient concentrations of such potent compounds are unlikely to be encountered *in vivo* in human tissues. It has been calculated that if DNA repair were working properly, the spontaneous mutation rate would have to be increased more than a thousandfold to account for the relatively short time necessary to generate the seven rate-limiting mutations necessary for colon carcinogenesis (Chapter 2). However, if DNA repair were defective, if an ancillary process such as proliferation increased or if cell death decreased, mutations that conferred selective advantages on the cells would accumulate at an accelerated rate.

A different form of instability becomes evident at later stages of carcinogenesis, especially during progression to more aggressive cancers. This involves gross increases in DNA content per nucleus (ploidy changes) or multiple amplifications of specific regions of certain chromosomes. Thus, the chromosome region containing the dihydrofolate reductase gene can be amplified more than a thousandfold in advanced cancers, so it becomes visible as a homogeneous staining region in chromosome preparations (Chapter 13).

Types of DNA damage

Figure 8.1 illustrates the main types of damage suffered by DNA and which, if not corrected, could result in the substitution of abnormal bases. Damaging agents can be categorised according to whether they are of endogenous (intracellular) origin or environmental origin. Chapter 7 details the mechanisms whereby oxidation, ionising radiation, UV light and chemical carcinogens modify DNA structure, and the mutational consequences are listed in Table 7.8. They will only be summarised here, but the additional processes identified in Figure 8.1 will be discussed.

Oxidation of guanine by reactive oxygen free radicals generated by ionising radiation or cell metabolism produces 8-hydroxyguanine (8-oxoguanine); DNA polymerase reads this as a thymine at the next round of synthesis (Figure 7.10). Ionising radiation also induces single- and double-strand breaks, which create deletions and gross chromosome abnormalities. UV light cross-links adjacent pyrimidines (cytosines or thymines, Figure 7.11) which are read as thymines. The effect of adducts consequent to carcinogen exposure is determined by the carcinogen involved. Small adducts such as those formed between guanine and dimethylnitrosamine (Figure 7.6) are read as adenines, whereas bulky guanine adducts such as those formed with benzopyrene (Figure 7.3) can either be treated as

Figure 8.1

Types of base change induced by different agents.

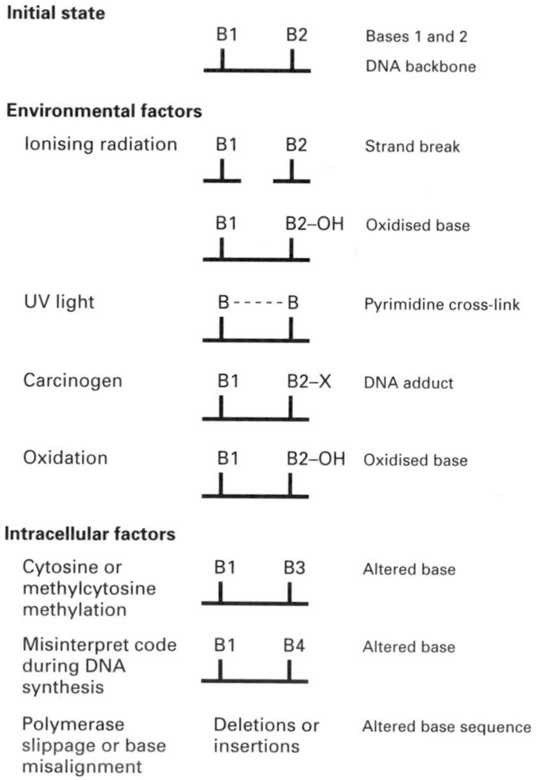

Initial state

| B1 | B2 | Bases 1 and 2 |
| | | DNA backbone |

Environmental factors

Ionising radiation — B1 B2 — Strand break

B1 B2–OH — Oxidised base

UV light — B - - - - - B — Pyrimidine cross-link

Carcinogen — B1 B2–X — DNA adduct

Oxidation — B1 B2–OH — Oxidised base

Intracellular factors

Cytosine or methylcytosine methylation — B1 B3 — Altered base

Misinterpret code during DNA synthesis — B1 B4 — Altered base

Polymerase slippage or base misalignment — Deletions or insertions — Altered base sequence thymines or they can distort the DNA structure so much that strand breaks occur. Several intracellular metabolic events generate mutations. Free radicals were mentioned above but a common change is the deamination of cytosine to form uracil, or 5-methylcytosine to form thymine (Figure 8.2); both are interpreted as thymines. DNA synthesis is an efficient process, with the base sequence of the template strand being converted with high fidelity (one error per 10^{10} nucleotides) into a complementary sequence on the daughter strand. This is largely due to the $3'-5'$ exonuclease (phosphodiesterase) activity of some of the DNA polymerases involved (Box 6.1 explains DNA terminology).

The commonest error of this type is a G pairing with a T instead of the normal G:C pattern. This is aptly called the proof-reading function of DNA polymerase. At least four DNA polymerases are involved in DNA synthesis (Box 9.1), two of which (α and β) have no attendant nuclease activity and therefore no proof-reading ability. Polymerases α and β can generate more than 100 errors for every million nucleotides incorporated. Fortunately, polymerases δ and ε have efficient exonuclease activities with good proof-reading functions, and the result is less than 20 errors per million nucleotides. Even if the overall fidelity of base incorporation were 99.99%, for a human genome of 10^{9} base pairs there would be 10^{5} misincorporated bases per cell at each round of DNA synthesis in the absence of additional repair processes. Given the other sources of damaged DNA, the experimental figure seems reasonable – 10^{4} bases per cell being repaired.

Replication of repeated base sequences presents special problems for the machinery responsible for their synthesis. The DNA polymerase can 'slip' on runs of similar base sequences and either incorporate additional bases into the daughter strand or leave out bases from the template strand. In each case the outcome is misaligned, single-strand loops of unpaired bases. If the loop is on the template strand, the daughter strand will contain a deletion; if the loop is on the daughter strand, the daughter strand will contain an insertion.

Figure 8.2

Deamination of cytosine and 5–methylcytosine as mutational events.

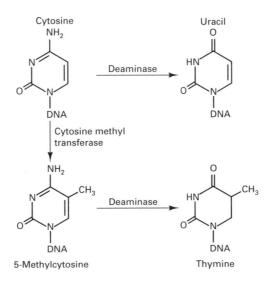

Gene amplifications

In advanced cancers, big regions of DNA can be replicated several thousandfold. Thus, the dihydrofolate reductase gene (Chapter 13) can be amplified together with large adjacent stretches of DNA. This complex process involves formation of multiple abnormal replication forks during DNA synthesis.

Clinical evidence that links DNA repair and carcinogenesis

Several inherited conditions exist that link DNA repair defects to a high risk of cancer. They are listed in Table 9.3 and described in Chapter 9. Patients with these inherited diseases often present with an ill-assorted collection of symptoms; these diseases were originally called syndromes to hide ignorance about their causes. Bloom's syndrome, ataxia telangiectasia and Franconi's syndrome have each been linked with increased risk of leukaemia and lymphoma whereas xeroderma pigmentosa is associated with a 2000-fold increased risk of skin cancer. All these conditions result in chromosome fragility and the molecular basis of the symptoms has been identified as inherited defects in genes coding for proteins that regulate DNA repair. Three other inherited conditions associated with DNA repair are linked with a different pattern of cancers, albeit at specific sites. Patients with Li–Fraumeni syndrome are at increased risk of bone cancers (sarcomas), breast cancers and brain cancers, whereas patients who have **h**ereditary **n**on-polyposis **c**oli **c**ancer (HNPCC, Lynch's syndrome) exhibit a different pattern of cancers – colon and endometrial (uterus), ovary and stomach. Inheritance of mutations in the breast cancer genes BRCA1 or BRCA2 confers yet another pattern of increased breast, prostate, ovary or colon cancers (Chapter 9). Compared with the general population, cancers appear at an earlier age in people with such defects. This fits with faster accumulation of errors because, having inherited the first mutation in a gene linked to DNA repair, other mutations will arise more rapidly. The defects are transferred to offspring through the germ cells (eggs or sperm), so all cells in the body carry the error; it is not clear, therefore, why cancer does not occur everywhere but only at a limited number of specific sites that can vary with the defect. The repair processes involved are common to all cells, which emphasises our ignorance about why the cell selectivity for cancer risk occurs. It might reflect repair efficiency or number and type of damaging events to which the cell is subjected.

HNPCC patients have defective mismatch repair (see below) whereas Li–Fraumeni individuals carry inactivating mutations in the p53 gene. This gene is not an immediate component of DNA repair but the p53 protein indirectly facilitates it. In normal cells, genotoxic damage such as ionising radiation increases the p53 content; this blocks proliferation and allows DNA repair to proceed. p53 also activates apoptosis, a suicide method of eliminating defective DNA (Chapter 10). Defective p53 does not block proliferation and apoptosis, so damage accumulates in daughter cells. The functions of the BRCA genes are not well understood but defective cells are sensitive to ionising radiation and genotoxic carcinogens; repair of strand breaks may be one of the normal actions of proteins from the BRCA genes (Chapter 9).

Mutations in the retinoblastoma (Rb) repressor gene can also contribute to error accumulation. When one Rb allele has mutated, the chance of the second allele becoming defective is increased (Chapter 9) and, when that occurs the G_1 block to the cell cycle is relieved, thereby decreasing the time available for repair (Chapter 10).

Repair mechanisms

With one exception (alkyl transferase), repair mechanisms use the principle of detection and excision of the damage followed by refilling the gaps. The main types of damage rectified by each of the following mechanisms are listed in Table 8.2.

Base excision repair

Basic excision repair is the primary way of removing nucleotides damaged by intracellular processes such as free radical oxidations or deamination of cytosine and 5-methylcytosine. It will also handle bases alkylated by exogenous agents such as nitrosamines. A family of N-glycosidases can hydrolyse the glycoside link between the N-9 of the purine base and deoxyribose, thereby releasing the damaged base and leaving an abasic site (**ap**urinic/**ap**yrimidinic, AP site) in the DNA chain (Figure 8.3). The deoxyribosephosphate chain is cleaved 5′ to the damaged base by an AP endonuclease and on the other side by exonuclease activity of DNA

Table 8.2 Repair mechanism and damage type.

Mechanism	Type of damage
Base excision repair	Abasic sites
	Free radical oxidations
	Deamination of cytosine/methylcytosine
	Alkylations
Base mismatch repair	Small adducts,
	Free radical oxidations
	Insertions/deletions
Nucleotide excision repair	Large adducts
	UV cross-links
Exonuclease component of DNA polymerase	Code misinterpretation (proof-reading function)
Alkyl transferase	Small alkyl adducts
Homologous recombination	Strand breaks
DNA end-joining	Strand breaks

Figure 8.3

Base excision repair: general situation. In the specific case of removing an 8-OH guanine this is accompanied by removal of three additional nucleotides 3′ to the damage site.

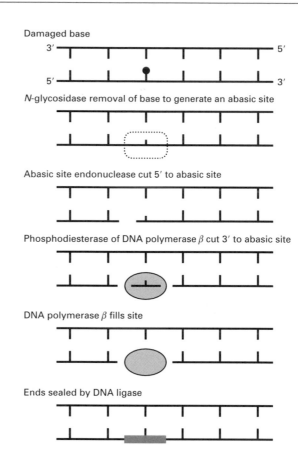

Damaged base

N-glycosidase removal of base to generate an abasic site

Abasic site endonuclease cut 5′ to abasic site

Phosphodiesterase of DNA polymerase β cut 3′ to abasic site

DNA polymerase β fills site

Ends sealed by DNA ligase

polymerase β; if an oxidised base is to be removed, a 4-nucleotide section is excised. The glycosidase responsible for excising 8-OH guanines is often deleted in lung cancers. DNA polymerase β fills the single nucleotide gap with a nucleotide determined by the sequence of the other strand; DNA ligase seals the nucleotide into the DNA strand.

The N-glycosidases repair uracil substitutions better than they repair thymines, which means that methylated cytosines are potentially more mutagenic than the parent cytosine. The relevance of this to DNA methylation, differentiation and carcinogenesis is discussed in Chapter 10.

Alkyl transferase (ATase)

A second type of base repair removes bases with small adducts such as O^6-methylguanine produced by alkylating mutagens such as N-methylnitrosourea (Figure 7.7). Although known as an enzymic mechanism, this is incorrect as the methyl group transferred to a cysteine on the protein renders the protein inactive (Figure 8.4).

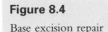

Figure 8.4

Base excision repair

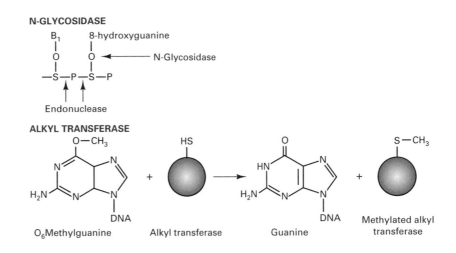

Nucleotide excision repair

Compared with base excision, nucleotide excision has a different specificity; it can remove mismatches as well as UV-induced pyrimidine dimers (Figure 7.11) and bulky adducts such as polycyclic aromatic hydrocarbons (Figure 7.4) and aflatoxin. In fact, it is the only method of removing bulky DNA adducts (Table 8.2).

The process is complex, involving proteins capable of recognising damaged regions and removing the defective segment. The remaining single-stranded, unaffected section is then used as a template to fill in the gap (Figure 8.5). All of this takes time, so proliferation is stopped by p53-mediated processes to allow repair to occur (see below). Interestingly, the repair mechanism uses the protein TFII, more usually associated with mRNA synthesis; thus the damaged cell can divert other functions to achieve repair.

The processes involved have largely been identified with cells obtained from patients with xeroderma pigmentosum or related disorders such as Cockayne's syndrome (see Figure 8.5). The presenting symptoms are due to hypersensitivity of skin to light, but affected individuals have a high probability of developing leukaemias and lymphomas. Xeroderma pigmentosum is a family of disorders in which one or more of the 20–30 proteins needed for nucleotide excision repair are defective. About 80% of patients with xeroderma pigmentosum have defects in at least one of seven proteins, labelled XPA to XPG, needed in the early stages of repair. Recognition and melting of the double-stranded damaged region is initiated by the DNA-binding proteins, XPA and XPC.

XPA is a DNA-binding protein that reacts with a second protein, RPA (**r**eplication **p**rotein **A**), and RPA interacts with single-stranded DNA. XPC is then recruited to the damaged site. The small region of single-stranded DNA is then enlarged by the **t**ranscription **f**actor **IIH** (TF-IIH) complex of 6–9 proteins that includes XPB and XPD. The latter proteins unwind the DNA helix (helicase activity) to generate the open region spanning 23–30 nucleotides. As the name

Figure 8.5

Nucleotide excision repair.

Damaged sequence distorts the helix

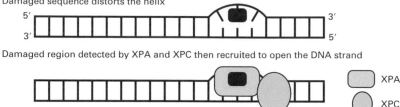

Damaged region detected by XPA and XPC then recruited to open the DNA strand

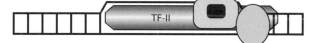

XPA

XPC

Single-stranded region of DNA extended by binding TF-II complex (contains XPB and XPD)

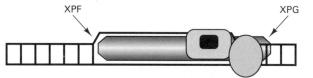

A 23–30 nucleotide section of the damged strand cut by XPF and XPG nucleases (part of TF-II)

XPF   XPG

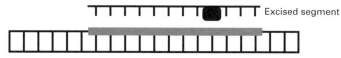

Gap left by excised nucleotides filled by DNA polymerase ε, ligase, PCNA and other proteins

Excised segment

implies, TF-IIH is also needed for gene transcription. This interrelationship between two important cell functions, repair and gene transcription, has beneficial functional relevance in that genes being transcribed at the time of damage are more likely to have rapid adverse effects on cell function. It is therefore helpful that actively transcribed genes are rapidly repaired, because the damage blocks RNA polymerase function and repair is facilitated by having TF-IIH already present at the site of damage. The single strand of damaged DNA is then excised by the endonuclease activities of XPF and XPG. Full nuclease activity of XPF requires the **e**xcision **r**epair **c**ontrol **c**omponent (ERCC1) protein. XPE participates with TF-IIH in repairing UV damage. The gap left by the excised nucleotides is then filled by a combination of DNA polymerase δ and/or ε, DNA ligase, **p**roliferation **c**ontrol **n**uclear **a**ntigen (PCNA) and other proteins.

The remaining 20% of patients with xeroderma pigmentosum have normal XPA–XPG proteins but have variants (XPV) defective in later stages, possibly due to an abnormal DNA polymerase subunit.

Mismatch repair

The repair processes described thus far are capable of repairing either DNA strand. If a mismatched base is incorporated into a newly synthesised daughter strand, it can

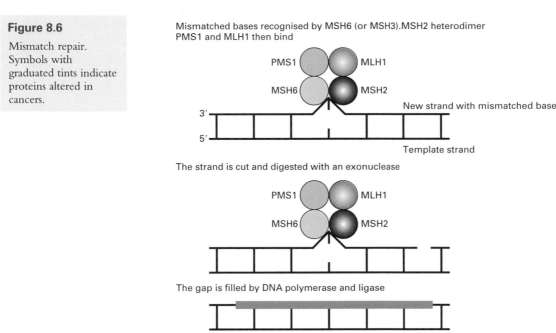

Figure 8.6

Mismatch repair. Symbols with graduated tints indicate proteins altered in cancers.

Mismatched bases recognised by MSH6 (or MSH3).MSH2 heterodimer PMS1 and MLH1 then bind

The strand is cut and digested with an exonuclease

The gap is filled by DNA polymerase and ligase

be repaired by mismatch repair (Figure 8.6). This is called post-replication repair. It can cope with a broad spectrum of small damage types. Misincorporated bases, alkyl adducts, small insertions or deletions and oxidations can be repaired but not bulky adducts or UV cross-linked pyrimidines (Table 8.2). The mismatched bases are recognised by a multiprotein complex, short regions of DNA sequence digested from the newly synthesised strand, and the gap filled by DNA polymerase δ and ligase. Recognition of the incorrect base(s) requires four proteins, two of which (MSH2, MLH1), cause HNPCC (Chapter 9) and are also altered in some sporadic cancers; PMS1 may even be a third. It is not known how strand specificity is achieved but initial recognition of the damage is by binding of an MSH2.MSH6 (or MSH3) protein heterodimer. MSH6 was called GT-binding protein because it has selectivity for guanine:thymine mismatches. MSH6 is preferentially recruited to single-base errors and MSH3 to those involving 2–4 bases but there is overlap of activities. PMS1 and MLH1 bind to the MSH2.MSH6 dimer and repair is effected by exonuclease cleavage and digestion of a limited number of nucleotides followed by gap filling with DNA polymerase and ligase. PCNA, which plays a coordinating role in DNA synthesis (Box 10.1), interacts with MLH1.PMS1 heterodimers, thus providing a link with the machinery needed to fill the excised gap.

HNPCC is an autosomal recessive condition in which both alleles of the affected gene must be inactivated. Normal cells from an HNPCC individual have a mismatch repair function one hundred times better than cancer cells from the same person. A single normal allele in an affected individual can result in effective mismatch repair; but when that normal allele is lost by somatic mutation, the repair mechanism is lost. This example of the two-hit model of carcinogenesis also provides evidence of a causal association between defective DNA repair and increased cancer risk. Over 40 different mutations have been identified in MLH1 and MSH2, only a single family has been identified with a PMS1 defect and none with MSH6 or MSH3 mutations. In most cases the mutations result in truncated proteins or inactivating amino acid substitutions.

Microsatellite instability   The multiple 2–4 base pair repeats in microsatellites are subject to misalignment during replication (see above) and in normal cells they are repaired by mismatch repair. Thus, defective mismatch repair increases the lengths of microsatellite sequences (microsatellite instability) which can be detected by gel electrophoresis. Microsatellite instability is a surrogate marker for defective mismatch repair; it is sometimes known as the **r**eplication **e**rror **r**epair phenotype (RER).

DNA strand breaks

Both single- and double-strand breaks occur as a consequence of ionising radiation or bulky adduct distortions of the DNA helix. If not repaired, the open-ended broken strands form promiscuous liaisons with inappropriate strands and this leads to chromosome abnormalities. Double-stranded breaks are particularly difficult for the cell to handle but they can be repaired by either homologous recombination with the undamaged second chromosome (Box 9.1) or by DNA end-joining of the broken strands.

Homologous recombination   Diploid cells contain two double helices of DNA (sister chromatids). A double-strand break occurs in only one helix that leaves the sister helix intact. Homologous recombination requires extensive regions of base homology on the undamaged helix to provide a template for repair (Figure 8.7). $5'–3'$ exonucleases digest damaged strands to expose single-stranded regions either side of the break. A complex series of proteins (RAD proteins) promote the sensing of homologies between single-stranded, damaged, DNA and homologous bases in the same region of the undamaged helix; resynthesis of the excised sequences is then determined by the base sequence of the undamaged strand of the sister helix. The functions of the RAD proteins are unclear but RAD51 polymerises onto the single-stranded DNA and searches for the homolgous sequence on the undamaged helix. The other RAD proteins plus the single-stranded DNA-binding protein RPA facilitate crossover between the strands (strand exchange). DNA polymerase, ligases and accessory proteins synthesise and ligate the four strands to reform two helices. RAD51 will also interact with p53, BRCA1 and BRCA2 proteins, providing a mechanistic link with proteins known to be involved in DNA repair. Cells deficient in any of these proteins are sensitive to agents such as ionising radiation that generate double-strand breaks and chromosome abnormalities (Chapter 9). There may be a role for the enzyme **p**oly(**A**DP-**r**ibose) **p**olymerase (PARP) in repair of strand breaks. PARP is recruited to the breaks and undergoes an autocatalytic modification by synthesis of poly(ADP-ribose). This plays an undefined, indirect role in repair.

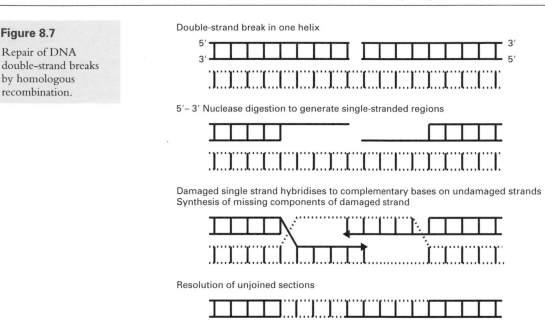

Figure 8.7

Repair of DNA double-strand breaks by homologous recombination.

DNA end-joining This needs only limited homologies to rejoin juxtaposed ends of broken strands; only the damaged helix is involved (Figure 8.8). Damaged strand ends are detected by protein heterodimers (KU70 plus XRCC5) which then recruit a **DNA**-dependent serine **p**rotein **k**inase (DNAPK). Additional proteins are incorporated into the complex, phosphorylated by DNAPK and rejoin the broken strands. The ATM gene, defective in ataxia telangiectasia, also influences strand repair and other types of repair but the mechanism is unclear. The ATM protein is a protein kinase that is vaguely said to regulate a signalling cascade responsive to DNA damage. It is activated by certain types of damage and is involved in p53 activation (see below).

Figure 8.8

Repair of DNA double-strand break by DNA end-joining.

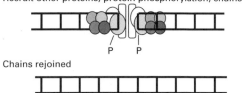

Coordination of DNA repair, proliferation and apoptosis

These three functions work in a coordinated fashion to ensure that damaged DNA does not adversely affect cell function; damage inhibits proliferation, and if too great to be repaired, the cell commits suicide by apoptosis. DNA damage activates the p53 repressor protein that plays a major role in coordinating these functions; it warrants the title of 'guardian of the genome'. Different types of damage activate p53 by different pathways (Figure 8.9), although post-transcriptional methods are used in each situation; protein synthesis is not required. Mechanistic details are sparse. Ionising radiation activates both DNAPK and ATM kinases, and ATM-deficient cells exhibit only a slow response to such radiation. The N-terminal phosphorylation sites of p53 are involved, but it is not clear whether there are direct or indirect interactions between the components shown in Figure 8.9. UV light-induced damage affects both N- and C-terminal domains of p53, although current details are confusing. The N-terminal phosphorylations generated by UV light are independent of ATM kinase, although the C-terminal changes require this enzyme. However, some of the C-terminal changes activated by UV light may eventually be mediated by a protein phosphatase that removes an inhibitory serine phosphate besides activating phosphorylations at other sites. Chapters 6 and 10 describe events downstream of p53 activation.

In normal cells, transient expression of p53 enables it to fulfil multiple functions primarily, but not exclusively, through its role as a transcription factor. It increases transcription from genes involved in the inhibition of DNA replication (p21, Gadd45) but has opposing effects on BAX and Bcl2, the two genes that regulate apoptosis. There is increased expression of the proapoptotic BAX and inhibition of the antiapoptotic Bcl2. This alteration in BAX:Bcl2 ratio relieves a block in the apoptosis pathway. The net result is blocked proliferation that enables repair to proceed and increased apoptosis that eliminates cells with damaged DNA.

Figure 8.9

Activation of p53 by DNA damage. UV damage also results in C-terminal phosphorylation (not shown).

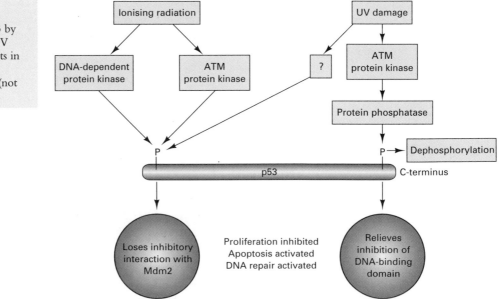

The p21 protein is an inhibitor of the cyclin-dependent kinases that are essential for progression through the cell cycle (Chapter 10). It also binds to PCNA, part of the active DNA polymerase complex required for both synthesis and repair. The p21–PCNA interaction inhibits DNA synthesis but not repair functions; this achieves coordinate inhibition of synthesis whilst allowing repair to proceed. p53 also facilitates repair by binding to two of the XP proteins (D and B).

Bcl2 inhibits apoptosis whereas BAX stimulates it, so in normal cells a p53-mediated block of Bcl2 and stimulation of BAX gene transcription synergistically promotes apoptosis. Mutated p53 has none of these functions, so proliferation continues in the absence of apoptosis and mutations are passed on to daughter cells.

Inactivation of p53 in cancer cells can be achieved by mutation of the gene or by interaction with other proteins (Chapter 6). The overall effect of such inactivation is loss of growth control and decreased repair of DNA damage. The biological effectiveness of this process is illustrated by the fact that cultured cells from patients with Li–Fraumeni syndrome are genetically unstable and are more sensitive to DNA-damaging agents than their normal counterparts. It is not known how p53 senses the damage but p53 inactivation favours genetic instability. There may be an autocatalytic loop operative such that codons in the p53 gene that are important for normal function of the protein are repaired only slowly. Therefore mutations in these codons are more likely to escape repair and decrease the efficiency of subsequent repair processes.

Key points

- Mutations inherited through germ cells contribute to a minority of cancers.
- At least two rate-limiting changes (hits) are required for tumour development. If the first hit is inherited through a germ cell, the cancer occurs earlier than if generated in a somatic cell.
- Germline mutations occur in repressor genes that can act in a recessive or dominant-negative way.
- Sporadic cancers often acquire mutations in the same genes as inherited cancers. In such situations, data from familial cancers have relevance to sporadic cancers. This is not universally true.
- Dissimilar germline mutations in one cell type can have a common end result, a cancer.
- Within one gene, germline mutations occur at different loci in different families.
- Germline mutations only generate cancers in selected cell types and in a limited number of cells of a common type.
- Defective DNA repair results in increased cancer risk.

Introduction

Three categories of cancer can be defined according to the degree to which inherited features are involved (Table 9.1). The great majority of cancers are of the sporadic type with no evidence of inherited links in cancer incidence within members of a family. These arise by mutations in somatic cells. However, a small percentage of the common cancers do arise because of inherited defects and a high proportion of rare cancers can result from inherited mutations. The inherited defects

Table 9.1 Categories of cancers.

Familial involvement	Percentage of all cancers	Examples
None (sporadic)	>90	All types of cancer
Involved	5–10	Colon, breast
Well-defined	0.1	Retinoblastoma, Wilms' (kidney)

are passed from parents to offspring via the egg or sperm. These germline mutations are confined to repressor genes. The probability of inheriting the same rare defect from both parents is very low, so the offspring from one affected parent are heterozygous, carrying one defective and one normal allele. The germline mutations are in genes coding for repressor proteins, so both alleles must usually be inactivated before an effect is seen (Chapter 6). Hence the one normal allele inherited from the unaffected parent must also be inactivated by a somatic cell mutation. The somatic cell mutation is usually different to the type present in the germ cells, although the gene and end effect are common.

Despite the rarity of familial cancers, genetic information obtained from their study is relevant to sporadic cancers. Thus, the Rb repressor gene was first identified by its absence in familial retinoblastoma and is now known to be a negative regulator of proliferation in many cell types (Chapter 10) and Rb mutations occur in several sporadic cancers. Likewise, the inherited mutation in the **a**denomatous **p**olyposis **c**oli (APC) gene is involved in both familial and sporadic forms of colon cancer (Chapter 2) but such generalisations cannot be taken too far. The germline mutation in genes linked to familial **br**east **c**ancer (BRCA1 and BRCA2 genes) is unaffected in sporadic cases. Before examining these points, consider some of the terms used to describe chromosome details.

Box 9.1 **Chromosome nomenclature and structure**

The normal diploid human genome is composed of two copies of each of 22 *autosomal* chromosomes plus two sex chromosomes, X and Y (male) or X and X (female). Chromosomes are numbered in descending order of size and each has a short arm (p) and a long arm (q) either side of the *centromere*, which is the point of attachment of mitotic spindles (Figure 9.1). These tubulin-containing spindles retract the chromosomes into daughter cells at mitosis. Each chromosome has a characteristic staining pattern that is used to divide a chromosome arm into numbered regions, so the Rb gene on the long arm of chromosome 13 at position14, is defined as having location 13q14. There is one copy (allele) of each gene per chromosome, so diploid cells have two alleles of each gene and are called *homozygous*. When one allele is lost and the other is unaffected, the cell is *heterozygous* for that allele. If the second, normal allele is lost there is *loss of heterozygosity (LOH)*. This is illustrated in Table 9.2. At the end of each chromosome is a *telomere* made up of a large number of

Figure 9.1

Chromosome structure.

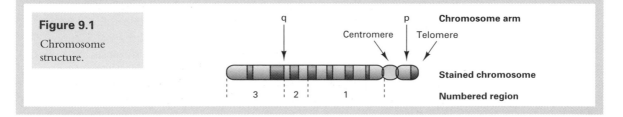

tandem (head to tail) TTAGGG repeats. These tandem repeats play an important role in determining the lifespan of cells (Chapter 10). The number, size and shape of a cell's chromosome complement define its *karyotype*.

One DNA double helix extends the length of the chromosome and is condensed into coils and supercoils; the lowest common denominator is the *nucleosome* in which 200 base pairs (bp) of DNA are wound round a histone protein core. The internucleosome bridges of DNA are sites of DNAase digestion during apoptosis (Chapter 10). Other proteins and RNAs are wrapped around the nucleosomes to form *chromatin*, sometimes called *interphase chromatin* in non-mitotic cells. At mitosis the chromatin rearranges into chromosomes. Interphase chromatin is attached to a cytoskeleton, the *nuclear matrix*. About 3% of human DNA base sequences code for proteins; the other 97% have complex regulatory and other poorly defined roles. One type of non-coding sequence, *microsatellite DNA*, consists of tandem 2–4 bp repeats and their length can increase if DNA mismatch repair is defective (Chapter 8); this is called *microsatellite instability*.

The sequence of bases in DNA can be altered in several ways, collectively known as *mutations*. Not all mutations have functional significance for the cell; non-significant mutations are called *silent mutations* or *neutral mutations*. Chromosome *translocations* occur commonly in cancers, especially leukaemias. *Heterologous or non-homologous recombination* involves exchanging segments of one chromosome with segments from a different chromosome. *Homologous recombination* between similar regions of two identical chromosomes is used to repair DNA strand breaks. Chronic myeloid leukaemia is characterised by a reciprocal translocation between chromosomes 22 and 9 (Chapter 2) and it is defined as having a t(9;22)(q34,q11) karyotype; the first set of parentheses contain the chromosome numbers and the second set contain the breakpoints. The **t** indicates a translocation; **del** indicates a deletion and **inv** an inversion. DNA deletions and inversions can sometimes be large enough to be detected by *cytogenetic* methods (chromosome staining). *Nonsense* and *frame shift mutations* involve base changes that alter the coding sequence to a non-coding one and prematurely terminate transcription; *truncated proteins* are produced. This can occur with Rb in retinoblastoma. Single *base substitutions* can result in the gene coding for a different amino acid (point mutations); this new amino acid may then alter the function of the overall protein. In colon cancer a guanine-to-adenine mutation in the ras oncogene leads to replacement of the normal glycine by aspartate and permanent activation of the ras protein (Figure 6.6). Not all base changes have adverse effects. *Polymorphisms* are neutral variations in base sequences between individuals and they have little effect on function. At a cleavage site for a restriction enzyme, polymorphisms alter the digestion pattern and this forms the basis of *restriction fragment length polymorphism* (RFLP) analysis for detecting mutations. RFLP changes can also be generated by any of the mutation types just described. Other relevant definitions are given in Box 10.1.

Strong familial link

Rare cancers that occur in childhood with high frequency in affected families are due to the inactivation of both alleles of key repressor genes. In Chapter 2 the tendency for common cancers to occur in older people was explained as being due to the time taken to accumulate the several genetic changes required for cancer formation. It follows that a cancer occurring in children indicates fewer changes. This is true for retinoblastoma (eye), the incidence of which can be explained by a two-hit model in which each allele is inactivated independently. Another less well characterised, more complex familial example is Wilms' tumour (kidney).

Retinoblastoma

Retinoblastoma occurs in unilateral and bilateral forms, with the bilateral form appearing in younger children. Over 90% of bilateral cases are diagnosed before the age of 2 years whereas the same point is reached by age 4 years with unilateral cancers. Children with bilateral cancers have a familial connection with retinoblastoma whereas the unilateral cases do not. These differences are explained by the number of mutations (hits) required to generate a cancer. Two hits are needed for both types of retinoblastoma but the first one is inherited in bilateral cases and acquired in unilateral ones (Table 9.2). The familial form is also characterised by having up to 10 individual cancers in each eye, each with a different type of second Rb mutation. This indicates that each cancer arose independently and provides evidence of the clonal origins of these cancers. With germline mutations, all cells in the body contain the first hit, which raises questions as to why many more cancers do not appear in such individuals given that Rb is so important in regulating proliferation of all cells (Chapter 10). The retina contains about 10^8 retinoblasts but even a severely affected child has less than 10 tumours, so unknown inhibitory influences must be operative. The same applies to other cell types. Familial retinoblastoma cases are at increased risk of developing bone cancers but not other types of cancer. On the other hand, once the first Rb allele has been inactivated there is a high probability of the second deletion occurring in the other copy. With 10^8 target cells, each with 10^9 nucleotide bases, random hits at a specific locus are extremely improbable. The first hit must generate genetic instability so as to increase the probability of generating the second event. This has been described as the creation of a mutator phenotype. How this is achieved is unclear but disruption of the balance between DNA synthesis, repair and cell death may be involved (Chapter 10).

A normal individual has cells with two Rb alleles (homozygous) whereas a carrier has only one copy (heterozygous); see Table 9.2. Loss of the remaining allele returns the cell to a homozygous state, albeit a different state than for a normal individual. If retinoblastoma cells are compared with normal cells from a carrier of the germline mutation, the retinoblastoma cells have no copies of the Rb gene whereas the normal cells have one copy. This provides convincing evidence that the cancer is due to loss of the second allele.

Rb was localised to chromosome 13q14 by means of karyotypic markers. Familial retinoblastoma cells were compared with normal cells from the same individual and

Table 9.2 Retinoblastoma characteristics.

1.

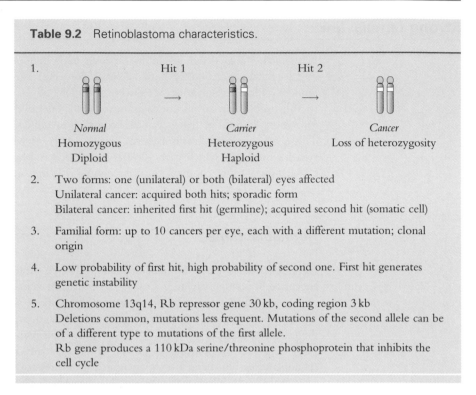

	Hit 1	Hit 2
Normal	*Carrier*	*Cancer*
Homozygous	Heterozygous	Loss of heterozygosity
Diploid	Haploid	

2. Two forms: one (unilateral) or both (bilateral) eyes affected
Unilateral cancer: acquired both hits; sporadic form
Bilateral cancer: inherited first hit (germline); acquired second hit (somatic cell)

3. Familial form: up to 10 cancers per eye, each with a different mutation; clonal origin

4. Low probability of first hit, high probability of second one. First hit generates genetic instability

5. Chromosome 13q14, Rb repressor gene 30 kb, coding region 3 kb
Deletions common, mutations less frequent. Mutations of the second allele can be of a different type to mutations of the first allele.
Rb gene produces a 110 kDa serine/threonine phosphoprotein that inhibits the cell cycle

found to have lost a number of markers from region 13q14 including the esterase D gene. Three separate retinoblastoma families were identified, each with a different chromosome 13q14 deletion. Two of the families had additionally lost the esterase gene whereas the third had not, thereby allowing precise localisation of Rb.

In normal cells, Rb codes for a phosphoprotein that inhibits proliferation at the G_1/S boundary of the cell cycle by binding to the transcription factor E2F (Chapter 10).

Rb alterations have been detected in other, non-familial cancers such as those of bone, breast, lung and bladder. Thus, identification of the Rb suppressor gene through a rare familial cancer has provided important clues about other cancers.

Wilms' tumour

This kidney tumour is the commonest abdominal tumour in children and exhibits some genetic similarities with retinoblastoma. It occurs in familial and sporadic forms, it is inherited as an autosomal trait and two hits are required for tumour formation. Furthermore, the sporadic form affects only one kidney whereas the inherited defect has bilateral effects. However, several forms of inherited defect have been identified with most information being available about the **W**ilms' **t**umour (WT1) gene on chromosome 11p13. This gene codes for a 49 kDa DNA-binding transcription factor that is only expressed in a limited number of cell types, which contrasts with the widespread distribution of Rb. Another difference to retinoblastoma is that the WT1 gene can act in a dominant-negative way similar to that observed with p53 (Chapter 6) so that both alleles need not be deleted. Genes influenced by WT1 include those for cytokines such as insulin-like growth factor II (IGF-II), epidermal growth factor (EGF) and platelet-derived growth factor (PDGF); cytokine receptors for IGF-I and transforming growth factor β); and other functions such as apoptosis (Bcl2). WT1 inhibits expression of both IGF-II and the IGF-I receptor through which that cytokine works (Chapter 11), which is one route through which WT1 could suppress growth.

Weaker familial link

Most cancers in this category involve genes that are directly implicated in the carcinogenic process, although some function indirectly through processes like immune response or metabolic defects.

There are families whose members have an elevated risk of developing one of several different types of tumour. In one example a mother who eventually died of liver cancer had 12 children, 9 of whom developed cancers or preneoplastic lesions of the breast (6 cases), cervix (2 cases) or bladder (1 case). Although increased risk may relate predominantly to one cell type, others can be affected. This is not surprising if the gene in question regulates a pathway common to many cell types, such as cell proliferation or transduction of signal from outside the cell to the nucleus, but it is important not to take too simplistic a view of a complex phenomenon. Thus, p53 is a regulator of cell proliferation but knocking out both alleles in all cells of a mouse generates abnormalities in only a limited range of cell types, and a similar cell-specific phenomenon is associated with Rb loss in humans (see above).

Conversely, it is clear that different genes contribute to formation of the same cancer (Table 9.3), implying that disruption of alternative pathways can generate the same apparent end result. The word 'apparent' is used because it has long been a view in clinical circles that a specific cancer, e.g. breast cancer, is really a collection of diseases with some common features.

Several familial conditions are known that carry an increased risk of getting specific multiple cancers. Many such cancers have the same morphological classification as sporadic cases, although their natural histories may be different. Thus, familial forms of breast cancer and colon cancer occur at earlier ages than their sporadic counterparts as anticipated from the acquisition of one of the required mutations through the germ cells.

The multiple endocrine neoplasias and neurofibromatosis are poorly understood but others listed in Table 9.3 are informative.

Colon cancer

This is a good example of the multiple routes to cancer formation because more than three inherited defects have been identified in different families on top of the sporadic cases. Their natural history is detailed in Chapter 2 but some of the points relevant to this chapter will be repeated here.

Table 9.3 Familial conditions associated with the genesis of specific cancers.

Condition	Gene	Chromosome	Cancer*	Function
Retinoblastoma	Rb	13q	Eye	Proliferation control
Wilms' tumour	WT1	11p	Kidney	Transcription
Familial adenomatous polyposis coli	APC	5q	Colon	Cell recognition
Hereditary non-polyposis colon cancer	MSH2	2p ⎫	Colon	DNA mismatch repair
	MLH1	3p ⎭		
Familial breast cancer	BRCA1	17q	Breast ⎱	DNA repair
	BRCA2	13q	Breast (male and female) ⎰	Transcription?
Li–Fraumeni syndrome	p53	17p	Breast	Transcription
Neurofibromatosis	NF1	17q	Neurosarcoma	Signal transduction
Multiple endocrine neoplasia type 1	?	11q	Parathyroid, pancreas, anterior pituitary	?
Familial melanoma	INK4A	9p	Skin	Proliferation control
Xeroderma pigmentosum	>7	–	Skin	DNA excision repair
Ataxia telangiectasia	AT	11q	Leukaemia, lymphoma	DNA repair
Bloom's syndrome	Helicase		Leukaemia, lymphoma	DNA repair
Drug metabolism	CYP2D6		Lung	Drug metabolism

* Not all listed here; see Table 9.5.

Familial **a**denomatous **p**olyposis **c**oli (FAP) patients inherit a defective APC repressor gene that results in multiple benign polyps within which cancers develop. The APC gene codes for a protein that mediates intracellular signalling pathways from contacts with other cells (Chapter 11). A second familial type of colon cancer is **h**ereditary **n**on-**p**olyposis **c**olon **c**ancer (HNPCC, Lynch's syndrome), in which polyp formation is not observed. Three subgroups of HNPCC have been identified depending on whether they have germline mutations in the MSH2 gene, the MLH1 gene or neither. The majority of HNPCC cases have inherited mutations in the MSH2 gene with smaller numbers in the MLH1 and in other genes. The genes involved code for nuclear proteins directly required to repair mismatched bases in the DNA double helix (Chapter 8). Different genetic disorders such as Gardner's syndrome, Peutz–Jeghers syndrome and flat-cell adenoma syndromes of unknown cause also increase colon cancer risk.

Breast cancer

Two main variants and several minor variants have been shown to increase risk. The important ones, familial breast cancer and Li–Fraumeni syndrome, make up less than 5% of all breast cancers.

Familial breast cancer Familial breast cancer is characterised by early age of onset and greater than 80% probability of developing breast cancer. This compares with a 10% lifetime risk of developing sporadic breast cancer. Two genes, **br**east **ca**ncer **1** and **2** (BRCA1 and BRCA2), are the inherited culprits. Of the affected families, about half carry a BRCA1 mutation and half the BRCA2 defect. Inheritance of either gene also confers an increased risk of developing cancer at other sites which differ according to the gene concerned (Table 9.5). The function of both alleles is lost in cancers, indicating that BRCA1 and BRCA2 are both repressors.

Whereas the APC gene advertises its presence by the many polyps and associated symptoms, the familial breast cancer genes generate no such phenotypic traits. BRCA1 was identified by detailed screening of DNA samples from different breast cancer families to identify the minimal region common to each family. Figure 9.2 shows the pedigree of one such family in which both daughters and four out of five granddaughters developed breast cancer. Epidemiological evidence has shown a two- to threefold increased risk of developing breast cancer if a mother or sister has the disease and this can increase to tenfold if several first-degree relatives are affected. Note that BRCA1 is autosomal and can therefore be inherited from either mother or father, and note that one male descendant in the above example developed breast cancer.

The BRCA1 gene codes for a 220 kDa nuclear phosphoprotein involved in DNA repair, although mechanistic detail is sparse. Interaction of BRCA1 protein with other proteins is important, one candidate (Rad51) being required to repair double-strand breaks in DNA (Chapter 8). The BRCA1 protein also has a domain common to many transcription factors and is serine/threonine phosphorylated but its functional significance is unknown. Many different mutations have been detected in different families carrying BRCA1 mutations, the majority being deletions, insertions, nonsense mutations or splice variants which result in truncated proteins being synthesised. In experimental systems, complete deletion of the BRCA1 gene is lethal whereas incomplete loss resulting in the production of a protein truncated at the C-terminal end is not. The truncated protein can support some development, albeit of an abnormal type. This suggests that different regions of the protein serve different functions. Ashkenazi families have a high incidence of specific point mutations in either BRCA1 (adenine.guanine deletion at position 185) or BRCA2 (deletion of thymine at position 6174). The close associations within such communities ensured that the initial mutation remained common within that population.

BRCA1 is expressed in many normal cells such as testis, breast and ovary, and in cell culture the expression is increased in the G_1 phase of the cell cycle by proliferative stimuli such as serum growth factors and the female sex hormone oestradiol. This is important given the stimulatory role of oestradiol in the genesis of breast cancer (Chapter 4) but the hormonal effect is indirect as the BRCA1 gene does not have a response element for the oestradiol receptor. Furthermore, BRCA1 expression can be

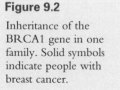

Figure 9.2

Inheritance of the BRCA1 gene in one family. Solid symbols indicate people with breast cancer.

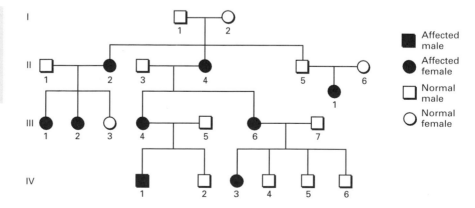

elevated by mitogens in oestradiol-insensitive cells. It is not clear why increased expression of the BRCA1 repressor protein results in increased rather than decreased proliferation. One explanation for this anomaly is that BRCA1 is not part of the DNA synthesis/mitosis pathway but regulates other processes such as DNA repair, associated with faithful replication of the DNA. Increased BRCA1 expression in normal cells would facilitate repair whereas loss would enhance damage accumulation. The decreased BRCA1 expression accompanying the transition from *in situ* to invasive breast carcinoma would fit with this hypothesis, as would the observation that BRCA2 mutations disrupt DNA repair but do not affect cell proliferation or apoptosis.

BRCA2 has been identified on a different chromosome to that of BRCA1. Loss of BRCA2 confers a modest increase in the risk of ovarian cancer plus an increased risk of breast cancer in men and women.

The BRCA2 gene sequence has low homology to that of BRCA1 but the proteins have functionally similar effects. They are coordinately regulated, they are expressed in many cell types and they are involved in DNA repair and transcription regulation; BRCA2 directly interacts with the DNA repair protein RAD51, whereas the latter's interaction with BRCA1 is indirect. Affected families have a diffuse pattern of mutations.

Li–Fraumeni syndrome   This disorder is due to germline mutations in the p53 gene that result in breast cancers and sarcomas but not other cancer types. The functions of p53 are fully described elsewhere (Chapters 6 and 10) but its universal involvement in normal pathways of proliferation and death raises the question of why its loss results in so few cancers. We do not know the answer to this question nor do we understand why an inherited Rb mutation quickly results in eye cancers whereas p53 mutations take much longer to develop. Familial eye cancers arise within 2 years of birth whereas Li–Fraumeni breast cancers take at least 20 years to appear.

The pattern of p53 mutations in Li–Fraumeni cells is different to the pattern in somatic cells (Figure 4.6).

DNA repair defects

DNA is subject to daily insults that require efficient repair mechanisms for their correction. Damaging agents include cosmic radiation, free radicals, ultraviolet light and a variety of chemicals (Chapter 7). There are familial conditions in which repair is defective and which are linked to increased cancer risk (Table 9.3). The HNPCC condition (see above) is in this category. Xeroderma pigmentosum is a complex condition caused by loss of a DNA-binding protein that identifies damaged regions of DNA prior to excision repair (Chapter 8). Affected people have a thousandfold greater risk of getting skin cancer when young, due to increased sensitivity to sunlight. Individuals with Bloom's syndrome and ataxia telangiectasia also have defective repair mechanisms, Bloom's patients because of DNA ligase deficiency and ataxia patients because of defective damage surveillance. The ataxia gene codes for a protein kinase involved in DNA repair (Chapter 8). The net result of these mutations is increased genomic instability and elevated error accumulation. Leukaemias and lymphomas most commonly arise in such patients but skin cancer can be a problem in individuals exposed to sunlight.

Drug metabolism

The cytochrome P450 (CYP) dependent hydroxylation of the drug debrisoquine by the CYP2D6 enzyme is genetically determined (autosomal recessive) and slow metabolisers may be at decreased risk of smoking-induced lung cancer, presumably due to slower activation of carcinogens in tobacco smoke (Chapter 7).

Connection with sporadic cancers

Mutations in the Rb gene are responsible for both familial and sporadic forms of retinoblastoma. The same is true for APC in colon cancer, but for other examples the picture is more complex (Table 9.4). The inherited HNPCC defects are only found in some sporadic colon cancers whereas mutations in the BRCA genes are not seen in sporadic cancers. These examples reinforce the point about there being multiple ways to generate one type of cancer. However, absence of mutations does not mean the gene plays no role in sporadic carcinogenesis; BRCA1 expression does decline in some cases (see above) so gene regulation rather than structure may be influential.

A different but related question is whether the genes identified from familial studies are relevant to sporadic cancers at sites other than the familial ones. In many cases the answer is yes but there are exceptions (Table 9.5).

Table 9.4   Inherited defects which also occur in sporadic cancers at same site.

Familial cancer	Gene	Altered in sporadic cancers
Retina	Rb	yes
Colon	APC	yes
	HNPCC	13% cases
Breast	BRCA1, BRCA2	no
Melanoma	INK4	yes

Table 9.5   Gene mutations identified in specific familial cancers that are changed in sporadic cancers at other sites.

Gene	Familial cancer*	Sporadic cancer
Rb	**Eye**, osteosarcoma	Many
APC	**Colon**, brain, thyroid	?
MSH2, MLH1	**Colon**, endometrium	Some
BRCA1	**Breast**, ovary, colon	None
BRCA2	**Breast (both sexes)**, prostate, ovary	None
INK4A	**Melanoma**	Many cancers
p53	**Breast**, sarcoma	Most cancers

* The major cancer associated with each defect is shown in bold type.

10 GROWTH: A BALANCE OF CELL PROLIFERATION, DEATH AND DIFFERENTIATION

Key points

- Growth can be altered by changing proliferation, apoptosis or differentiation.
- Different cancers use different options to achieve uncontrolled growth.
- Proliferation is regulated at several checkpoints in the cell cycle.
- The G_1 checkpoint is the focus of negative and positive extracellular signals.
- In normal cells, hypophosphorylated Rb blocks transit through the checkpoint. This inhibition is relieved by cyclin-dependent serine/threonine protein kinases (CDKs).
- CDKs are subject to stimulatory (cyclin) and inhibitory (CKI) controls mediated by protein–protein complexes. Protein phosphorylations modulate these interactions.
- The cell cycle is regulated at different stages by altered activities of specific CDKs, CKIs and cyclins.
- Alterations in cyclins and CKIs have been detected in cancers.
- There are two types of cell death. Apoptosis (programmed cell death) requires RNA and protein synthesis whereas necrosis does not.
- Apoptosis is activated by DNA damage, withdrawal of growth stimulatory cytokines or addition of death-promoting cytokines.
- Diverse apoptotic signals converge to alter mitochondrial function. Proapoptotic (BAX, Bad) and antiapoptic (Bcl2) proteins regulate the release of mitochondrial cytochrome C.
- Apoptosis can be regulated by altering the relative proportions of proapoptotic and antiapoptotic proteins.
- Cytochrome C activates proteases of the caspase family.
- Proliferation and apoptosis are integrated by mechanisms involving p53 and Rb.
- Leukaemias result from blocked differentiation.
- Methylation of cytosine bases in regulatory regions of DNA contributes to differentiation.

Introduction

Growth is a general term indicating alteration in size of a cell mass and is the end product of several interrelated influences, such as proliferation, differentiation, cell death, cell contacts and blood supply. This chapter will deal with three of those

Table 10.1 Doubling times of human tumour cells.

Cell type	Tumours	Doubling times (days)	
		In patient*	Cell lines
Colon	Primary	700	3
	Metastasis	100	
Breast	Primary	200	3
	Metastasis	20	
Lymphoma		5	1

* This is an average that covers a wide range of values.

influences: proliferation, death and differentiation. If the time taken for cultured cells to double their number is compared with the time required for a tumour to double its volume in a patient, there is a discrepancy – cultures double in days whereas months or years are required in patients (Table 10.1). Regulatory processes are present in solid cell masses that are absent in dispersed cells in culture. Cell culture conditions have been designed to maximise proliferation and minimise negative influences such as cell death. In patients, changes in cell number represent a balance between proliferation and death so alteration of either parameter can influence the size of a cellular mass. Additionally, if cells differentiate their proliferation potential decreases, so differentiation has a negative influence on growth kinetics. Thus, in a normal tissue, cell number remains constant because of a balance between proliferation, death and differentiation (Figure 10.1). In abnormal situations, increased cell number can result from either blocked death and/or differentiation or increased proliferation with no change in the other two properties. Each of these routes is used in carcinogenesis.

Cancer cells are often said to proliferate faster than their normal counterparts but this is far from true. Proliferation rates of well-differentiated tumours are not

Figure 10.1

Growth can be regulated by altering proliferation, death or differentiation.

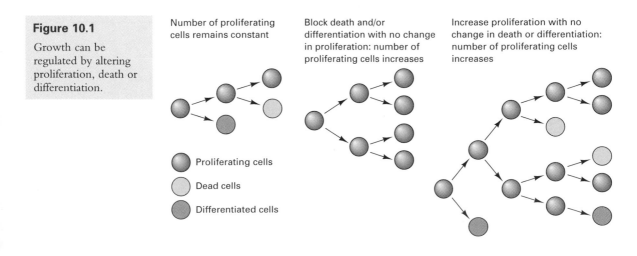

Number of proliferating cells remains constant

Block death and/or differentiation with no change in proliferation: number of proliferating cells increases

Increase proliferation with no change in death or differentiation: number of proliferating cells increases

Proliferating cells

Dead cells

Differentiated cells

dissimilar to those seen in progenitor normal cells. What is different is the lack of stop signals in the cancer that maintain normal tissue stasis. As tumour cells progress from differentiated to dedifferentiated, the situation changes and proliferation rates increase. This is seen in the much shorter doubling times of metastases compared with those of primary tumours (Table 10.1).

Two types of cell death exist, necrotic and apoptotic; necrotic cell death is passive whereas apoptotic cell death requires macromolecular synthesis. A third mechanism, whereby cancer cells are lost from a tumour mass, is migration of live cells into blood and lymphatic vessels during metastasis.

As cells multiply they accumulate errors in their DNA that result in senescence after about 40 doublings; if this was the only factor involved, all cells would eventually die. However, in some cases cell division is asymmetrical in that one daughter cell proceeds along the development and senescence pathway whilst the other retains the potential of unlimited proliferation and is called a stem cell. Thus, in the small intestine, epithelial stem cells are located in the base of the crypts; the number of proliferating cells decreases as they differentiate and move towards the mouth of the crypt. The molecular mechanisms behind this asymmetric division are unknown.

This chapter will consider each of the processes mentioned above on the assumption that a single cell type is involved and that factors such as the extracellular matrix (ECM) do not contribute to regulation. Although incorrect it is a necessary simplification. The influence of cell–cell and cell–ECM interactions on growth are dealt with in Chapters 11 and 12. Most of the biological and molecular features of growth control in mammalian cells have been elucidated with experimental systems involving cell culture and animal models. This data has been very informative but it sometimes requires caution when applied to cancers in patients. Cultured cell lines proliferate much faster than cancers in people (Table 10.1) – tumours doubling in size once per year may have additional mechanisms to those detected in cells doubling once per day.

Normal proliferation and its regulation

The cell cycle

For a cell to divide, the DNA must be replicated and distributed equally to the daughter cells. These processes of DNA synthesis and mitosis are separated by gaps, during which RNA and protein are made and the cell reorganises itself for the next round of division. This series of events is called the cell cycle and the first letters of each of these events are used for its description (Figure 10.2). The first gap (G_1) is sometimes divided to include a G_0 phase in order to distinguish quiescent cells from those preparing to enter the next phase of the cycle. Differentiation takes cells out of cycle and can be represented as an exit from G_1. Normal cells have a diploid DNA content; as DNA content doubles during the next phase of the cycle, exit beyond G_1 generates non-diploid cells. For example, exit in the second gap (G_2) between DNA synthesis and mitosis produces

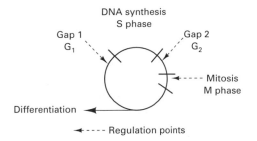

Figure 10.2

The cell cycle and its regulation. In rapidly dividing cells the various phases have the following durations: M lasts 1 h, G_1 lasts 8–30 h, S lasts 8 h, G_2 lasts 3 h, and the whole cycle lasts 20–50 h.

tetraploid cells. During the complex series of events leading to cancer formation, chromosomal (DNA) changes occur that generate DNA contents per cell that are simple multiples of those in diploid cells. Such cells are said to be polyploid. Frequently the altered DNA content is not a simple multiple and the cells are said to be aneuploid. Although doubling the amount of DNA is the major biochemical feature of normal cell proliferation, the other components that contribute to the mass of a single cell must also be coordinately replicated so that the two daughter cells are viable.

Careful regulation is needed for the complex series of events by which cells amplify their synthetic machinery (G_1) in preparation for the synthesis of DNA and other macromolecules (S) and then reorganise their interphase chromatin into chromosomes (G_2) prior to mitosis (M). Three main checkpoints have been identified in G_1, G_2 and M that must be traversed for accurate cell reproduction. For simplicity, each of these will be dealt with as though they were single entities, which is not the true situation. Thus, within the G_1 checkpoint, different controls exist for commitment to DNA synthesis and transition of the G_1/S boundary.

G_1 transition requires a critical level of regulatory macromolecules, some of which relieve the inhibitory effect of the Rb repressor protein. Growth stimuli such as hormones, growth factors and cell contacts act via this checkpoint. These stimuli increase the probability that cells cross this barrier, and as such is said to be a stochastic event. The G_1 checkpoint or regulation point ensures two functions: adequate machinery for future events and accurate transmission of genetic information. Adequate machinery involves relief of Rb inhibition by sequential and synchronised changes in gene activity resulting in protein synthesis. Phosphorylation of serine and threonine hydroxyl groups by protein kinases is a key feature of these regulatory events. Fidelity of genetic information transfer is maintained by three mechanisms for detecting and eliminating damaged DNA. Cells have a delay process mediated by the p53 repressor protein, which is activated when DNA damage is detected. On the other hand, cells with unrepairable DNA are killed. In fact, p53 and Rb act in concert to ensure transition through this stage of the cycle.

The G_2 checkpoint ensures the elimination of damaged cells that may have escaped G_1 control or which have not accurately duplicated their DNA. The spindle assembly checkpoint in the M phase monitors accurate chromosome alignment and retraction into the two daughter cells.

Each stage of the cell cycle will be separately described.

G_1: the first gap phase

G_1 is the most variable of the cycle phases, its length being the major determinant of cycle time. It is also the period in which future commitment to division, differentiation or death is made and is the focal point for important regulatory signals. It follows that if these signals are altered, the cell cycle is affected. Many changes in gene products have been identified in G_1 and it is convenient to classify these changes into early and late events. Late events include enzymes such as the DNA polymerases and those needed for nucleotide synthesis, e.g. dihydrofolate reductase, and whose levels increase at the G_1/S boundary. The stimuli for these changes come from earlier events, and typically there is a time interval of several hours between addition of a proliferation signal like serum to cultured cells and the onset of DNA synthesis. This delay reflects the time required for both signal transduction from the cell membrane to nucleus and the altered gene activity that results. Transcriptional changes in early genes like c-fos can be detected within minutes of adding serum, indicating that the signalling pathway from membrane to nucleus is fast and the overall lag in DNA synthesis is due to other events. Other examples of early gene activation common to most cell types include the oncogenes, c-myc and c-jun, which code for transcription factors that amplify regulatory signals (Chapter 11). Jun is a component of several signalling pathways, including the ras pathway (Figure 11.11) whereas the transcription factor formed by heterodimerisation of myc and max directly activates genes required for DNA synthesis (ornithine decarboxylase, carbamyl phosphate synthetase) or cyclin–dependent kinase activation (Cdc25, a tyrosine phosphatase). Additional cell-specific oncogene products like c-myb in haemopoietic cells can also be detected at this time. It should be noted that regulation is not confined to the transcriptional level as the half-life of c-fos mRNA can be extended and the activity of its protein product modulated by phosphorylation (see below).

Primary regulation of the G_1 checkpoint involves three protein families: (i) cyclins, (ii) **c**yclin–**d**ependent serine/threonine protein **k**inases (CDKs) and (iii) **c**yclin-dependent **k**inase **i**nhibitors (CKIs) (Figure 10.3). Their molecular features are detailed later as they are also important at the G_2 and M checkpoints.

Figure 10.3

The cyclin–dependent protein kinase system.

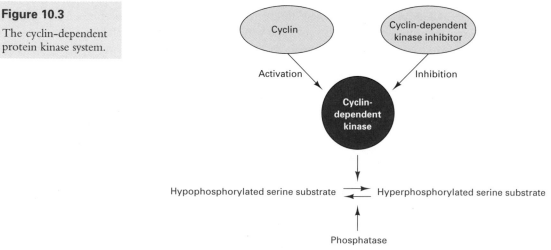

The kinases alter the biological functions of regulatory proteins; thus phosphorylation is one general way of regulating function, the other being the presence of activating (cyclin) and inhibitory (CKI) proteins that enable fine-tuning of this checkpoint. In fact, CKIs have all the properties of repressors.

One key substrate of the kinase is the protein product of the retinoblastoma gene Rb. This protein blocks cell proliferation at the G_1 checkpoint; this repression is released by protein phosphorylation and regained by dephosphorylation via protein phosphatases. The phosphorylation/dephosphorylation cycle therefore provides a rapidly reversible switch mechanism for altering proliferation rates (see later).

The second element of G_1 regulation involves DNA repair. DNA damaged by ultraviolet (UV) light or X-irradiation (Chapter 8) is detected by a mechanism involving the repressor protein p53, which blocks cycle progression until repair is completed. In normal cells, p53 levels are low but its transcription is increased by DNA damage.

Box 10.1   DNA synthesis and telomere length

DNA synthesis

Double-stranded DNA has a polarity; one strand is orientated in a $5'$ to $3'$ direction and the other strand in a $3'$ to $5'$ orientation (Box 6.1 gives details of DNA structure and base pairings to form the genetic code). DNA replication requires opening and unwinding of the helix to generate single-stranded regions of DNA (Figure 10.4). DNA polymerases join the deoxyribonucleotides to form the new chains; the base sequence of the chains is determined by the base sequence of the *parent* strand, also called the *template, coding* or *non-transcribed* strand. DNA polymerases only add nucleotides to hydroxyl groups at $3'$ ends, which is fine for the new *daughter* (*primer*) strand, being lengthened in a $5'$ to $3'$ direction; this is called the *leading* strand. The other daughter strand, the *lagging* strand, has the wrong orientation to be made in a $5'$ to $3'$ direction; it is synthesised as discontinuous, small (30–50 nucleotide) $5'$ to $3'$ segments called *Okazaki fragments*. The Okazaki fragments are then joined by ligases.

The protein complex involved in this series of events is the *replisome* situated at the *growing fork* of the DNA. The replisome contains enzymes and structural components. The enzymes include helicases that generate single-stranded DNA regions, DNA polymerases that synthesise the daughter strands, DNA ligases that join the Okazaki fragments into a continuous strand, and topoisomerases that release conformational constraints generated during passage of DNA strands through the replisome. At least five DNA polymerases (α, β, γ, δ, ε) are used in different circumstances (Chapter 6) but the δ and ε enzymes are primarily involved in chain elongation during DNA synthesis. DNA polymerases δ and ε possess $3'$ to $5'$ exonuclease activities that remove

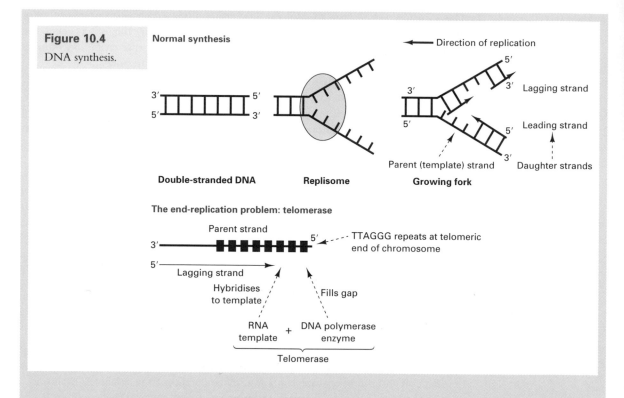

Figure 10.4
DNA synthesis.

Normal synthesis

← Direction of replication

Double-stranded DNA   Replisome   Growing fork

3′   5′
5′   3′

5′
3′ Lagging strand

5′ Leading strand

3′
5′

Parent (template) strand   Daughter strands

The end-replication problem: telomerase

Parent strand

3′
5′ ---- TTAGGG repeats at telomeric end of chromosome

5′ —————
Lagging strand

Hybridises to template   Fills gap

RNA template + DNA polymerase enzyme

Telomerase

incorrect, misaligned bases to minimise errors (mutations) of base insertion during synthesis; this is called the *proof-reading* function.

The structural components provide a scaffold to which other regulatory proteins can attach; one of these proteins is **p**roliferating **c**ell **n**uclear **a**ntigen (PCNA). As its name implies, it is only detected in the nucleus of proliferating cells. One of its scaffolding functions is to hold together replicated, double-stranded DNA, and as the protein is ring-shaped, the DNA passes through the central hole. PCNA has additional functions mediated through its binding of regulatory proteins such as p21 (a cyclin-dependent protein kinase inhibitor), GADD45 (regulation of proliferation), MSH2 and MLH1 (DNA excision repair), several cyclin/cyclin-dependent protein kinase complexes (cell cycle control) and DNA polymerases (DNA synthesis). The involvement of PCNA with these proteins makes it a key player not only in DNA synthesis but also in cell cycle control and DNA repair. It is unclear how these processes are coordinated by PCNA.

Telomeres and the end-replication problem

DNA polymerase initiates synthesis by hybridisiation of its RNA with the 3′ regions of the parent strand. This creates a problem at the final 3′ end of the lagging strand: when the RNA is released, a single-stranded stretch of parent strand nucleotides remains at the *telomeric* end of the chromosome (Box 8.1). It is known as the end-replication problem. Embryonic cells contain the enzyme *telomerase*, consisting of an RNA template and a DNA polymerase; telomerase completes the 3′ chain elongation so the length of the telomere remains constant (Figure 10.4). If telomerase is inactivated, as in normal adult cells, the single-stranded region is removed at each round of DNA synthesis and the telomere shortens; the consequences include chromosome instability, senescence and death.

S: the DNA synthesis phase

DNA synthesis is largely controlled at the level of its initiation and the build-up of enzymes, regulatory proteins and nucleotide triphosphates at the G_1/S boundary provides that control. During S, when the DNA strands are separated, bases are exposed and therefore sensitive to external agents such as drugs and mutagens so it is understandable that synthesis should be completed as fast as possible once it has started. Given the fundamental importance of DNA replication, defects in synthesis would be lethal, so it is not surprising that alterations have not been detected that lead to cancers. On the other hand, many cancer treatments are directed at disrupting DNA synthesis (Chapter 13). A related process, DNA repair, occurs in S and plays an important role in preventing the more widespread generation of cancers (Chapter 8).

G_2: the second gap phase

Several reorganisational and synthetic events occur in G_2. The double complement of DNA and chromatin proteins formed during S condense and are packaged into sister chromatids. DNA synthesis also leads to unwanted intertwining of chromosomes, which must be untangled by topoisomerases. Mitosis can be blocked by unreplicated DNA or by damaged DNA that has escaped repair, so these defects must also be rectified; p53 is involved in monitoring this checkpoint. All these processes are monitored at the G_2 checkpoint, probably in different ways, but the cyclin/CDK/CKI system is required.

M: mitosis

Sister chromatids must be aligned correctly so that they are retracted to opposite poles of the dividing cell; this is monitored at the spindle assembly checkpoint. Limited data indicate that regulation is achieved at the point of attachment of microtubules to the centromere. This occurs through a chromosome structure known as a kinetochore, which attaches to the microtubules. If any centromeres are not attached to microtubules, mitosis is delayed. Additional regulation occurs if inappropriate tension or abnormal dynamics of the microtubule are detected. Once again, CDKs are required for these events. If any of these events go wrong such that cells traverse S but not M, increases in ploidy occur.

The cyclin-dependent kinase system

ATP-dependent phosphorylation of serine/threonine residues in proteins such as Rb alter the function of the protein. Changes in activity of protein kinases can therefore regulate the cell cycle. The kinases involved in this control are called cyclin-dependent kinases because they are activated by cyclins. Another family of regulatory proteins, the cycle-dependent kinase inhibitors (CKIs) have the opposite effect. Interactions between these three classes of protein regulate the checkpoints of the cell cycle.

Each of the three components of the kinase system represents a family of molecules, the members of which are activated at different periods of the cell cycle (Figure 10.5). Cyclins E, A and B are highest in late G_1, G_2 and M respectively, and their presence contributes to checkpoint regulation during those periods. Cyclin D, on the other hand, rises early in G_1 and remains constant thereafter. Cyclins are increased through the transcriptional machinery and destroyed by ubiquitin-mediated proteolysis. CDKs are inactive on their own because their catalytic site, where ATP and substrate bind, is blocked by the C-terminal tail of the CDK; cyclin binding relieves that block. Phosphorylation of CDKs also has an important but poorly understood role in that a threonine phosphorylation activates enzyme activity and tyrosine phosphorylation inhibits enzyme activity. Each cyclin preferentially binds to specific CDKs, as illustrated in Figure 10.5. The presence or absence of specific cyclins and CDKs at different periods of the cell cycle determines which kinase is active during any one period.

An important protein substrate for CDKs is Rb which, in its hypophosphorylated state, binds to and inactivates the E2F transcription factor. Phosphorylation releases E2F, which is thus available to increase transcription from genes such as DNA polymerase α, and thymidine kinase (Figures 10.6 and 6.9). Rb phosphorylation also releases blocks on the synthesis of other RNA species required to increase the mass of a cell (Figure 6.10).

CDKs are activated by mitogenic growth factors. A complex series of changes involving multiple pathways (Chapter 11) forms a jun–fos transcription complex that binds to regulatory DNA sequences known as AP1 sites (Figure 10.7). Activation of genes containing an AP1 site results in increased cyclin and CDK function although details are sparse on how this is achieved.

Inhibitory signals involve the CKI family of proteins, with different signals using different methods to increase CKI activity. There are two main families of CKIs, both of which block the kinases involved in the G_1 checkpoint. The INK4

Figure 10.5

Changes in cycle-dependent kinases during the cell cycle.

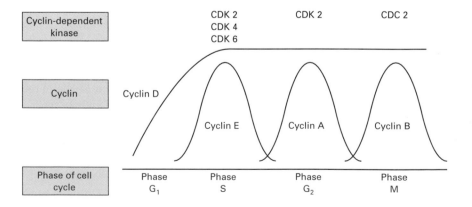

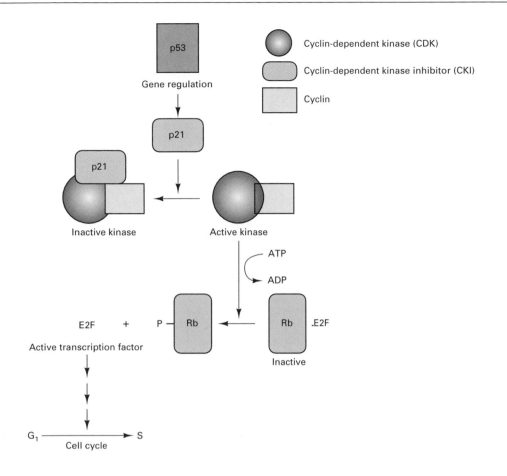

Figure 10.6

Inhibition of the cell cycle by p53 and Rb. Each of the 'boxed' proteins can be altered in cancers.

(**in**hibitor of cyclin-dependent **k**inase **4**) family (p15, p16, p18, p19) specifically bind to CDK4 and CDK6, thus preventing attachment of the cyclin. The other family (p21, p27, p57) have a wider specificity and bind to the cyclin–CDK complex rather than the CDK alone. Expression of the various CKIs is cell type specific. Thus, strong expression of p21 occurs in colon and prostate epithelium whereas p57 predominates in kidney and skeletal muscle. Figure 10.6 shows an important example of how a CKI functions when binding to a cyclin–CKD complex. The p53 protein blocks proliferation by switching on the synthesis of a 21 kDa CKI (p21, *not* the same as the ras p21 product). This binds and inactivates the cyclin D–CDK4 complex that phosphorylates Rb.

This figure also illustrates the key role that the Rb protein plays in regulating the G_1 checkpoint. Thus, p53 activation results in hypophosphorylation of Rb which binds and inactivates the E2F transcription factor; growth stimulatory genes are switched off (Chapter 6). Rb phosphorylation/dephosphorylation provides the chemical basis of the G_1 checkpoint. Phosphorylation is activated by growth factors (see above). An example of the INK family of CKIs is provided by p16 that specifically interacts with CDK4 and CDK6, thus preventing the CDK6 from interacting with cyclins. p16 is involved in a novel mechanism whereby the INK4

Figure 10.7

Growth factor stimulation of growth-related genes.

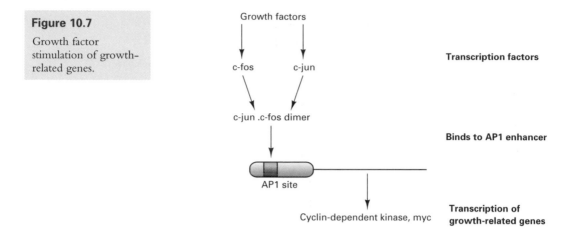

gene can code for two completely different proteins, p16^{INK4} and p19^{ARF} (Figure 10.8). The INK4 gene can be transcribed into mRNA at two different start sites; the larger transcript codes for a 19 kDa protein and the smaller transcript codes for a 16 kDa product. Some of the DNA base sequences coding for p19 are also used for p16, but because the sequences have separate start sites, the bases are read in different reading frames (Box 6.1) and the two products do not have the same amino acid sequence. This creates terminology problems. The proteins are named according to their size but are sometimes further categorised with superscripts. p16^{INK4} indicates that p16 is a product of the INK4 gene whereas p19^{ARF} indicates that p19 is produced from an **a**lternate **r**eading **f**rame (ARF) within the INK4 gene. The situation is further confused in that p19 is the size of the rodent product whereas in the human it is smaller (p14). The term ARF will be used here for both

Figure 10.8

INK4^{ARF}: one gene, two products that inhibit different functions.

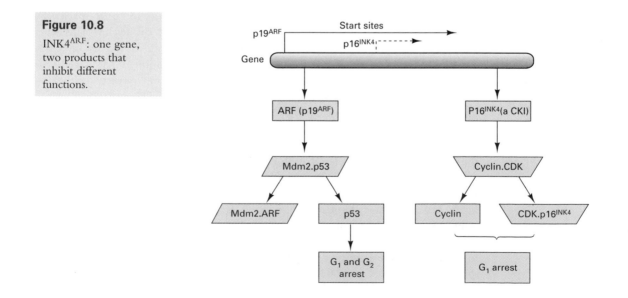

p14 and p19. Important features of the INK4 gene structure are that the two mRNAs are independently regulated and the protein products have different functions. p16 is a CKI that blocks Rb phosphorylation whereas ARF has a different function. It binds Mdm2 thereby releasing p53 bound to Mdm2; p53 is activated by this process (Figure 6.14). One gene transcript can thus generate products that enhance Rb inhibitory effects and augment p53 responses.

This is reminiscent of some of the carcinogenic DNA viruses that code for proteins influencing both pathways. Any agent that alters both Rb and p53 responses will have major effects so it is noteworthy that deletions in the INK4 gene have been detected in many cancers (see below). Further molecular details of Rb and p53 interactions are given in Figures 6.9 and 6.13 respectively.

Part of the growth inhibitory effect of the cytokine TGF-β (Chapter 11) may be mediated by stimulation of a member of the INK family of CKIs. Also cell–cell contacts (contact inhibition, Chapter 2) inhibit proliferation by a CKI-mediated process whereas differentiated cells with limited proliferative potential often have high levels of the p27 CKI.

Cancer cells

Proliferation

Cancer cells are characterised by their unregulated proliferation; this means they have a lower requirement for growth factors and they do not respond to negative environmental stimuli like contact with other cells. These changes, detailed in Chapter 11, mainly feed into the system via the G_1 checkpoint and many of the mechanistic variations used by different cancers occur in those pathways. Figure 10.9 shows examples of changes in CDK/cyclin/CKI/Rb that have been detected in human cancers and which illustrate the general point that different cancers use alternative pathways to achieve a similar end result, in this case increased Rb phosphorylation. Mechanistic details of these events are given in Figures 10.6 and 10.8. Cyclin and CKI changes are common whereas activating mutations in CDKs are rare (melanoma, sarcomas, gliomas). The CDK4 mutation in some melanomas destroys its p16^{INK4} CKI-binding property. The cyclin D gene is rearranged in

Figure 10.9

Cyclin, CDK and CKI: how their levels change in cancers.

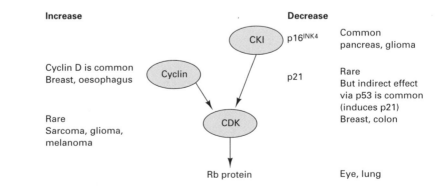

Increase

Cyclin D is common
Breast, oesophagus

Rare
Sarcoma, glioma,
melanoma

Decrease

p16^{INK4} — Common pancreas, glioma

p21 — Rare
But indirect effect
via p53 is common
(induces p21)
Breast, colon

Rb protein — Eye, lung

human parathyroid adenomas and amplified and overexpressed in a proportion of breast and oesophageal cell tumours, thereby providing a method of upregulating proliferation. Inactivating changes in the p16^{INK4} CKI are common, particularly in pancreatic cancers and gliomas. They are mainly deletions and mutations. Such changes could diminish inhibitory signals.

Alterations in cyclin and CKI genes are important for the genesis of certain cancers but the two genes most frequently altered in cancers are p53 and Rb, especially p53. Functional inactivation of the p53 and Rb genes can be achieved by mutation or deletion of the gene itself, or by binding of the normal product to other proteins. At a simplistic level, changes in p53 are more dangerous because alteration of only one allele will result in derepression due to the dominant-negative effect of heterodimerisation (Chapter 6).

Several features of the cell cycle, especially during the S and M phases, are exploited in the treatment of cancers (Chapter 13).

Senescence, cell mortality and telomerase

A major distinction between cancer cells and normal cells is that, prior to senescence, cancer cells undergo more cycles of proliferation than normal cells (Figure 2.7). Cancer cells are said to be immortal, although this is not strictly true as they do eventually die. This prolonged life provides more time to accumulate genetic errors with their attendant effects on cell function. Normal cells must therefore have a mechanism for limiting the life of a cell lineage that is lost in cancers. A major component of this process is the enzyme telomerase that fills the single-stranded gaps at the 3' ends of newly synthesised lagging strands of DNA (Figure 10.4, Box 10.1). In germ cells, fetal somatic cells and adult stem cells, enzyme activity is high with no problem in completing the full resynthesis of DNA. In adult somatic cells, telomerase declines (Figure 10.10) with the consequence that telomere length progressively shortens at each round of DNA synthesis. This results in chromosome instability which, at a telomere length of about 4 kb, disrupts cell function sufficiently to cause senescence.

Figure 10.10

Telomere length and cell function in culture.

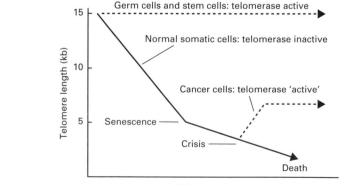

In this state the cells are alive but arrested in the G_1 phase of the cell cycle. There is not an absolute block to their transition into S phase (Figure 2.7) until the further telomere shortening results in apoptotic cell death. The term 'crisis' is sometimes used to define this stage; it originated when cultured cell lines (prolonged lifespan) were being produced from primary cultures (limited lifespan). The primary cultures eventually stopped proliferating (senescence) but foci (clones) of cells would spontaneously be reactivated and could be recultured as cell lines. These cell lines were said to have passed through 'crisis' and been immortalised. We now know that successful transition of the crisis period is associated with reactivation of telomerase. The link between this enzyme and chromosome instability is exemplified by the fact that primary cell cultures often become polyploid.

In cancer cells, telomerase is frequently reactivated by unknown mechanisms although not to the levels seen in germ cells. This extends their lifespan by preventing further loss of telomeric repeats but does not lengthen those repeats to the original levels. Hence a degree of chromosome instability remains. It is unclear as to what stage of carcinogenesis is linked to elevated telomerase. It is high in malignant colon but undetectable in polyps and adenomas at that site. On the other hand, about half of gastric adenomas and pre-invasive prostate cancers are telomerase-positive compared to all their invasive counterparts. The enzyme is also elevated in pre-invasive lung and neck cancers. If a telomerase-positive cell is hybridised with a normal cell that is telomerase-negative, the hybrid has a normal phenotype; normal cells have a mechanism for inhibiting telomerase. That mechanism remains obscure, although inactivation of a repressor process is involved. Important regulatory processes are usually controlled by multiple pathways, so it is not surprising that telomerase-independent mechanisms exist for maintaining telomere length. The exact nature of those mechanisms and their importance are still unknown.

It is not clear why single-stranded 3' ends of DNA should result in chromosome instability, although there is a causal link between the two processes. The link is vaguely described as being due to 'sticky ends' causing abnormal separation of DNA strands or chromosomes. The term 'sticky' refers to the single strand being able to inappropriately hybridise with single strands on other chromosomes. Cytogenetic abnormalities frequently accompany senescence and crisis. Senescence is associated with polyploidy whereas chromosome aberrations and aneuploidy characterise the crisis period.

The biochemical consequences of these major chromosomal changes are poorly defined. Senescent cells are arrested in the late G_1 stage of the cycle but there is no clear picture for the cause of that arrest. Growth factors (serum) can still elevate transcription of some growth-related genes such as myc and jun, but not fos, in senescent cells. Receptors for growth cytokines like epidermal growth factor and platelet-derived growth factor are normal but signal transduction therefrom may be impaired. Cyclin–CDK complexes actually accumulate at senescence but downstream phosphorylations do not occur.

Attempts are being made to develop inhibitors of telomerase for clinical use and it is possible that either telomerase or telomere length might become a predictive tool for determining how far a cancer has advanced or the future outcome (prognosis) for patients with cancer.

Ploidy changes and gene amplification

Advanced cancers often have an increased DNA content per nucleus. Unbalanced DNA synthesis and incorrect separation of chromosomes to daughter cells during mitosis are two contributing factors but amplification of specific DNA segments also occurs. The net result is a DNA content per cell that is not a simple multiple of 2 (diploid) or 4 (tetraploid). This is known as an aneuploid DNA content. Aneuploid tumours kill their host faster than diploid tumours, and amplification of growth factor receptors like those for epidermal growth factor (Chapter 11) or amplification of the multidrug resistance gene (Chapter 13) have been recorded in many tumours. These DNA changes occur because of errors in mitosis or because of unscheduled DNA synthesis.

Cell death

Cell death is a normal process that serves two functions: tissue remodelling and removal of damaged cells that might otherwise harm the rest of the body. DNA is constantly being damaged (Chapter 7) and although efficient repair mechanisms exist, they are not wholly effective. To prevent unwanted consequences, cells have a method for detecting such defects and committing suicide. In embryogenesis, extensive remodelling occurs in which some cells are removed and others expanded. Removal is achieved by cell death and the process continues into adult life. In skin the basal keratinocyte stem cells proliferate; as they move towards the surface, proliferation stops, differentiation (keratin production) occurs and the cells die leaving the keratin. Integration of proliferation and death is essential for normal homeostasis and they are tightly linked such that death occurs even in rapidly proliferating cells. Conversely, regressing tumours contain mitotic cells. It follows that if the equilibrium between proliferation and death is altered, abnormal growth occurs. In carcinogenesis, unregulated proliferation or decreased cell death will generate a tumour; the objective of cancer treatments, be they chemical or physical, is to achieve the converse.

There are two types of cell death, apoptosis and necrosis, with different morphological and molecular features (Table 10.2).

Apoptosis

Also called programmed cell death or cell suicide, apoptosis requires mRNA and protein synthesis. Apoptosis is a normal process involved in any situation requiring tissue remodelling. An extreme example is embryogenesis but adult tissues undergo the same process. Growth stimuli tend to be of variable strength, which leads to periods of low and high exposure. The consequences of this variability are best illustrated with cultured cells (Figure 10.11) in which addition of a growth factor stimulates proliferation. If that was all that happened, stimulus withdrawal would

Table 10.2 Features of apoptotic and necrotic cell death.

	Apoptosis	Necrosis
Causes	Programmed tissue remodelling, cell turnover, DNA damage, withdrawal of growth signals	Hypoxia, nutrient shortage, changes in pH and temperature
Morphology		
Affected cells	Single	Groups
Cell volume	Decreased	Increased
Chromatin	Dense	Fragmented
Lysosomes	Intact	Abnormal
Mitochondria	'Normal'	Abnormal
Inflammatory response	No	Yes
Cell fate	Apoptotic bodies	Lysis
Molecular changes		
Gene activity	Required	Not required
DNA cleavage	Specific	Random
Intracellular Ca^{2+}	Increased	No change
Ion pumps	Retained	Lost

Figure 10.11

How growth factor affects cell number.

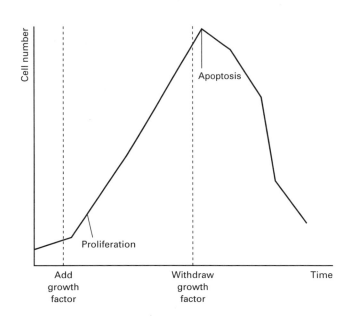

result in a cell number plateau whereas they actually fall; cell death by apoptosis is increased. An analogous phenomenon occurs *in vivo*, in that waves of proliferation are always followed by a pulse of apoptosis. Thus, cells must have the ability to coordinate proliferation and apoptosis in response to external stimuli. This occurs in both normal cells and cancer cells, but in many cancers the gene changes lead to decreased apoptotic death, which contributes to an increase in cell numbers. In tumours, apoptosis is still a major determinant of size, with individual cells being eliminated in about 3 hours; in regressing tumours, volume can decrease by about one-quarter in 1 day. However, apoptosis is not confined to regressing tumours and it is a balance between proliferation and death that determines whether a cancer gets bigger or smaller. Apoptosis is also important in determining response to treatments like chemotherapy and radiation (Chapter 13).

Cellular features of apoptosis

The main cellular features of apoptosis are given in Table 10.2. Under the microscope, the most striking features are the pattern of chromatin condensation and the appearance of membrane-bounded apoptotic vesicles representing cell remnants that are removed by phagocytosis. A major biochemical feature of apoptosis is the sequential activation of the caspases (see below), a family of proteases whose substrates include large protein precursors of enzymes capable of destroying DNA (endonucleases); lamin and actin (proteases); as well as proteins involved in DNA repair, RNA splicing, signal transduction and transcription factors. Endonuclease digestion at internucleosome bridges generates a ladder of DNA fragments that are multiples of 200 base-pair units characteristic of a nucleosome (Figure 10.12). The nucleases involved are sensitive to Ca^{2+} ions; an increase in Ca^{2+} is another characteristic of apoptosis.

Figure 10.12

Pathways promoting apoptosis.

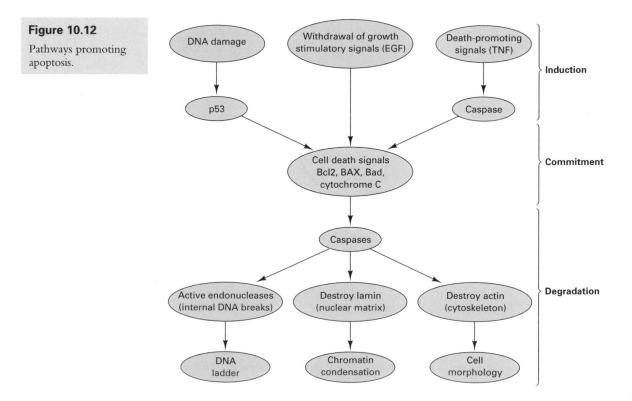

The Ca^{2+} released from mitochondria may be a consequence of their altered permeability (see below). Lamin, a component of the nuclear matrix, provides a structural framework for chromatin so its loss leads to chromatin condensation. Cytoplasmic collapse and decreased cell volume result from loss of cytoskeletal elements such as actin-containing microfilaments. The membrane-bounded apoptotic vesicles are unusual in that phosphatidylserine, normally occluded within the vesicles, becomes exposed on the surface and this marks them for elimination by phagocytosis.

A wide range of external events activate apoptosis, such as withdrawal of growth cytokines (TGF-α, IGF, PDGF), addition of apoptotic cytokines (TNF), ionising radiation (via free radicals), genotoxic chemicals (via DNA damage) and drugs used for chemotherapy (disruption of various cell functions).

Untransformed cells in culture require a substrate on which to grow (monolayer culture) plus growth factors. Anchorage is commonly prevented by putting cells into suspension culture (Chapter 2); they stop in G_1 and eventually undergo apoptosis. This may reflect the conflicting signals received by the cell. The positive signals from the serum conflict with the negative signals due to lack of substratum. In solid tumours, confusion can arise because unregulated proliferation is in conflict with a lack of synchrony between the multiple signalling pathways involved.

Apoptosis can be divided into three phases (Figure 10.12). The induction phase is initiated by diverse pathways described elsewhere – radiation and genotoxic agents (Chapter 7), cytokines and anchorage independence (Chapter 11), chemotherapy (Chapter 13) – although the pathways are outlined below (Figure 10.16). These pathways converge to a common series of molecular events required for cell death signals to be translated into morphological changes. After induction the cells enter a commitment phase, with no obvious morphological features, in which they are committed to apoptosis but from which they can be rescued. They then pass into the irreversible degradation and execution phase with the morphological changes described in Table 10.2.

A process as important as apoptosis has to be carefully regulated and integrated with other cell functions. How this is achieved requires an understanding of the molecular events involved, primarily related to two categories of protein: caspases, with proteolytic functions, and regulatory proteins of the Bcl2, BAX and Bad families capable of dimerising with themselves and with each other.

Molecular features

All the essential signals for apoptosis arise outside the nucleus, although the culminating event is nuclear destruction. The induction phase ends with the activation of a family of proteases called caspases, so-called because they all need a **c**ysteine at their catalytic site and their substrates are cleaved at **asp**artate residues (Figure 10.13). These caspases alter mitochondrial function to release cytochrome C into the cytoplasm, where it activates additional caspases and initiates the final degradation phase.

Caspases These proteases are synthesised as large, inactive precursors (procaspases) from which the active enzyme is released by cleavage at aspartate residues. This

Figure 10.13

Caspase activation.

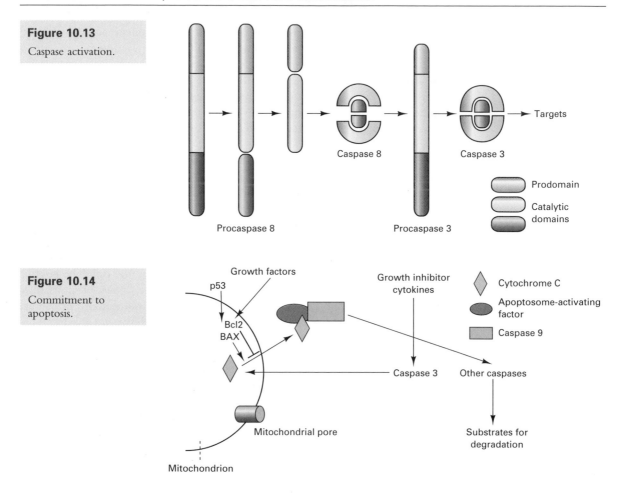

Procaspase 8

Caspase 8

Procaspase 3

Caspase 3

Targets

Prodomain

Catalytic
domains

Figure 10.14

Commitment to
apoptosis.

Growth factors

p53

Bcl2

BAX

Mitochondrial pore

Mitochondrion

Growth inhibitor
cytokines

Caspase 3

Other caspases

Substrates for
degradation

Cytochrome C

Apoptosome-activating
factor

Caspase 9

means that the activating proteases are themselves caspases, so a cascade of proteolytic events occurs with the sequential appearance of different caspase activities. An example is given in Figure 10.13. Two successive autocatalytic cleavages release the prodomain polypeptide plus two proteins that aggregate to form the active caspase 8. This catalyses a similar set of events on procaspase 3 which can either alter mitochondrial function (Figure 10.14) or activate other caspases. The mitochondrial changes (see below) release cytochrome C that activates procaspase 9 by binding to **ap**optosis-**a**ctivating **f**actor (Apaf). This complex of procaspase 9, Apaf and cytochrome C is called an apoptosome. Caspase 9 activates downstream caspases responsible for the degradation phase; caspase 1 digests actin, caspase 6 digests nuclear lamin and caspase 3 cleaves and activates a protein which then activates DNAase.

Mitochondrial events: Bcl2, BAX and cytochrome C   These proteins form the core of the commitment phase of apoptosis. The mitochondrial membranes enclose proteins that either activate apoptosis (proapoptotic proteins, BAX) or inhibit apoptosis (antiapoptotic proteins, Bcl2). These proteins are important, along with cytochrome C and the formation of mitochondrial pores, but certain aspects are unclear. The increased mitochondrial permeability is associated with cytochrome C release into the cytoplasm but it is poorly understood how upstream signals generate that release. Cytokines like tumour necrosis factor signal via caspase 3 but it is not clear how caspase 3 releases cytochrome C. Likewise p53 and growth factor withdrawal alter the balance of Bcl2 and BAX such that BAX stimulates cytochrome C release, but details of that link are unknown. The same ignorance applies to the inhibitory effect of Bcl2 on cytochrome C release (Figure 10.14). Bcl2 was first identified in a **B c**ell **l**ymphoma as a chromosome translocation that moved the Bcl2 gene from chromosome 18 to 14, (t14;18), adjacent to a strong immunoglobulin promotor, analogous to events in Burkitt's lymphoma with c-myc (Figure 6.5). The Bcl2 gene codes for a 26 kDa protein found mainly in the outer mitochondrial membrane, although the protein is coded by a nuclear and not a mitochondrial gene. It can also be detected in nuclear envelope membranes and endoplasmic reticulum. Constitutive overexpression of Bcl2 blocks apoptosis and thus protects cells against ionising radiations, ultraviolet light, viral infection and chemotherapeutic agents. A consequence of this effect is that cancers with elevated Bcl2 are resistant to drugs used for treating cancers (Chapter 13). Skin melanocytes, whose function is to make melanin as a protection against UV damage, express high levels of Bcl2 protein so they are resistant to the killing effect of the UV light. Mice in which both alleles have been destroyed would be expected to die *in utero* because of excess apoptosis. Somewhat surprisingly, this does not happen but they do die within a few weeks of birth with extensive destruction of lymphoid cells and kidney disease.

Like so many growth regulators, Bcl2 is just one member of a family which includes proteins that either block or induce apoptosis. Members of the anti-apoptosis group include Bcl2 and Bcl$_x$ and BAX, Bad, Bak and Bik form the proapoptosis members. Whether apoptosis is induced or blocked depends on the relative ratios of family members and reflects the dimerisation state of those members (Figure 10.15). Homodimers of Bcl2 block apoptosis whereas BAX homodimers elicit the opposite effect; Bcl2.BAX heterodimers are inactive. The relative proportions of the two proteins in the cell determine the nature of the

Figure 10.15

Response is determined by the dimerisation state of Bcl2 and BAX. Relative concentrations of Bcl2 and BAX determine the dimerisation state. The proapoptotic protein Bad (not shown) influences this equilibrium by forming heterodimers with Bcl2.

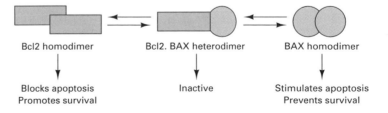

Bcl2 homodimer	Bcl2. BAX heterodimer	BAX homodimer
Blocks apoptosis Promotes survival	Inactive	Stimulates apoptosis Prevents survival

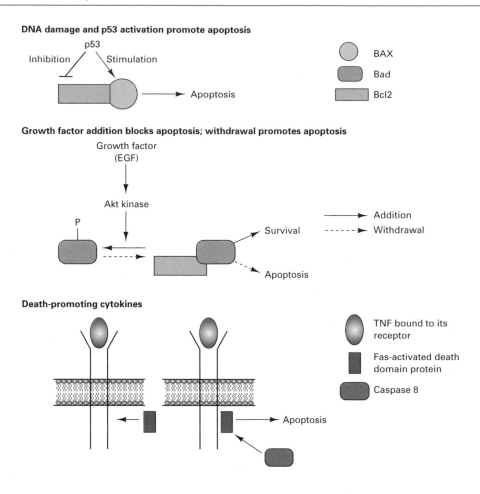

DNA damage and p53 activation promote apoptosis

Growth factor addition blocks apoptosis; withdrawal promotes apoptosis

Death-promoting cytokines

Figure 10.16

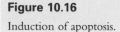

Induction of apoptosis.

response; high Bcl2 blocks apoptosis and favours cell survival whereas high BAX levels have the opposite effect.

Proapoptotic Bad forms heterodimers with antiapoptotic Bcl2, decreasing the concentration of active Bcl2 (see below). This stimulates apoptosis by altering the equilibrium in favour of BAX dimers. This has important consequences for the regulation of apoptosis because alterations in relative levels of the two proteins can determine whether or not apoptosis occurs. It is known that apoptosis is more easily activated in some cells than in others. Thus, cortical lymphocytes are very sensitive to apoptotic signals whereas medullary lymphocytes are not. The different sensitivities could be explained by a chemostat mechanism in which different cell types have different settings at which apoptosis is switched on or off. The relative levels of Bcl2 and BAX could provide the molecular basis for such a chemostat.

p53 activates transcription from the BAX gene and inhibits transcription from the Bcl2 gene (Figures 6.13 and 10.16); the net result is that the equilibrium alters in favour of the proapoptotic BAX complex. Cell death triggered by withdrawal of growth stimulatory factors is mediated by a third member of the family, Bad (Figure 10.16). In proliferating cells, phosphorylated (serine) Bad is bound to a cytoplasmic protein, enigmatically named 14-3-3, that removes Bad from the apoptosis picture. Growth-promoting factors indirectly promote Bad phosphorylation via a pathway involving phosphoinositols and protein kinase B (Akt, Figure 11.14). Growth factor withdrawal results in Bad dephosphorylation, dissociation from 14-3-3, heterodimerisation with Bcl2 and blockade of the Bcl2's inhibitory effect on cell death. The end result of growth factor removal is Bcl2 inactivation and apoptosis. Growth factor addition reverses these changes and cell survival is enhanced.

Necrosis

Necrosis is commonly seen in central regions of solid tumours; the trigger is poor nutrient supply leading to disruption of energy-dependent, membrane-mediated ion channels. The resultant increase in cell volume and loss of membrane integrity cause the release of lysomal lytic enzymes such as proteases and nucleases; cell lysis is accompanied by an inflammatory response associated with the cell damage (Table 10.2). Supply of nutrients is via the blood supply, and tumours growing around blood vessels exhibit a progressive decrease in proliferation the further they are from the vessel; at $200\,\mu$m the cells are static and necrosis sets in. Thus, necrosis is also linked with proliferation albeit for very different reasons than apply to apoptosis. This link between blood supply and tumour growth is also seen in very early stages of cancer growth (Chapter 2) and during metastasis (Chapter 12).

Apoptosis and cancer

Apoptosis is important at several stages of carcinogenesis, some of which have already been described. Transgenic mice that overexpress Bcl2 develop normally but exhibit hyperproliferation of haemopoietic cells and eventually succumb to lymphomas due to the absence of apoptosis. This example of malfunctioning apoptosis in the early stages of carcinogenesis is complemented by the p53 data indicating that genetic defects predispose towards high cancer risk (Chapter 9). Loss of the p53 brake on the cell cycle to allow apoptotic removal of abnormal cells results in cancer.

Apoptotic defects are also influential in established cancer. In both solid (e.g. prostate) and non-solid (e.g. leukaemia) tumours, Bcl2 overexpression indicates a poor prognosis, presumably because of proliferation in the absence of death. It is also involved in treatment responses; an approximate but far from universal observation is that tumours with high Bcl2 expression are resistant to chemotherapy (Chapter 13). An ironic example of generalities about cancer being wrong is that the original cancer in which Bcl2 overexpression was detected (follicular B-cell lymphoma) is in fact chemosensitive!

Integration of proliferation, apoptosis and DNA repair

In normal adult tissues proliferation, apoptosis and DNA repair are in equilibrium and maintain a steady-state level of healthy cells. But the DNA in these tissues is constantly being damaged (Chapter 7); it can either be repaired or, if damage is extensive, cells enter the apoptotic death pathway (Figure 10.17). For repair to occur, proliferation is stopped to ensure the damage is not transmitted to daughter cells. If repair is successful, additional cells are not required whereas cell death warrants further proliferation to maintain a steady-state mass of cells. Molecular mechanisms exist to ensure that the equilibrium is not altered. If the number of cells in a mass is increased by altering control of proliferation, death or both, then hyperplasias or benign lumps will result but not a malignant cancer capable of invasion and metastasis (Chapter 3).

For carcinogenesis to proceed, the link between DNA repair and blocked proliferation must be broken so that errors in the DNA base sequence are passed on to daughter cells. If such an error blocks DNA repair, increases proliferation or inhibits apoptosis, further errors will be propagated. An autocatalytic loop will have been created which could be the engine (Chapter 6) that generates the additional changes associated with the malignant phenotype. Different cancers use different options to achieve error propagation and frequently one cancer will acquire changes in each of the three properties at different stages of carcinogenesis. Thus, the primary driving force for retinoblastoma formation is increased proliferation (Figure 6.9 and Chapter 9); in hereditary non-polyposis colon cancer it is defective repair (Chapter 8); and one form of B-cell lymphoma results from decreased apoptosis (see above). In sporadic colon cancer, altered proliferation, DNA repair and apoptosis are acquired sequentially (Chapter 2).

The p53 repressor protein is a key factor in integrating responses from the DNA synthesis, repair and apoptosis pathways (Figure 10.18), which accounts for the observation that defective p53 exists in so many cancers. Normal p53, acting as a transcription factor for several genes, inhibits proliferation by inducing p21, a cyclin-dependent kinase inhibitor; it stimulates DNA repair by a poorly understood route and it promotes apoptotic death by increasing BAX and decreasing Bcl2 levels (Figure 6.13). Provided these pathways are intact, DNA damage elicits the coordinated changes just described, allowing the formation of normal daughter cells at mitosis. Defective p53 disrupts all three downstream pathways and its deleterious

Figure 10.17

The link between DNA damage, repair, proliferation and apoptosis.

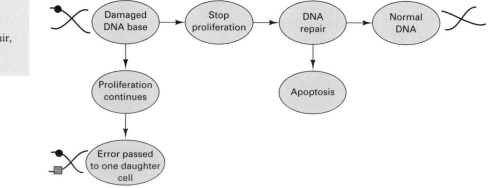

Figure 10.18

Coordination of DNA synthesis, repair and apoptosis.

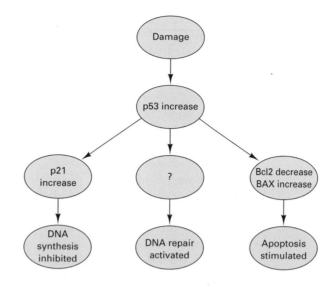

effects are being enhanced by the fact it is a dominant-negative gene, so only one allele needs to be damaged to generate a functional effect (Chapter 6).

Alterations to the DNA repair pathways can explain the carcinogenicity of genotoxic agents such as tobacco smoke and ionising radiation, but more problematic are non-genotoxic agents like the sex hormones associated with increased risk of common cancers such as breast and prostate. Oestrogens (breast) and androgens (prostate) are potent mitogens (Chapter 12) and may disrupt the repair/proliferation/death equilibrium by this route. But proliferation alone will not generate malignant cells; additional changes are required. It is significant that inheritance of the BRCA genes greatly increases the risk of developing breast cancer as compared to the normal population and these genes may be involved in DNA repair (Chapter 6). The additional changes needed for the formation of sporadic breast cancers are of unknown origin.

These views on how disruption of these pathways contributes to carcinogenesis are backed by a solid body of experimental evidence but they do not rule out the involvement of other processes. Several experiments involving genetic alterations in key genes in the above pathways indicate that we do not have all the answers. If defective p53 is so carcinogenic for all cells, why is it that patients with inherited p53 defects in all their cells (Li–Fraumeni syndrome) only get cancers in a few cell types such as breast and fibroblasts (sarcomas)?

The same question arises from studies with mice that have had both p53 alleles deleted. As anticipated, such mice are prone to tumour formation but certain types predominate, lymphomas in one strain and sarcomas in another. Additional unknown controls clearly exist to prevent cancers appearing everywhere. Another anomaly has been identified in Rb-regulated pathways. This protein exerts its antiproliferative effects by inhibiting the E2F transcription factor (Chapter 6), so genetic elimination of E2F expression would be expected to result in hypoproliferation and malfunctions of embryogenesis. In fact, embryogenesis is completed and some cell types are actually hyperplastic. Once again, answers that are too simplistic usually prove to be wrong when generalised to cancers.

Differentiation

The inverse relationship between differentiation and proliferation is valid if one compares the two features at the beginning and end of a developmental sequence, although they can occur simultaneously at intermediate stages. Thus, in the haemopoietic system the pluripotent stem cell commits itself to certain cell lineages at an early stage but those cells must be amplified (Figure 10.19). A similar process occurs in solid tissues such as mammary gland, which during pregnancy undergoes both differentiation in readiness for milk production and proliferation to generate the requisite number of specialist cells. As illustrated below with leukaemias, this temporary synergy of increased proliferation plus differentiation can be achieved by the production of growth factors. Cells at one stage of differentiation are sensitive to one growth factor whilst cells at another stage are stimulated by a different growth factor. These comments are relevant to the early stages of carcinogenesis whereas in later stages, where established tumours progress to dedifferentiated or anaplastic states, there exists the simpler relationship of faster growth, poorer differentiation.

Older models of carcinogenesis referred to reverse differentiation but this is inappropriate as differentiation is an irreversible process. The dedifferentiation seen in many tumours reflects loss of functions by mechanisms different to those involved in their acquisition.

Leukaemias result from blocked differentiation (see below) and the same may be partially true for some of the solid tumours. Thus, a full-term pregnancy in young women (<30 years) protects against later development of breast cancer, which is compatible with differentiation (pregnancy) hindering carcinogenesis. Cows, despite the large number of potential target cells, do not get breast cancer because of continuous maintenance of the udder in a differentiated, milk-producing state. Another notable example of the inverse link between carcinogenesis and differentiation comes from the loss of tumour properties when a cancer cell is hybridised with a normal cell. The differentiation properties of the normal cell are

Figure 10.19

Cytokines and myeloid cell differentiation. Changed differentiation status is represented by altered tinting of the cell symbols.

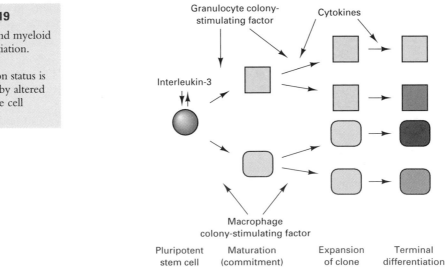

retained by the hybrid until, with chromosome loss, return of tumorigenicity is accompanied by loss of differentiation (Figure 2.6).

Leukaemia as a model for blocked differentiation

Cancers of the haemopoietic system occur in many forms and their generation can be explained as blocked maturation at variable stages of differentiation. Each step in the normal differentiation represents a balance between self-renewal and maturation. Leukaemias result from increased self-renewal at the expense of maturation. In normal haemopoiesis, a family of glycoprotein growth factors has been identified that integrate the proliferation and differentiation signals (Figure 10.19). These growth factors are collectively known as cytokines, individual members having names that describe their functions, e.g. **c**olony-**s**timulating **f**actors (CSFs) and interleukins. These proteins alter cell kinetics by reacting with specific cell membrane receptors. In the case of myeloid cell differentiation, the pluripotent stem cell proliferates under the autocrine influence of interleukin 3 (IL-3), also known as multi-CSF because of its broad cell specificity. More specific CSFs are switched on that initiate both differentiation and proliferation: granulocyte CSF promotes granulocyte development whereas macrophage CSF induces a macrophage lineage. The crucial events in the genesis of leukaemia occur at this maturation stage; the exact point at which the abnormality occurs determines the resultant type of leukaemia (Figure A.4).

Autocrine production of cytokines is an important feature of self-renewal, but it does not entirely explain carcinogenesis. For unknown reasons, chromosome translocations are a common cause of leukaemias, although none of the translocations involve cytokine genes and overexpression of cytokines generates hyperplasias not cancers. Cytokines act via cell surface receptors (Chapter 11), at least one of which, c-fms, the proto-oncogene receptor for macrophage CSF, is altered in some animal leukaemias.

Normal differentiation can be regulated by low molecular weight signalling molecules such as retinoic acid. This pathway can be altered in some cancers; an example is acute promyelocytic leukaemia (Figures 6.7 and 11.20), in which the retinoic acid receptor α gene is disrupted such that it does not function at normal ligand concentrations. Differentiation is arrested at the stage where the myeloid cells continue to proliferate. Another case of altered differentiation due to uncoupled signal transduction is chronic myeloid leukaemia (Figure 2.10). Chromosome translocation results in a constitutively active mitogenic signal from the c-abl tyrosine kinase oncogene (Figure 11.8) that stimulates proliferation at the expense of further differentiation.

It is not known how the signals described here contribute to differentiation. Both the cytokines and retinoic acids influence the activity of proteins that regulate gene transcription (Chapter 11) so part of the answer must lie in this area of biology. Many transcription factors have been identified at various stages of myeloid differentiation. Current evidence suggests that multiple selective interactions between these factors determine which genes are activated or repressed

Figure 10.20

Transcription factor rearrangements during differentiation. Each shape is a different transcription factor.

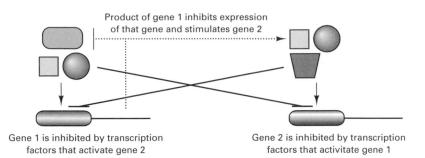

Gene 1 is inhibited by transcription factors that activate gene 2

Gene 2 is inhibited by transcription factors that activitate gene 1

(Figure 10.20). At an early stage of myeloid differentiation, the model proposes that transcription factors A, B and C are present and form a complex that activates gene 1 and represses gene 2. A consequence of gene 1 activation is that C is switched off and D is switched on. The new complex can activate gene 2 and repress gene 1. This chain reaction would continue until the fully differentiated state was reached; interference with specific transcription would block differentiation at the stage requiring that factor. This model accounts for many features associated with differentiation but identifies neither the genes nor the transcription factors involved; the retinoic acid receptor α (see above) is one of many candidates.

DNA methylation and differentiation

Differentiation involves the coordinated switching on and off of genes specific to the cell type concerned. These changes in gene activity require altered regulation of transcription involving DNA–protein interactions. As commitment to differentiation also necessitates proliferation, those transcriptional alterations must be passed on to the daughter cells. DNA methylation is involved in the process.

Cytosine–guanine (CpG) dinucleotide sequences in DNA can be enzymically methylated at the 5-position of cytosine. Transcription factors will not bind to such methylated sites and transcription of the gene is therefore diminished. Such methylations on one strand of DNA are passed on to the daughter strand because DNA methylases preferentially act on hemimethylated DNA (one strand). This method of inheritance is called epigenetic, although it is functionally equivalent to an inactivating mutation. DNA can be demethylated by drugs such as 5-azacytidine, which is incorporated during DNA synthesis, blocks methylase activity and induces differentiation in some cells. Cytosine methylation is inherently mutagenic as thymine, the product of 5-methylcytosine deamination, is repaired less readily than deaminated cytosine (uracil; see Chapter 8).

Although DNA methylation provides a mechanism to account for the three requirements of differentiation, altered transcription and inheritance, it is not certain whether its importance is as a causal event or whether it has a secondary role in maintaining the changed phenotype.

If hypermethylation is linked with differentiation, hypomethylation should be associated with the dedifferentiation occurring during carcinogenesis and progression. The promoter region of the MAGE tumour antigen gene (Chapter 5) is hypomethylated and there is a sixfold decrease in methylation of the α globin gene in colon cancer as compared to adjacent, normal colon. Hypomethylation has also been noted in metastases as compared to primary tumours, suggestive of increased activity of certain genes. Mice in which both cytosine methyl transferase (CMT) alleles have been lost die during fetal life, so DNA methylation is required for tissue remodelling and differentiation of individual cell types during that period. Other mice strains have been bred with diminished CMT activity and they have proved useful in determining biological factors influenced by CMT, particularly in relation to colon carcinogenesis. The Min mouse has a germline, inactivating mutation in the equivalent of the human APC gene that is inactivated in human colon carcinogenesis. Min mice mimic humans in that they spontaneously develop multiple intestinal cancers. When Min mice are cross-bred with CMT-deficient animals, the offspring get no intestinal cancers; decreased cytosine methylation switches off carcinogenesis.

11 RESPONDING TO THE ENVIRONMENT: GROWTH REGULATION AND SIGNAL TRANSDUCTION

Key points

- Extracellular influences alter cell function via receptor binding and signal transduction to the cell nucleus. The efficiency of this machinery is altered in cancer cells.
- Extracellular signals can be stimulatory (growth factors, hormones) or inhibitory (other cells, extracellular matrix, growth factors, hormones).
- Cancers escape from control by their environment through having (i) decreased sensitivity to inhibitory signals from adjacent cells and the extracellular matrix and (ii) decreased requirement for growth stimulatory factors.
- Endocrine, autocrine and paracrine stimuli are important.
- Polypeptide growth factors have local, autocrine and paracrine effects on multiple cell types.
- Hormones and related, low molecular weight, hydrophobic molecules have endocrine and autocrine actions.
- Cancers can either produce more ligand or become independent of the ligand.
- Signalling pathways use multifunctional proteins at several points to regulate diverse (pleiotropic) functions.
- Cancer cells often alter the functions of these pleiotropic molecules in order to gain a growth advantage.
- Transmembrane receptors alter their conformation in response to extracellular ligands and relay signals to within the cell.
- Membrane receptors can be qualitatively or quantitatively altered in cancer cells.
- Membrane receptors use enzymic (tyrosine kinase, serine/threonine kinase, adenyl cyclase) and non-enzymic methods to transduce signals.
- Protein phosphorylation is widely used to alter protein function.
- Membrane receptors whose intrinsic tyrosine kinase activity is activated by ligands are especially important for growth control.
- Proteins with tyrosine phosphates bind to other proteins with SH domains. This mechanism is used to pass information between proteins.
- Protein phosphatases reverse the effects of protein phosphorylation.
- A cascade of serine/threonine phosphorylations, involving several cellular oncogenes, carries signals to the cell nucleus.
- There is extensive crosstalk between signalling pathways.

- Alterations in ras oncogene activity, either by mutation of ras or a protein that regulates its function, are common in cancer cells.
- Extracellular, low molecular weight, lipophilic molecules bind and activate intracellular receptors that are gene transcription factors.
- These receptors can be altered in cancer cells.
- Signals from cell–cell and cell–ECM interactions are transduced by four classes of cell adhesion molecules: integrins, cadherins, selectins and members of the immunoglobulin superfamily. The transmembrane receptors relay signals to the cytoskeleton and the cell nucleus.
- Cell recognition receptors are altered in cancers.
- Activation of genes coding for growth-regulatory proteins results from all these signalling events. Activation is achieved by altering the phosphorylation status or amount of transcription factor.

General features

Cancer cells attain a degree of autonomy from external regulatory signals that renders them less subject to such signals than normal cells. This autonomy is reflected in a lower requirement for growth-stimulatory molecules such as growth factors and a diminished sensitivity to inhibitory signals provided by adjacent cells and the extracellular matrix (ECM). These stimulatory and inhibitory extracellular stimuli are recognised by receptors and conveyed to the nucleus by complex, multiple pathways with communication (crosstalk) between individual pathways (Figure 11.1). The altered transcriptional activity is directed at obtaining a growth advantage over adjacent cells and is achieved by increasing the efficiency of the intracellular machinery directed at proliferation and by production of secreted growth factors. Additionally, proteases are produced that facilitate invasion (Chapter 12). The growth factors can modulate functions of the producing cells and functions in the immediate vicinity. This chapter will mainly discuss extranuclear events, nuclear changes having been dealt with in Chapters 6 and 10.

Figure 11.1

The cancer cell and its environment.

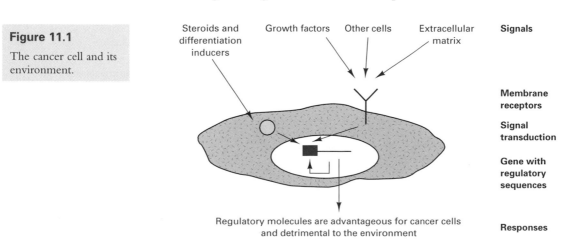

Steroids and differentiation inducers — Growth factors — Other cells — Extracellular matrix — Signals

Membrane receptors

Signal transduction

Gene with regulatory sequences

Regulatory molecules are advantageous for cancer cells and detrimental to the environment — Responses

Versatility of response pathways

In normal cells there is a need for versatility and specificity of responses such that different cell types can perform their own specialist functions while utilising common signalling pathways. This is achieved by having key intermediary regulators, usually proteins, common to all cells (Figure 11.2). These *pleiotropic* (multiple function) proteins receive upstream signals by reaction with one set of proteins and relay the signal by influencing the function of another set of downstream effectors. Specificity is provided by the presence or absence of different upstream and downstream molecules in different cells. This cascade of response pathways between upstream regulators and downstream effectors generates the versatility and specificity required.

Pleiotropic regulation is used at a number of points in the signalling pathway. The ras oncogene is one such key intermediate, receiving input signals from extracellular molecules via their receptors and transmitting signals to a variety of pathways, determined by the differentiation status of the particular cell type. Another example is the membrane receptor for epidermal growth factor (EGF). The gene ErbB1, also known as an oncogene, codes for a protein that binds either EGF or transforming growth factor α (TGF-α) as its upstream regulator, whilst downstream effectors determine responses via the cytoplasmic tail of the receptor. As some of these effectors are upstream regulators of the ras pathway with its multiplicity of effectors, the potential complexity of responses from a limited number of extracellular signals becomes apparent. In this way, one growth factor can elicit multiple effects in one cell type and different responses in different cell types.

The versatility of response pathways exhibits itself in another way – extensive crosstalk between signalling pathways. In simplistic terms, this means there are many routes by which a single extracellular signal can elicit a given response and whereby different signals synergise to generate a response. Anchorage-dependent growth of normal cells (Chapter 2) illustrates the latter point, because growth factors will only function if adhesion receptors are also operational; this synergy is lost in many cancer cells.

Figure 11.2

How one protein can regulate different functions (pleiotropic effect).

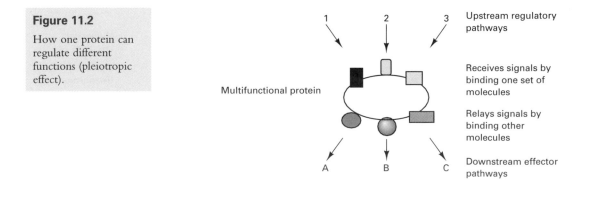

Oncogenes and protein phosphorylation

The complexity of the signalling pathways makes it difficult to generalise about changes involved in carcinogenesis but two principles can be identified: (i) the key regulatory proteins are coded for by oncogenes rather than repressors; and (ii) protein phosphorylation is a common method whereby function is altered without requiring *de novo* protein synthesis. Different cancer types use different ways to become autonomous so that no single change in a gene or signalling pathway predominates. Of the oncogenes involved in signal transduction, ras is the one most frequently altered in cancers but many others are also changed. Examples of proteins involved in both signal transduction and carcinogenesis are shown in Table 11.1. They are described in greater detail below but the point to note here is that several cell compartments are implicated.

Extracellular signals that influence cell growth

Signalling molecules can be large or small, charged or uncharged, and to a large extent their chemical characteristics determine the choice of signal transduction pathway (Figure 11.1). The large molecules are polypeptides (growth factors) or proteins (membranes of other cells, extracellular matrix), with polysaccharides providing important post-translational modifications in some cases such as extracellular matrix

Table 11.1 Signal transduction molecules that are influential in cancers.

Type of molecule	Function
Growth factor	
EGF, IGF	Mitogenic
TGF-β	Inhibits proliferation
	Chemotaxis
	Promotes differentiation
Growth factor receptor	
EGF and IGF receptors	Tyrosine kinase
TGF-β receptor	Serine kinase
Cell recognition	
Integrins	Cytoskeleton
Cadherins	Cell contacts
Signal transduction	
ras	GTP binding
raf	Serine kinase
Transcription factor	
fos, jun, myc	Early replication genes
Oestrogen receptor	Mitogenic
Retinoic acid receptors	Differentiation

EGF = epidermal growth factor; IGF = insulin-like growth factor; TGF-β = transforming growth factor β.

Figure 11.3

Types of extracellular signal.

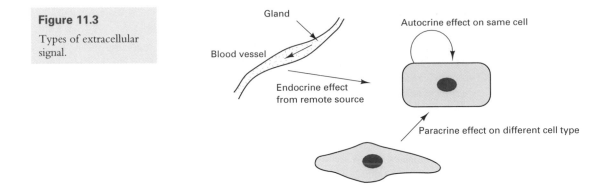

proteins. Extracellular polypeptides and proteins act via cell membrane receptors whose signals must be transduced to the nucleus by intermediary events involving processes as diverse as protein–protein interactions, cytoskeletal changes and movement of macromolecules within intracellular compartments.

Low molecular weight, lipid-soluble regulators such as steroid hormones and retinoic acid readily traverse the cell membrane and bind to intracellular receptors that are gene transcription factors.

Endocrine, autocrine and paracrine regulation

Extracellular signals can be categorised according to the source of the signal (Figure 11.3). *Endocrine* control, mainly involving hormones, is exerted via molecules transported in the bloodstream from producing glands, whereas the other two processes refer to molecules produced locally, either from the same cell (*autocrine*) or from different cells (*paracrine*). Some transmembrane proteins interact with receptors on adjacent cells; this is called juxtacrine regulation. Each type of signal is important in carcinogenesis.

Three categories of extracellular signal will be described: the polypeptide growth factors, the larger glycoproteins involved in cell interactions with other components of the cell's immediate environment such as the extracellular matrix, and low molecular weight, hydrophobic molecules.

Growth factors

Nomenclature

Nomenclature of growth factors reflects historical events associated with their discovery and can be confusing as the name does not convey current knowledge about their actions. **P**latelet-**d**erived **g**rowth **f**actor (PDGF) was named after its identification as the factor released from platelets in serum formation but it is now known to be produced by a variety of cell types. Likewise TGF-α and TGF-β were first characterised as a combined entity capable of promoting anchorage–independent growth (transformation) of cultured cells. TGF-α is mitogenic for a wide spectrum of normal and neoplastic cells such as those of colon, breast and ovary. TGF-β is growth inhibitory for epithelial cells but stimulatory for fibroblasts. It also has potent chemotactic (cell attractant) properties and can induce production of extracellular matrix proteins such as collagen and fibronectin. Therefore, TGF-β provides a multifunctional defence mechanism by inhibiting proliferation, recruiting antagonistic cells (lymphocytes) and promoting differentiation. The use of the term 'growth factor' to describe the actions of TGF-β indicates that inhibitory as well as stimulatory actions are mediated by this class of molecule. The term 'cytokine' is in some ways better as it does not imply stimulatory effects on proliferation. Both terms will be used but 'cytokine' will be used predominantly for polypeptides that promote differentiation and death with secondary effects on growth inhibition; 'growth factor' will be applied mostly to growth stimulatory molecules, although the interleukins can be mitogenic for white blood cells even though they are designated as cytokines.

Local actions on many cell types

Growth factors are most commonly synthesised and act locally within a tumour although external, endocrine routes are also used by insulin in the pancreas and insulin-like growth factor I (IGF-I) in the liver. The multiple effects of TGF-β just described indicate that, within a tumour, growth factor synthesis and effects are not confined to cancer cells and that growth of solid cell collections involves interaction between multiple cell types and with the extracellular matrix. Other examples of multiple effects are provided by PDGF and fibroblast growth factor (FGF). Many tumour cells produce these growth factors, both of which are mitogenic for endothelial cells of blood vessels and for normal stromal cells either surrounding or within a tumour mass. Tumour-stimulated angiogenesis at early stages of growth facilitates transition from the avascular state to the vascular state (Chapter 2) and is also important during metastatic growth (Chapter 12). Stromal growth is a common feature of epithelial tumours partly due to paracrine effects of tumour-produced factors. Thus, breast cancer cells can produce PDGF but they do not have PDGF receptors, whereas the stromal cells are receptor positive and can respond. The converse situation also occurs in which stromal cells produce the growth factor (ligand) that binds to a receptor on the neoplastic epithelial cells; a good example is IGF and the IGF2 receptor.

Synthesis

Polypeptide growth factors are synthesised as large precursors that are cleaved by proteases to give final products whose monomer size varies from 6 kDa (TGF-α) to 12 kDa (PDGF, TGF-β). Each growth factor in fact represents a family of molecules, individual members of which can be produced in a tissue-specific way. Thus, for the insulin family, insulin is synthesised in the pancreas and IGF-I in the liver (endocrine action) or locally (autocrine or paracrine action) by many cells. IGF-II on the other hand is produced predominantly by foetal cells, although it has been identified in some cancers (Wilms' tumour, sarcomas).

Cancer

Abnormal production of growth factors by tumours has been identified in several situations. The monkey viral oncogene v-sis codes for the B subunit of PDGF, the factor responsible for sarcoma production. Patients with pituitary tumours that secrete growth hormone have increased serum IGF-I due to the growth hormone effect on the liver, but other cancers generate local IGF-I changes. Small-cell lung cancers produce the autocrine, mitogenic polypeptide, **g**astrin-**r**eleasing **p**eptide (GRP), also known as bombesin. Blockading bombesin disrupts tumour growth. Indeed, various agents that block growth factor receptors are being tested as potential treatments for advanced cancer (Chapter 13). In cancers such as lung and ovary, increased production of the mitogenic growth factor TGF-α is associated with poor survival of the patient.

Increased production of normal growth factor by cancer cells commonly results from altered signal transduction consequent to carcinogenic events (see below). This establishes an autonomous loop between the growth factor and gene transcription that contributes to unregulated growth.

Growth factor receptors

General features

Membrane receptors recognise the growth factor at the external face of the cell membrane and relay the signal to the intracellular side; this is how cells recognise and react to these types of external signal. Ligand binding induces conformational changes in the transmembrane protein that activate its cytoplasmic tail; the consequences depend on the receptor concerned. Different cell types display characteristic profiles of receptors that determine the response potential of the cell concerned. As receptors recognise only specific types of growth factor this provides an extra degree of specificity as to which cells will respond to a given signal.

For events as important as proliferation, fine control of on/off signals is essential; this is achieved by ensuring that small changes in ligand concentration maximise signal response. Growth factor receptors have dissociation constants in the 10^{-10} M range, which means that they can respond to growth factor concentrations in the same low range. Magnitude of response is determined by the law of mass action, such that both ligand and receptor levels determine the end result and both are manipulated by cancers to achieve a growth advantage.

Cancers have adopted several stratagems to influence receptor activity, ranging from gene amplification (EGF receptor) to mutations that generate constitutively active molecules (neu oncogene). Receptor numbers can also be increased by normal events, as is the case with breast cells in which IGF-I receptors are increased by oestrogens and the cells are therefore more sensitive to a given concentration of ligand. Receptors for inhibitory pathways, such as those for TGF-β, can be inactivated by mutations; this occurs in colon cancers and lymphoma.

A receptor is a molecule that binds a ligand and generates a biological response. Other ligand-binding proteins exist that do not directly generate a response and are therefore not receptors. In most cases such binding proteins provide a means of reversibly inactivating the growth factor. This second category of binding protein usually inactivates the ligand but because of the reversibility of the interaction, the protein-bound ligand can act as a pool of readily available ligand. Several IGF-binding proteins in serum and tissues fall into this category. Sometimes such protein interaction is important for biological activity of the ligand. Thus, TGF-β is synthesised and secreted in a latent form from which the active polypeptide can be released by low pH or proteases. FGFs bind avidly to heparin-containing proteoglycans of the extracellular matrix, which therefore provide a reservoir of the polypeptide, but additional proteins in the cell membrane may function as a means of recruiting growth factors such as TGF-β and FGF to their receptors. Proteins that do not directly transduce signals but contribute to the overall response are called *type II receptors*; whereas *type I receptors* transduce the signal across the plasma membrane.

Growth factor receptors can be divided into two groups depending on whether tyrosine kinases or serine/threonine kinases mediate immediate post-ligand binding events.

Tyrosine kinase receptors

Proteins modified by phosphorylation of tyrosine residues represent less than 1% of those modified by serine/threonine phosphorylation. The former are involved predominantly in early growth-related events with subsequent changes in the transduction pathway being dominated by serine/threonine phosphorylations. Although typically involved with membrane events, intracellular tyrosine kinases are also important.

Kinase receptors will be divided into those that contain a tyrosine kinase activity as an integral part of the receptor molecule and those that are inactive in this respect but which can recruit a kinase as a result of ligand binding. The EGF receptor is an example of the first kind and cytokine receptors predominate among the second kind (Figure 11.4).

Receptors with integral kinase activity

Receptors with integral kinase activity have an extracellular ligand-binding domain, a transmembrane region and a multifunctional cytoplasmic tail. The tail has an ATP-binding site plus tyrosine kinase activity capable of phosphorylating itself (autophosphorylation) as well as other proteins. Autophosphorylation of the cytoplasmic face of the receptor generates a docking site for intracellular proteins that provide the next step in the signal transduction route.

The receptors must be in a dimeric form to be active, because the kinase on one chain cannot phosphorylate itself and an interchain phosphorylation is required (Figure 11.5). Different members of the tyrosine kinase receptor family use different methods of achieving dimerisation. TGF-α binds to the EGF receptor in a 1:1 ratio that then dimerises, whereas the IGF-I receptor pre-exists as a dimer and the ligand

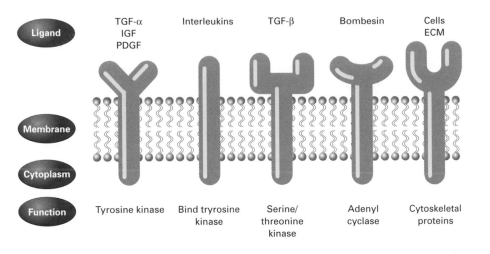

Figure 11.4

Transmembrane receptors involved in growth regulation. The receptors are dimers in reality.

alters the conformation of the dimer. The PDGF receptor is ligand-dimerised by virtue of the ligand itself being a dimer, each monomer binding to one receptor chain. Members of the EGF receptor family can form functionally important heterodimers with each other. The family contains four subgroups, erbB1 to erbB4 (**er**ythro**b**lastosis virus protein **B**), each with a distinct ligand specificity. Thus, the EGF receptor (erbB1, HER-1) will bind EGF, TGF-α and amphiregulin polypeptides whereas erbB2 (HER-2, neu) has no obvious ligands. As ligands activate conformational changes in the receptors, it is important to identify the activating mechanism for erbB2. The EGF receptor achieves this, as growth factor (ligand) binding to the EGF receptor can activate the erbB2 tyrosine kinase pathway by a process called *transmodulation*. A monomer of EGF receptor plus ligand will heterodimerise and tyrosine phosphorylate an erbB2 monomer. Tyrosine

Figure 11.5

Tyrosine kinase receptor signalling.

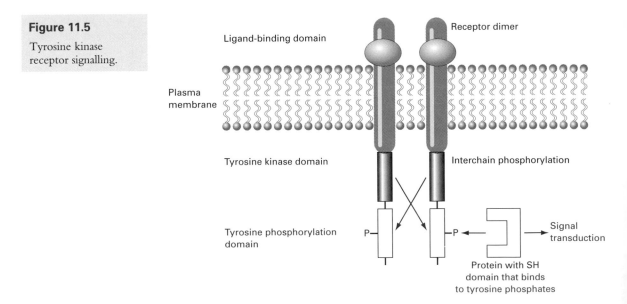

phosphorylation generates a docking signal for proteins having a **src h**omology (SH) domain (see below).

Receptors that recruit tyrosine kinases

Transmembrane receptors for cytokines such as interleukins, haematopoietic growth factors (e.g. colony stimulating factor) and interferons activate tyrosine kinases indirectly by ligand-dependent dimerisation and binding of cytoplasmic kinases (Figure 11.6). These **Ja**nus **k**inases (JAKs) – 'Janus' means 'two-faced' – phosphorylate nuclear transcription factors called STATs. Additionally, the JAK can phosphorylate the adjacent chain of the dimerised receptor and activate other mitogenic pathways via ras (Figure 11.12) and phosphoinositols (Figure 11.14). This class of receptor is critically important in haemopoiesis, disruption of which can result in leukaemia. This requires coordinate changes in differentiation plus proliferation (Chapters 2 and 10), each of which is regulated by different regions of the cytoplasmic domain of the cytokine receptor.

Integrins are a second class of receptor that recruit tyrosine kinases. Integrins mediate cell–cell and cell-ECM interactions (see below); they activate a **f**ocal **a**dhesion **k**inase (FAK) localised to such points of contact (Figure 11.17). FAK can be autophosphorylated and bind other proteins including the tyrosine kinase from the src oncogene.

Proteins with domains that bind to tyrosine phosphates

Phosphorylated tyrosines are recognised by amino acid motifs on other proteins called SH (**src h**omology) domains. This type of interaction mediates the next step in ligand-induced signal transduction. The amino acids on the C-terminal side of the phosphorylated tyrosine determine the type of SH domain to be recognised, although the whole domain involves a sequence of about 100 amino acids. The type and number of SH domains determine which proteins will bind to the receptor and thereby influence

Figure 11.6

Cytokine receptor: recruitment of a tyrosine kinase. Janus kinase (JAK) phosphorylates tyrosines on an adjacent subunit of the STAT transcription factor.

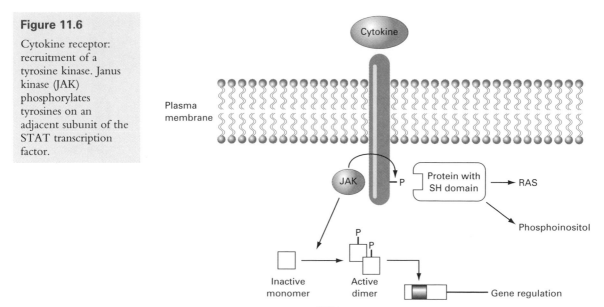

specificity of effect; the other determinant being the presence or absence of the binding protein itself (Figure 11.7). Thus, the PDGF receptor has several autophosphorylation sites capable of binding SH domains of proteins like src, **p**hosphatidyl **i**nositol **k**inase (PIK), **p**hospho**l**ipase **C** (PLC), **G**TPase-**a**ctivating protein (GAP) and tyrosine **p**hosphat**ase** (Pase). Depending on the availability of these proteins, several signalling pathways can be activated. PIK is a heterodimer of an 85 kDa adaptor protein that binds to the receptor and a 110 kDa catalytic subunit. PIK contributes to the phosphoinositol pathway and PLC releases diacylglycerol, the natural ligand for protein kinase C (see below). GAP is a bifunctional regulator of ras (see below) and Pase provides a mechanism for inactivating the whole process by hydrolysing the tyrosine phosphates.

The EGF receptor follows a similar pattern, with some SH domains binding similar proteins (PLC) to that of the PDGF receptor and others binding different proteins. The EGF receptor activates ras by a different pathway involving GRB (**g**rowth factor **r**elated **b**inding protein); see Figure 11.7.

Some SH-containing proteins have their own tyrosine residues capable of phosphorylation by the receptor. GRB becomes tyrosine phosphorylated and is recognised by the next SH-containing protein in the reaction sequence. Hence the initial autophosphorylation of the receptor activates a sequence of protein–protein interactions.

Protein tyrosine phosphatases

Several tyrosine phosphatases have been characterised that reverse the biological effects of tyrosine phosphorylations. Some of these phosphatases have SH domains;

Figure 11.7

Signalling events at the cytoplasmic face of tyrosine kinase receptors. Multiple SH domains can dock with tyrosine phosphates on the receptors and activate alternative pathways. The receptors are dimers in reality.

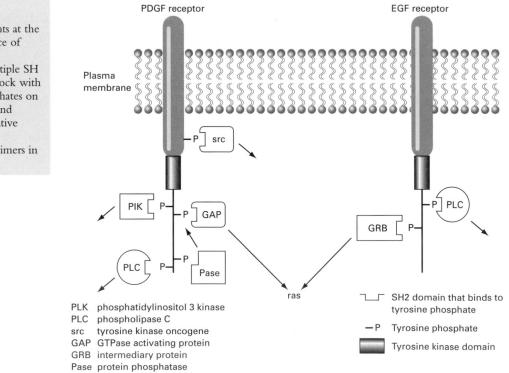

PLK phosphatidylinositol 3 kinase
PLC phospholipase C
src tyrosine kinase oncogene
GAP GTPase activating protein
GRB intermediary protein
Pase protein phosphatase

they can therefore bind to tyrosine-phosphorylated sites on receptors and dephosphorylate adjacent sites (Figure 11.7).

Cancer

Tyrosine kinases are altered in many cancers (Table 11.2). Several viral oncogenes code for tyrosine kinases – rat neuroblastoma results from a point mutation in the neu oncogene that generates a constitutively active kinase. This mutation changes a valine to a glutamate in the transmembrane domain, which causes the kinase to dimerise in the absence of ligand. In human cancers, tyrosine kinase alterations have been identified at several stages of tumour development. A translocation between chromosomes 5 and 12 activates the PDGF receptor B chain, which is an early event in the development of chronic myelomonocytic leukaemia; this is a separate leukaemia from the chronic myeloid leukaemia (CML) described in Chapter 2. Kinase involvement in later stages of carcinogenesis has been identified in several epithelial cancers, although the relationship between kinase activity and stage of carcinogenesis is not always a simple one. In cervical cancer, EGF receptor activity increases with tumour aggressiveness and mitotic activity; the same is true for lung and ovarian cancers. With each of these examples, increased receptor is associated with decreased likelihood of prolonged survival, which is to be expected given the involvement of these receptors in mitogenic pathways (see below). The picture with breast is more complex; ErbB2 activity increases at early stages of carcinogenesis (well-differentiated, *in situ* carcinomas) then declines and rises again in poorly differentiated, invasive cancers. Gene amplification accounts for some cases of higher expression, but not all of them. A chromosome rearrangement in CML results in the production of a fusion protein in which a tyrosine phosphate in one partner (bcr, chromosome 22) binds an SH domain of the other partner (abl, chromosome 9) thereby activating the abl kinase (Figure 11.8). The bcr tyrosine phosphate also spontaneously binds the SH domain of GRB resulting in ras activation. An additional feature of the bcr–abl fusion is that it alters the intracellular location (nucleus to cytoplasm) of the kinase that brings it in contact with novel substrates.

Manipulation of tyrosine kinases/phosphatase activities are being tested as potential treatment regimens (Chapter 13).

Table 11.2 Tyrosine kinases altered in cancers.

Kinase	Function	Cancer
Animal		
neu	Membrane receptor	Rat neuroblastoma
v-kit (virus)	Cytokine receptor	Cat sarcoma
v-src (virus)	Membrane protein	Chicken sarcoma
Human		
EGF receptor	Growth factor receptor	Epithelia
TRK	Growth factor receptor	Thyroid
PDGF receptor	Growth factor receptor	Myeloid leukaemia

EGF = epidermal growth factor; PDGF = platelet-derived growth factor.

Figure 11.8

CML: combined SH domain and tyrosine kinase activation. The chromosome translocation t(9,22) leads to the production of a protein with functions derived from both chromosomes.

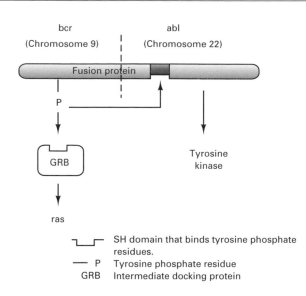

Receptors that act via serine/threonine kinases

Both stimulatory (phorbol ester) and inhibitory (TGF-β) proliferation signals can be relayed by serine/threonine kinase receptors. The principles are similar to those used by tyrosine kinases except the SH domains do not provide the docking mechanism with other proteins.

TGF-β receptor is present in all cells except retinoblastoma cells and thus has widespread functions. These functions can be as varied as inhibition of proliferation, induction of extracellular matrix proteins, chemotaxis and stimulation of another growth factor, such as PDGF. TGF-β initially binds to a type II receptor, which then dimerises with a type I receptor (Figure 11.9). The type II kinase domain phosphorylates and activates the type I kinase domain, which transduces the signal by phosphorylating intracellular proteins of the SMAD family (originally called MAD – **m**others **a**gainst **d**ecapentaplegic). All these phosphorylations are on serine/threonine. Phosphorylation of cytoplasmic SMAD1 or SMAD2 promotes nuclear entry and heterodimerisation with another family member, SMAD4. This oligomeric complex will not bind to specific DNA sequences in regulatory regions of genes until joined by a third protein, Fast. Genes directly activated by this pathway are involved in extracellular matrix production (collagen), inhibition of proliferation (the cyclin–dependent kinase inhibitor p21, transcription factor jun), metastasis (plasminogen activator inhibitor) and differentiation (bone formation). Indirectly, genes requiring the **CREB-b**inding **p**rotein (CBP) coactivator are also inhibited because CBP binds with SMAD2 and SMAD4, so it is not available to activate those other genes (see below).

The membrane-bound protein kinase C is normally activated by diacylglycerol but the tumour promotor, phorbol ester is also an effective ligand.

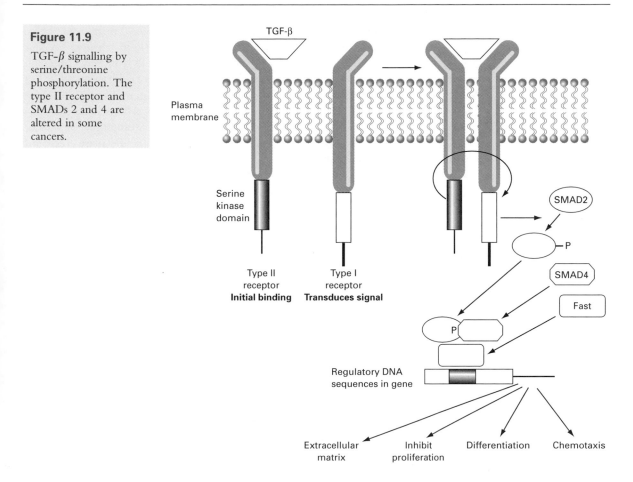

Figure 11.9

TGF-β signalling by serine/threonine phosphorylation. The type II receptor and SMADs 2 and 4 are altered in some cancers.

Serine/threonine phosphatases

Serine/threonine phosphatases reverse the phosphorylation effects. Several have been identified with different substrate specificities.

Cancer

Various components of the TGF-β signalling pathway can be altered in different cancers. The gene coding for the type II receptor contains dinucleotide repeats analogous to those occuring in microsatellites and which are therefore sensitive to DNA mismatch repair defects (Chapters 8 and 9). Hence colon cancers with such defects sometimes contain truncated, inactive type II receptors. Missense mutations in type II receptors have also been detected in T-cell lymphomas and head/neck cancers. SMAD mutations are more frequent with SMAD4 being inactivated in some cancers of the pancreas, colon, breast, ovary and lung; SMAD2 function is lost in colon cancers. The net result of these changes is loss of differentiation, increased proliferation and altered cell adhesion. In mice, type I and type II receptors are normally expressed in the luminal (upper) region of colon crypts where differentiation occurs. Mice with homozygous knock-out deletions of SMAD3 have a high incidence of invasive colon cancers, but up to now no SMAD3 mutations have been detected in humans. These facts about SMADs provide an interesting example of how changes in our understanding of molecular events can alter previously held concepts. In colon carcinogenesis the DCC repressor gene was originally detected as a deletion by its loss of heterozygocity (LOH) and was said to code for a cell adhesion molecule. It was later identified as a receptor (semaphorin) for extracellular chemotactic peptides (netrins) involved in cell migration. It is now known that the LOH at chromosome 18q (Table 2.1) also applied to the SMAD4 gene adjacent to the gene for the netrin receptor. SMAD was identified as the relevant gene for colon carcinogenesis by experiments with knock-out mice; homozygous deletions of the SMAD gene resulted in colon cancers whereas DCC-deleted mice remained cancer-free.

Adenyl cyclase linked receptors

Adenyl cyclase linked receptors have a single protein chain that loops across the membrane seven times and a cytoplasmic domain that interacts with two regulatory proteins to form the active adenyl cyclase complex (Figure 11.10). Ligand binding

Figure 11.10

Pathways activated by adenyl cyclase linked receptors.

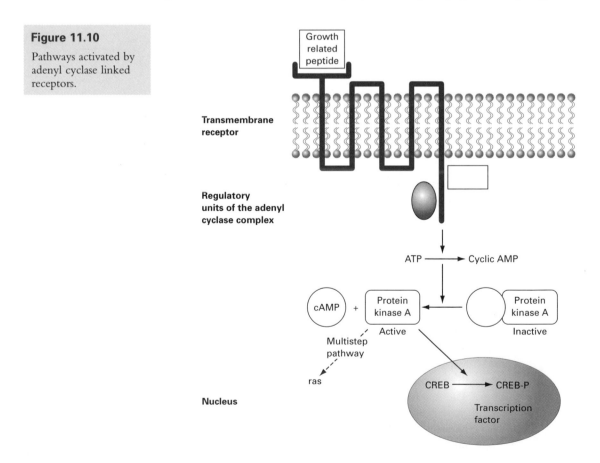

activates the adenyl cyclase and increases intracellular cyclic AMP formation from ATP. This type of receptor is used by polypeptides such as hypothalamic **go**nadotrophin-**r**eleasing **h**ormone (GnRH), whose normal function is to regulate pituitary secretion of gonadotrophins that modulate ovarian and testicular steroid hormone production. These hormones have major causal influences on the development of breast and prostate cancer. Additionally, GnRH receptors have been identified on tumour cells and their growth is influenced by the appropriate ligands. Synthetic ligands of this type are used in the treatment of hormone-sensitive cancers (Chapter 13). GRP, a growth-related mitogen secreted by certain lung tumours also uses an adenyl cyclase receptor.

Cyclic AMP binds to and dissociates a dimeric cytoplasmic complex made up of a cyclic AMP binding protein and serine/threonine **p**rotein **k**inase **A** (PKA). On translocation to the nucleus, PKA phosphorylates and activates the transcription factor CREB (**c**yclic AMP **r**esponse **e**lement **b**inding protein); see Figure 11.10.

Growth factors: from membrane to nucleus

General features

The multiple pathways used by tyrosine and serine kinase receptors to convey their signals are dominated by one feature: a cascade of serine/threonine phosphorylations that alter the functional activities of the proteins involved. These phosphorylations can be reversed by protein phosphatases.

The events involved in this series of reactions are also characterised by a versatility achieved by divergence and convergence of pathways, which goes some way towards explaining how messages from different initial signals converge on a common route and how different cell types can respond in cell-specific ways to a common signal (Figure 11.2). The ras oncogene acts as one of the pleiotropic modulators capable of redirecting input signals from the receptors to alternative pathways.

The end result of this cascade is transcriptional activation achieved by altering either the amount or functional activity of transcription factors (Figure 11.1). Several such factors are involved, but c-fos and c-jun have been particularly well studied. They were originally identified as viral oncogenes that activate growth-related genes. Increasing the amount of protein upregulates c-fos, whereas serine/threonine phosphorylation and dephosphorylation of c-jun are its main activating events. The c-fos and c-jun proteins form a heterodimer that binds to regulatory DNA base sequences (AP1 sites) of genes coding for proliferation-related proteins.

The checkpoints that regulate the cell cycle (Chapter 10) are the main focus of this sequence of changes with the G_1 checkpoint being particularly involved. The repressor activity of Rb is exerted at this focal point and it is inactivated by serine/threonine phosphorylation (Chapters 6 and 10) resulting from the events described here.

Although regulating proliferation is an important feature of kinase receptor activation, other cell functions such as the cytoskeletal arrangement, apoptosis, invasion and metastasis are also affected.

The ras GTP-binding protein

Normal function

The 21 kDa GTP-binding protein that is attached to the cytoplasmic face of the cell membrane receives input signals from several pathways and relays them to an equally diverse set of effectors (Figure 11.11). Its molecular details were described earlier (Figure 6.6). Ras is active when bound to GTP and inactive with GDP. The intrinsic GTPase activity of the protein mediates the inactivation step but an additional protein, GAP, is needed for this process. Activation involves exchanging GDP for GTP, which requires the exchange protein SOS (son of sevenless). Input signals from PDGF modulate the activity of GAP in a poorly understood way. GAP is usually described as an inhibitor of ras activation so its designation as an activator in conjunction with PDGF is confusing. It is postulated that GAP has two separate functions with opposing effects. IGF and TGF-α/EGF growth factors increase SOS function via an intermediary protein, GRB (Figure 11.7). The protein–protein complexes required for this set of events involve SH domain interactions.

Ras is synthesised as a precursor with a C-terminal CAAX motif (C = cysteine, A = aliphatic amino acid, X = variable) that loses its three C-terminal amino acids by proteolysis. This leaves a cysteine as the terminal amino acid that is modified by attachment of a hydrophobic chain (prenylation is the general term) which facilitates attachment of ras to the inner wall of the cell membrane (Figure 11.11). Prenylation and membrane insertion are essential for ras activity. The carboxyl of the terminal cysteine is then methylated. The hydrophobic chain is usually a 15-carbon isoprenyl (farnesyl) group, but sometimes a 20-carbon geranylgeranyl chain can be substituted. The main enzyme responsible for farnesyl modification, farnesyl diphosphate protein transferase (farnesyl transferase), is much more active than the equivalent geranylgeranyl transferase, which accounts for the predominance of the farnesyl reaction. These events are discussed in more detail in Chapter 13 as they are targets for new types of drug therapy.

Downstream effectors include phosphoinositols, cytoskeletal proteins and raf, a serine/threonine kinase (Figure 11.11). Two members of the ras superfamily of GTP-binding proteins, rho and rac, modulate actin polymerisation and therefore affect the cytoskeleton (Figure 11.14). Hence the ras family of proteins provide a route whereby proliferation and cytoskeletal changes can be coordinately linked.

As far as proliferation is concerned, the most important consequence of ras activation is its attachment to raf, a cytoplasmic serine/threonine kinase, thus recruiting it to the cell membrane where it effects the next step in the response cascade (see below).

Altered function in cancer cells

The ras gene is mutated in about 40% of all human cancers, although mutations can be as high as 90% in pancreatic cancer. Besides this data, experimental evidence from transfection studies, transgenic mice and site-directed mutagenesis indicates that the carcinogenic mutations destroy the GTPase activity of ras and it is therefore maintained in an active, GTP-bound form. Molecular details of the ras mutations are detailed elsewhere (Figure 6.5 and Table 6.4). Different ras alleles are activated in different cancers – K-ras in most cancers, H-ras in colon and head/neck cancers. Some cancers have normal ras but alterations in other molecules that influence its function. Genes that are mutated in human cancers and which code for proteins

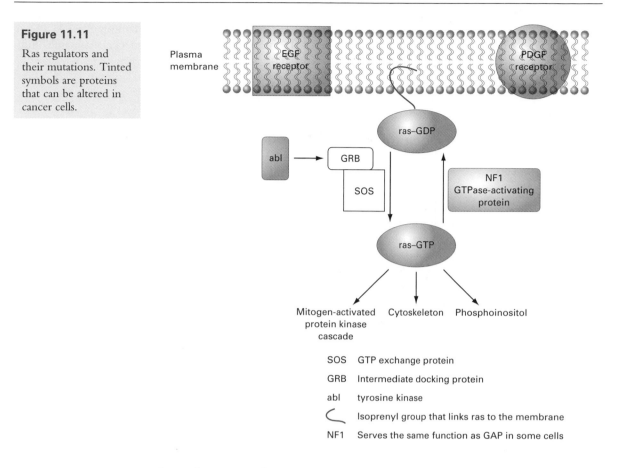

Figure 11.11

Ras regulators and their mutations. Tinted symbols are proteins that can be altered in cancer cells.

SOS   GTP exchange protein

GRB   Intermediate docking protein

abl   tyrosine kinase

⌒   Isoprenyl group that links ras to the membrane

NF1   Serves the same function as GAP in some cells

that influence ras function have been specially designated in Figure 11.11. In addition to the tyrosine kinase receptor mutations described above, some cells contain NF1, a protein that has similar actions to those of GAP. Defects in NF1 increase the risk of sarcomas and childhood chronic myeloid leukaemia (CML) due to loss of its GTPase-activating potential. This effectively maintains ras in a GTP-bound state. NF1 therefore has the properties of a repressor protein.

The varied ways in which cancers can alter one regulatory pathway is illustrated by changes in ras in myeloid leukaemias (Table 11.3). Blocked differentiation of myeloid cells in these leukaemias can result from the disruption of ras itself or indirectly by

Table 11.3 Mutations in human myeloid leukaemia (ML) that activate ras.

Gene	Type of change	Function	Leukaemia
Ras	Point mutations	GTPase lost	Acute ML
PDGF receptor	Chromosome translocation t(5;12)	GTP binding prolonged	Chronic mono ML
Abl	Chromosome translocation t(9;22)	GTP binding prolonged	Chronic ML
NF1	Inactivation	GTPase lost	Childhood chronic ML

altering ancillary proteins. NF1 inactivation decreases GTP hydrolysis while PDGF receptor activation prolongs GTP binding. In CML increased GTP–ras results from elevated GTP exchange (Figures 11.8 and 11.11). It is not clear why ras activation by different mechanisms should generate different types of myeloid leukaemia.

Raf and the MAP kinase cascade

GTP–ras will bind raf and translocate it from the cytoplasm to the plasma membrane (Figure 11.12). The serine kinase activity of raf is normally inhibited by sequences at the N-terminal of the protein. When GTP–ras binds to this N-terminal sequence, inhibition is lost and the raf kinase becomes functional. Raf was originally identified as a viral oncogene in which the inhibitory sequences were lost and the serine kinase was constitutively active.

Raf is the first of a series of kinases that activate subsequent members of a cascade, culminating in the phosphorylation of transcription factor c-jun. The general term for these kinases is **m**itogen-**a**ctivated **p**rotein kinase (MAP kinase), so named because it is activated (phosphorylated) by many mitogens, such as the polypeptide growth factors, serum, phorbol esters and hormones. Individual members of the MAP kinase cascade include, in order of activation, raf (MAP kinase kinase kinase), MEK (MAP kinase kinase) and ERK (**e**xtracellular signal **r**elated **k**inase, MAP

Figure 11.12

Ras activation of jun transcription factor.

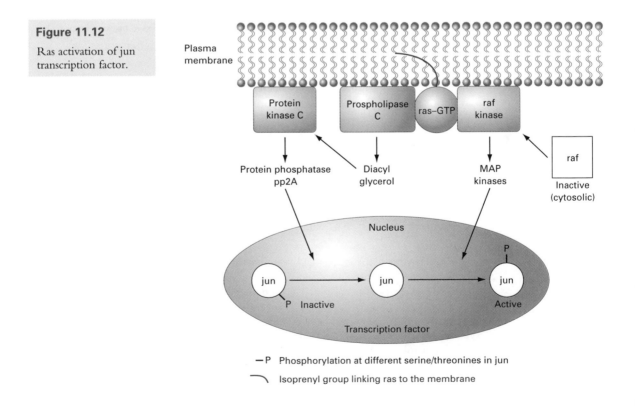

−P Phosphorylation at different serine/threonines in jun

⌒ Isoprenyl group linking ras to the membrane

kinase). ERK phosphorylates the ELK transcription factor needed for fos induction (see below). Ionising radiations and free radicals (Chapter 7) alter serine/threonine protein kinase activity. These **stress-activated protein kinases** (SAPKs) such as JNK are included within the general category of MAP kinases.

Signalling molecules derived from phosphoinositol

Cell membranes contain **phosphatidyl inositol** (PtdIn) lipids made up of inositol linked by a phosphate to glycerol esterified with a long-chain, saturated fatty acid and an unsaturated (4 double bonds) fatty acid, arachidonic acid (Figure 11.13). Separate **PtIn kinases**, PIKs 3, 4 and 5, add additional phosphate to the inositol moiety. **Phospholipase C** (PLC) releases these phosphoinositols together with **diacylglycerol** (DAG), the activator of protein kinase C (Figure 11.12). Phospholipase A2 can release arachidonic acid from PtdIns to serve as a substrate for prostaglandin and ceramide synthesis (Figure 11.22). Thus, through these hydrolytic

Figure 11.13

Phosphatidyl inositol metabolism.

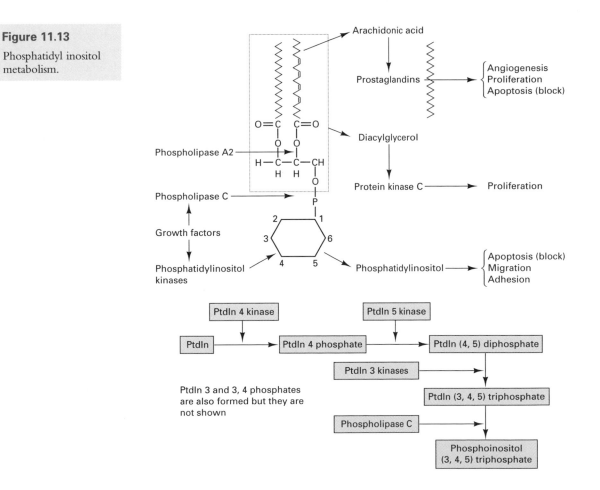

and phosphorylation reactions, phosphatidyl inositol can generate three sets of secondary messengers – DAG, arachidonic acid and phosphoinositols – each of which can influence a spectrum of intracellular pathways.

Of the PIKs, the 3-kinase family, referred to here as PIK3, is particularly important in influencing cancer-related events (Figure 11.14). PIK3 is made up of an 85 kDa adaptor subunit with an SH domain and a 100 kDa catalytic subunit. The SH domain binds to tyrosine phosphates on tyrosine kinase receptors (Figure 11.7). PIK3 can also interact with adenyl cyclase receptors (via GTP binding adaptors) and possibly with GTP–ras. PIK3 is activated by these interactions and increases the intracellular concentrations of rate-limiting PtdIns; PtdIn (4,5) diphosphate and PtdIn (3,4,5) triphosphate are likely to be the more important compounds that activate downstream events. The PtdIns are inactivated by phosphatases. PtdIns bind to and activate proteins with lipophilic **p**leckstrin **h**omology (PH) domains that include serine/ threonine kinases such as Akt (protein kinase B), p70 and protein kinase C. Akt phosphorylates the proapoptotic protein Bad. In its unphosphorylated form, this protein binds and inactivates the antiapoptotic protein Bcl2 (Chapter 10), thus activating apoptosis. Phosphorylation of Bad releases Bcl2 thereby inhibiting apoptosis (Figure 10.16). Phosphorylated Bad is sequestered in the cytoplasm as a heterodimer with the strangely named 14-3-3 protein. Akt also phosphorylates **g**lycogen **s**ynthase **k**inase (GSK) which activates several proteins involved in regulating cell proliferation. p70 phosphorylates a ribosomal protein (S6) that helps regulate the G_1 checkpoint of the cell cycle (Figure 10.2). The way in which phosphoinositols influence migration is less clear but it functions downstream of integrins and rho/rac (Figure 11.14).

Adhesion of cells to the extracellular matrix also promotes survival by blocking apoptosis via the ras/phosphoinositol/Akt pathway. Activated forms of ras keep this pathway open, which represents a major contribution to the phenomenon of anchorage independence (Chapter 2).

Figure 11.14

Effects of phosphoinositols.

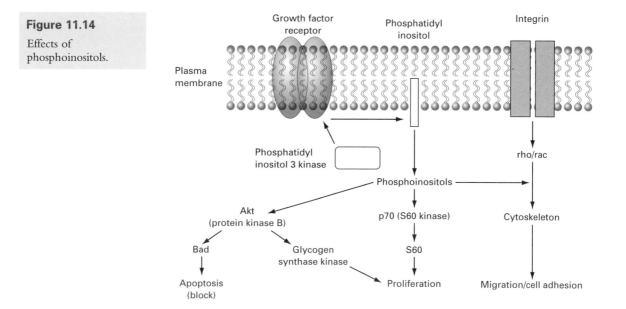

Nuclear events stimulated by growth factors

The net result of the kinase cascade is altered activity of transcription factors such as fos and jun that, in dimeric form, bind to specific DNA base sequences called response elements in the regulatory regions of growth-related genes (Figure 6.1). A particularly important example of such an element is the AP1 site that binds AP1 protein complexes made up of dimeric complexes of the fos and jun families (Figure 11.15). Each of these oncogenes can be independently regulated by events described in the preceding section.

Activation of jun involves two ras-related pathways (Figure 11.12). The activating serine/threonine phosphorylation of jun is mediated by the MAP kinase route but a different, inhibitory phosphate must be removed first by a protein phosphatase 2A that is itself activated by a PKC phosphorylation. Thus, activation of jun is accomplished by post-translational phosphorylations but fos is transcriptionally regulated. The promotor region of this gene has several regulatory sites; one of them is the **s**erum **r**esponse **e**lement (SRE, Figure 11.15), so called because the growth factors present in serum exert their effects via these DNA base sequences. The SRE binds a dimeric complex made up of one ubiquitous transcription factor, **s**erum **r**esponse **f**actor (SRF) and another, ELK, that is only active when it is serine/threonine phosphorylated. This activating phosphorylation occurs via the MAP kinase route.

Figure 11.15

Gene regulation via transcription factors affected by MAP kinases.

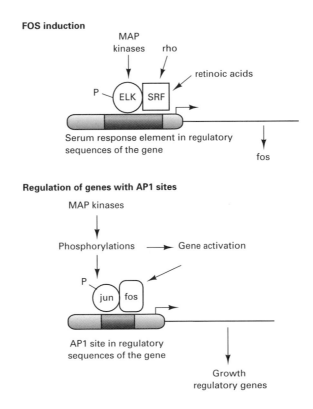

195

Proteins additional to ELK and SRF are required to form the active transcription complex; these **t**ernary **c**omplex **f**actors (TCFs) include additional serine/threonine kinase such as **j**un **N**-terminal **k**inase (JNK) and the coactivator **CREB-b**inding **p**rotein (CBP). Transcription of fos can rapidly be altered by lipophilic factors such as retinoic acid and vitamin D that induce differentiation; response elements for their nuclear receptors (see below) are present in the regulatory sequences of the fos gene. SRF can also be indirectly activated by the GTP-binding proteins rho and rac. Details are sparse but histone acetylation is important and gene transcription may be stimulated via structural changes in the chromatin. Existence of the rho/rac pathway means that cell adhesions can influence fos transcription (see below). Growth factors that increase proliferation also inhibit apoptosis (Chapter 10), and this inhibition is mediated via phosphoinositol pathways (Figure 11.14).

There are several MAP kinase signalling pathways that respond to different external signals. The growth factor responsive pathway has been described above; another MAP kinase pathway is poorly activated by growth factors but sensitive to stress such as low oxygen levels (hypoxia). These kinases, exemplified by JNK, are called **s**tress-**a**ctivated **p**rotein **k**inases (SAPKs). It is not clear how the various kinases are assembled so as to respond to these different stimuli. A multiprotein scaffold may exist to which kinases can be attached and spatially organised so as to confer specificity of response; putative scaffold proteins such as JIP (**j**un **N**-terminal kinase **i**nteracting **p**rotein) and MPI (**MAP** kinase **i**nteracting **p**rotein) have been identified. The oxygen-sensing mechanism involves a flavoprotein

Figure 11.16

Hypoxia and gene transcription.

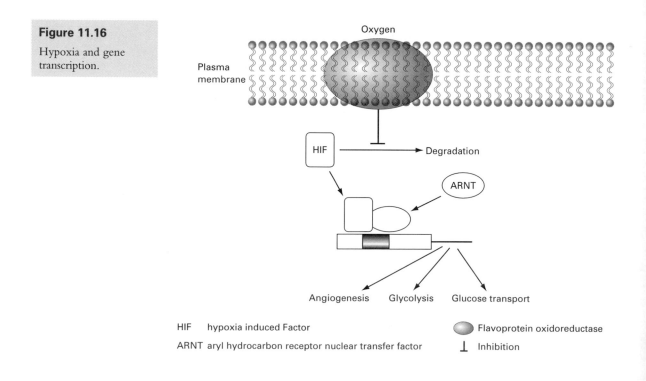

HIF   hypoxia induced Factor

ARNT   aryl hydrocarbon receptor nuclear transfer factor

Flavoprotein oxidoreductase

⊥   Inhibition

oxidoreductase, with the oxygen tension determining whether the flavin cofactor is in an oxidised or reduced state. Another pathway influenced by low oxygen tension is gene activation by **h**ypoxia-**i**nduced transcription **f**actor (HIF); see Figure 11.16. Details are sparse but involve post-transcriptional stabilisation of HIF. This increases HIF concentration and the protein heterodimerises with **ar**yl hydrocarbon **n**uclear **t**ransporter (ARNT) which activates genes with the appropriate enhancer sequences. Additional hypoxia-sensitive, HIF-independent mechanisms exist that stabilise mRNAs transcribed from these genes such as for vascular endothelial growth factor (Chapter 12). This can activate angiogenesis (Chapter 12), anaerobic glycolysis and glucose transport. All of these responses help the cell survive in a low-oxygen environment.

Oncogenic forms of both fos and jun have been identified in virus-infected cells. They are usually constitutively expressed under the influence of the viral promoter but additional deletions in the $3'$ untranslated region of the mRNA increases its half-life. Although regulation of fos and jun is important in human cells, gene defects have not been identified in human cancers.

Another set of DNA bases present in regulatory genes binds proteins phosphorylated by the cyclic AMP/PKA pathway (Figure 11.10). TGF-β signalling via SMAD and Fast transcription factors (Figure 11.9) was described earlier.

Cell adhesion molecules

Cancers differ from benign growths in their ability to invade surrounding tissues and metastasise to other parts of the body. For epithelial cancers, this involves breaking links with adjacent epithelial cells, migration through the **e**xtra**c**ellular glycoprotein **m**atrix (ECM) and invasion of blood vessels (Chapter 12). The **c**ell **a**dhesion **m**olecules involved are called CAMs. These varied functions require the recognition of proteins on other cells and the ECM. The changes in recognition patterns that occur during carcinogenesis cannot be defined in simple terms of increased or decreased activity because of the complexity of the processes involved. For example, cell migration, as a factor in metastasis, requires alternate attachment and detachment of the cell to the ECM so that retention of recognition mechanisms is essential. On the other hand, invasive epithelial cancer cells must lose their attachment to other epithelial cells and to the basement membrane. The one generalisation that can be made is that cancer cells have a different profile of receptors to their normal counterparts.

The ability to recognise similar (*homotypic*) or dissimilar (*heterotypic*) cell types or ECM proteins such as collagen, fibronectin or laminin is mediated by four classes of membrane receptor: integrins, cadherins, immunoglobulin family and selectins (Figure 11.17). Additional membrane glycoproteins include syndecans and CD44. All these CAMs are in effect membrane receptors whose extracellular domains bind ligands that generate conformational changes in the cytoplasmic tail, enabling it to bind specific cytoplasmic proteins. These adaptor molecules link with various signalling pathways that influence cell proliferation, migration,

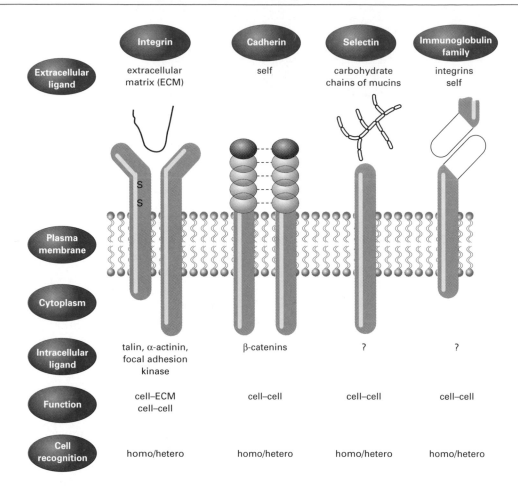

Figure 11.17

Cell adhesion molecules and their functions. Homo = same cell type; hetero = different cell types.

differentiation and apoptosis. Changes in the cytoskeleton (Box 11.1) are of special importance for these events. Anchorage-independent growth in culture is a hallmark of cancer cells (Chapter 2). This property confers a selective advantage on the cancer cells because they become less dependent on their environment, and for a solid tissue the environment means the surrounding ECM and other cells.

Box 11.9

How a cell interacts with its environment

General   Within a tissue, cells interact with other cells of the same (homophilic) or different (heterophilic) types as well as with the glycoproteins and proteoglycans of the **e**xtra**c**ellular **m**atrix (ECM). These interactions are mediated by transmembrane, glycoprotein **c**ell **a**dhesion **m**olecules (CAMs). There are four CAM families, integrins, cadherins, selectins and immunoglobulin-like proteins (see text for details). Additional membrane components include syndecans and the **c**luster of **d**ifferentiation protein CD44. The ECM glycoproteins include several types of collagen, laminin, fibronectin, vitronectin and thrombospondin.

Glycoproteins have various carbohydrate chains covalently attached to the protein through either the −OH of serines and threonines (O-linked) or the −NH$_2$ of asparagine (N-linked). Additional modifications can include sulphations and phosphorylations. Proteoglycans have a core protein with glycosaminoglycan side chains made up of disaccharide repeats of two different sugars (usually hexuronate and hexosamine); tyrosine −OH groups may be sulphated. Important proteoglycans include heparin (heparin sulphate) and chrondroitin sulphate.

CAMs are transmembrane proteins whose external domains function as receptors for ligands that can be ECM proteins or CAMs on other cells. CAMs on other cells can create a terminology problem in deciding which CAM is the receptor and which the ligand. The term 'counter-receptor' is sometimes used to overcome the problem. The cytoplasmic domain interacts with cytoplasmic proteins which transmit (transduce) the extracellular signals to the cell's interior. This process can also function in reverse with intracellular signals being transmitted to the exterior.

Intracellular structures   Cells contain networks of polymerised proteins that provide both elasticity and rigidity when required. This cytoskeleton is primarily composed of three such networks each identified by one of their major proteins: the actin cytoskeleton, the tubulin microfilaments, and intermediate filaments containing cytokeratins (epithelia) or vimentin (other cell types). The actin cytoskeleton, in conjunction with the motor protein myosin and associated proteins, provides contractile structures essential for cell migration and shape. Through ancillary proteins like talin and α-actinin, the actin cytoskeleton is linked to integrin-containing focal adhesions. Microtubules also polymerise/depolymerise and contribute to the polarity of epithelial cells. Microtubules emanate from a cytoplasmic structure, the centrosome, within which is the centriole. The centriole divides prior to mitosis and provides an anchorage point in each potential daughter cell for microtubules. These tubulin-containing filaments are linked to individual chromosomes, so filament contraction retracts each complement of chromosomes into the daughter cells. This retraction requires tubulin depolymerisation, and drugs used in cancer treatment can prevent this by stabilising (taxol) or destabilising (vinca alkaloids) the microtubules (Chapter 13). Intermediate filaments provide mechanical stability to the cell. There are many members of the cytokeratin family: cytokeratins in epithelia, vimentin in other cells and lamin in nuclei. Each type of epithelial cell has a characteristic pattern of cytokeratin expression which can be used for diagnostic purposes in determining origins of cells in cancers.

Cell junctions   Epithelial cells have several junctional complexes. Those involved in cell–cell contacts include tight (occluding) junctions, gap junctions and desmosomes, all of which can be detected by light microscopy, as well as more diffuse contacts. Cell–ECM interactions are mediated by hemidesmosomes, focal adhesions and other non-junctional contacts. All these interactions must be perturbed in order that cancerous epithelial cells can escape their immediate environment, invade the surrounding tissue and metastasise to remote parts of the body. Each type of junction contains CAMs characteristic of that junction. Cadherins occur in desmosomes and diffuse contacts; integrins occur in hemidesmosomes, focal contacts and elsewhere; the immunoglobulin family and selectins are linked with non-junctional interactions. Non-epithelial cells have different arrangements of macromolecules but the CAMs involved have similar mechanistic properties (see text for details). The membrane CAMs interact with the cytoskeleton through adaptor proteins. The nature of these proteins is determined by the CAMs and the cytoskeletal components involved.

Cell migration   Cell migration occurs on the ECM. The front end of the cell extends and attaches to the ECM; this is followed by cell contraction and release at the rear end; the process is then repeated. The intracellular processes are centred on the cytoskeleton, linking through integrins in the plasma membrane (focal adhesions) to the ECM. The on signal for integrin–ECM attachment includes ligand (ECM) interaction, protein phosphorylations and integrin clustering. The off signal involves the internal forces generated by the cytoskeleton and dephosphorylation of focal adhesion proteins. The actin plus myosin cytoskeleton generates the necessary contractile forces; GTP binding proteins such as rho and rac are needed to mediate integrin–actin cytoskeleton linkage.

Extracellular matrix   In this book the ECM can be considered as two structural entities, basement membrane and extracellular stroma. Basement membrane is a distinct structure surrounding collections of epithelial cells and it is composed of glycoproteins such as collagen IV, laminin, fibronectin, proteoglycans and other proteins. It provides a structural framework on which epithelial cells can function but it is also involved in bidirectional signalling between epithelium and stroma. Basement membrane is composed of a basal lamina containing the aforementioned components adjacent to the epithelium and a reticular lamina of other collagen types and proteoglycans. Extracellular stroma is a heterogeneous mixture of proteoglycans and glycoproteins.

Some of these properties are due to indirect interactions between growth factor receptors and CAMs. Thus, the effects of liganded growth factor receptors such as those for EGF or PDGF in normal cells, necessitate the occupancy of CAMs by ECM molecules. In the absence of such occupancy, growth factor binds to its receptor but the mitogenic signal is not transduced to the nucleus; proliferation is blocked at the G_1 checkpoint of the cell cycle (Chapter 10). Anchorage independence reflects CAM changes that allow the mitogenic signals to reach the nucleus. However, signalling by CAMs is a bidirectional process so it can also be viewed as a mechanism that translates genetic information into a three-dimensional pattern of cells in tissues; a major feature of cancer is the disruption of that pattern (Chapter 3). During normal embryogenesis, considerable cell migration occurs involving contractile changes in the cytoskeleton directed by components of the ECM. Although cell migration is diminished in adult life, it is regained by cancer cells when they become invasive and metastasise. Again, the migratory property of cancer cells is related to CAM and ECM changes. Cell migration is also important in the formation of new blood capillaries around cancers (Chapter 12).

Integrins

Integrins promote the assembly of protein complexes containing cytoskeletal elements in response to ligands provided by the ECM or other cells. Tyrosine phosphorylations are required for the formation of those complexes.

This class of receptor is composed of one α and one β protein chain, both of which contribute to ligand binding. Thus far, 15 different α and 9 β chains have been identified; it is the combination of different α and β chains that determines ligand specificity, with divalent metal ions such as Ca^{2+} and Mg^{2+} acting as a bridge between the α subunit and the ligand. Table 11.4 provides examples of ligand specificities of various integrins. Arginine–glycine–aspartate (RGD) motifs commonly, but not universally, form part of the ECM binding domain. Thus, $\alpha_V\beta_3$ favours an asparagine.proline.any amino acid.tyrosine (NPXY) sequence in its ligands. This ubiquitous integrin interacts with a broad range of ligands, enabling it to signal in many different environments. Although ECM molecules predominate in the list of ligands, other CAMs and extracellular proteins (metalloproteinases) also participate. Functions of those integrins linked with metastasis and angiogenesis are described in Chapter 12.

Ligand binding initially causes clustering of several integrins, which increases the overall strength of cell attachment to the ECM. Structural changes in the

Table 11.4 Integrin specificity: changes relevant to cancer.

Integrin	Ligand	Function
$\alpha_2\beta_1$	Laminin, collagen	Lost in anchorage-independent cells, lost in breast cancer
$\alpha_3\beta_1$	Laminin, collagen, fibronectin	High in some metastases
$\alpha_4\beta_1$	V-CAM, fibronectin	Arrest of cells in capillaries
$\alpha_5\beta_1$	Fibronectin	Angiogenesis, extravasation of cells from capillaries
$\alpha_6\beta_1$ or $\alpha_6\beta_4$	Laminin	High in cancers of bladder, lung, colon
$\alpha_V\beta_3$	Most ECM proteins Matrix metalloproteinase-2	High in metastatic melanoma, angiogenesis
LFA1 ($\alpha_L\beta_2$)	ICAM	Immune response (Figure 5.4)

cytoplasmic domain of the integrin β subunit, including serine/threonine phosphorylations, facilitate its interaction with proteins such as talin, **f**ocal **a**dhesion **k**inase (FAK) and α-actinin, which transduce signals to intracellular processes (Figure 11.18). In unliganded integrins, the α-subunit blocks the binding sites on the β-subunit for these cytoplasmic proteins; ligand binding relieves that inhibition. FAK can tyrosine phosphorylate some of the attached proteins as well as itself, and these phosphorylations are essential for signal transduction. Those signals promote cell migration, stimulate proliferation and inhibit apoptosis.

Effects on proliferation involve the ras, PLC (Figure 11.12) and phosphoinositol (Figure 11.14) pathways. Integrin–ECM interaction recruits FAK that activates GTP-binding proteins, ras, rho and rac. Ras stimulates cell proliferation via the MAP kinase pathway (Figure 11.12) whereas rho and rac act by phosphoinositol-mediated steps (Figure 11.14). Growth factors such as EGF and PDGF also stimulate both these pathways, but in normal cells they are inactive in the absence of cell adhesion (anchorage dependence). The molecular details involved are unclear but, in the case of PDGF effects on fibroblasts, they are related to concentrations of phosphoinositol intermediates. In the absence of integrin occupancy, PDGF activates (tyrosine phosphorylation) phospholipase C but the enzyme

Figure 11.18

Integrin structure and function. Signal transduction involves clustering of multiple integrin dimers.

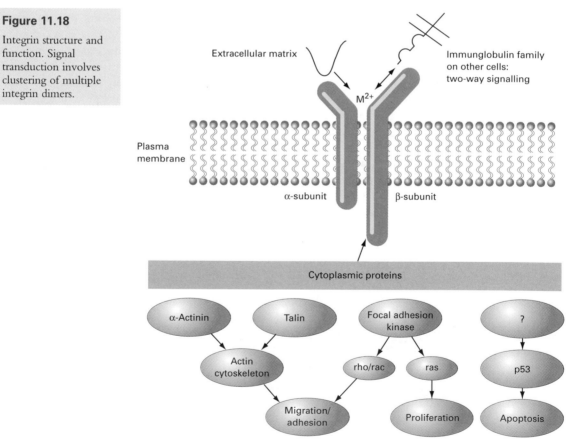

phosphatidylinositol 3 kinase is rate limiting; ECM–integrin interaction activates this enzyme and relieves the block.

Inhibition of apoptosis by integrin-mediated cell adhesion occurs by blocking p53-activated events (Figure 10.18) but mechanistic details are sparse.

Cancer

The integrin repertoire is altered in cancer cells but the changes are complex. An approximation would be that integrins involved in tissue organisation are decreased whereas those needed for migration are not. Thus, in breast cancers the $\alpha_5\beta_1$ integrin that recognises fibronectin is decreased whereas melanomas express increased levels of $\alpha_3\beta_1$ integrin that binds laminin, fibronectin and collagen. The $\alpha_V\beta_3$ integrin is of special interest because it influences several processes important for carcinogenesis. It binds a wide range of ECM glycoproteins as well as a metalloproteinase. $\alpha_V\beta_3$ is poorly expressed on normal cells such as capillary endothelial cells and skin melanocytes but is elevated in metastasising cancers such as melanomas. Migration is determined by the ECM on which the cells move and therefore on the cell receptors that recognise the ECM; the wide specificity of $\alpha_V\beta_3$ means that cell migration can proceed over almost any ECM substrate, a property that facilitates invasion and metastasis (Chapter 12). Its additional property of binding a metalloproteinase to digest a path through the ECM further contributes to invasive potential. Two other processes influenced by $\alpha_V\beta_3$ are apoptosis and angiogenesis. Interaction of this integrin with an ECM ligand promotes cell survival by inhibiting apoptosis (Figure 11.18). The $\alpha_V\beta_3$ integrin is also elevated in normal capillary endothelial cells participating in angiogenesis. The three properties just described – wide ligand specificity, binding metalloproteinases and inhibition of apoptosis – all facilitate formation of new capillaries (Chapter 12). Both the antiapoptotic and angiogenic effects have adverse consequences for the patient and they are now being targeted as potential forms of treatment. Monoclonal antibodies against $\alpha_V\beta_3$ inhibit its function, thus promoting apoptosis and blocking angiogenesis (Chapter 13).

Cadherins

Cadherins represent the 'glue' by which adjacent epithelial cells are attached to each other; they are important in determining the pattern of cells in a tissue. The extracellular domain of a cadherin monomer has five repeat sequences that dimerise with similar repeats on the adjacent monomer in the same cell; Ca^{2+} is needed for this interaction (Figure 11.19). The most distal repeat interacts with the analogous repeat of cadherins on the next cell. The names of individual members of this family can be frequently prefixed with a letter derived from the cell type in which it was first identified, such as E-cadherin from an epithelial member of the family.

Cadherins transduce the extracellular signals by recruiting β-catenin to their cytoplasmic face. This activates a series of changes centred on changing the pool of available β-catenin in the cytoplasm (Figure 11.19). This pool serves a dual role of regulating both the cytoskeleton and nuclear transcription. The central region of β-

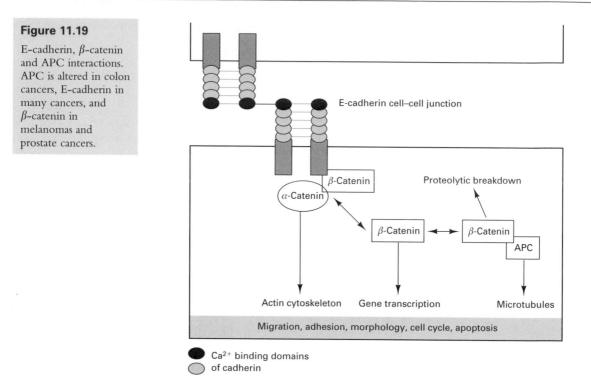

Figure 11.19

E-cadherin, β-catenin and APC interactions. APC is altered in colon cancers, E-cadherin in many cancers, and β-catenin in melanomas and prostate cancers.

catenin contains 13 tandem amino acid repeats (Armadillo repeats from fruit fly terminology) required for both cadherin and transcription factor interaction. The genes whose transcription is influenced by these events in humans are poorly defined other than the observation that β-catenin interacts with transcription factors Tcf and Lef. In insects, β-catenin signals to the Wnt pathway involved in wing formation. More information is available about cytoskeletal responses; β-catenin interacts with α-catenin on the actin cytoskeleton and with the normal **a**denomatous **p**olyposis **c**oli (APC) protein which in turn binds to microtubules. There are two pools of β-catenin, one bound to the actin and microtubule cytoskeletons, the other free and available for downstream effects on gene transcription. APC may play a role in cell movement but additionally its interaction with β-catenin accelerates ubiquitin-mediated proteolytic destruction of β-catenin. As APC is a key protein in carcinogenesis (see below), its modulation of β-catenin availability indicates an important but indeterminate role for the β-catenin in cell function.

β-catenin can be tyrosine phosphorylated by the src oncogene and by growth factor receptors such as EGF (Figure 11.11). This dissociates APC and alters the cytoskeleton as well as activating gene transcription (Figure 11.19).

Cadherins, APC and cancer

Disruption of tissue organisation associated with carcinogenesis is often accompanied by loss of cadherins, which act as repressor molecules. Metastases from epithelial cancers often lose E-cadherin expression thereby facilitating escape of cells from one part of the body to another (Chapter 12). Loss of E-cadherin expression is sometimes due to hypermethylation of regulatory regions of the gene (Chapter 10), but in familial stomach cancer there is a germline, inactivating mutation in the coding region of the gene.

A defective APC gene is inherited in adenomatous polyposis coli cancer patients and both alleles are lost by somatic mutations in sporadic colon cancers (Chapter 9). Loss of APC repressor function is thus a key (gatekeeper) event in the formation of this type of cancer (Chapter 2). About a thousand different mutations have been mapped, all of which result in the synthesis of truncated, inactive proteins. All the somatic and most of the germline mutations occur in the middle region of the gene that codes for the β-catenin binding domain. Loss of the β-catenin binding site of APC results in less degradation and higher concentrations of β-catenin in colon cancer cells than the normal counterparts. The truncated APC protein will still bind microtubules. The importance of β-catenin in carcinogenesis is further emphasised by the observation that a limited number of melanomas, endometrial cancers and prostate cancers have mutations in its gene, as do a limited number of colon cancers with no APC defects. In most cases these β-catenin mutations stabilise the protein against degradation.

Immunoglobulin superfamily

Immunoglobulin superfamily proteins are single-chain proteins; they have extracellular domains with repeated sequences homologous to those in the recognition domains of immunoglobulins. These repeats recognise similar sequences on adjacent cells. The number of repeats is variable in different members of the family but the terminal two repeats determine the specificity of interactions. Overlapping terminologies are again a problem in that members of this family are called CAMS, which is also the general term for cell adhesion molecules. Individual members of the immunoglobulin CAM family are prefixed with the letter derived from the cell type in which it was first identified. Thus, N-CAM is of neural origin whilst V-CAM relates to blood vasculature, but their expression is not confined to these cell types.

N-CAM mediates homotypic cell–cell recognition in normal colon epithelium and its loss represents one of the rate-limiting steps in colon carcinogenesis (see Chapter 2). V-CAM is induced by cytokines in vascular endothelia, where its binding to integrins on metastatic cancer cells helps arrest the cells prior to extravasation (Chapter 12). ICAM is a third member of this family that has a role in cancer biology. It has similar properties to V-CAM including its induction by cytokines, but it is also expressed in cancer cells, such as those of the colon, pancreas and kidney. It is not present in the normal progenitor cells in those sites.

Other members of the immunoglobulin family include a membrane receptor (semaphorin) for extracellular chemotactic peptides (netrins) that provide directional stimuli for cell movement, and carcinoembryonic antigen used for diagnostic purposes (Chapter 13).

Selectins

Selectins are single-chain receptors that recognise carbohydrate side chains of ECM, mucins and cell proteins. They are confined to vascular cells and may play a part in metastasis by arresting cell movement within blood vessels (Chapter 12).

CD44

Over 20 variants of CD44 are translated from a single mRNA by splicing out different introns. Normal CD44 is a receptor for ECM proteins containing hyaluronic acid. CD44 is widely expressed in normal cells but it is downregulated in metastatic cancers of the colon, ovary and prostate. Expression of variant CD44s is complex and no general picture is evident. Thus, variant 6 is not found in normal colon epithelium but increases in amount through the polyp stage until all the cancer cells express it. Variant overexpression also correlates with metastasis in other cases like melanoma. It is not known how these effects are achieved.

Syndecans

Syndecans are transmembrane glycoproteins that bind heparin proteoglycans on their extracellular surface and facilitate the function (coreceptor) of other adhesion receptors such as integrins and cadherins. Their cytoplasmic domains can bind enzymes such as protein kinase C and cofactors like phosphoinositols.

Hydrophobic growth regulatory molecules

Low molecular weight hydrophobic molecules such as steroid hormones, retinoic acids and thyroid hormone, influence several aspects of tumour development. This section will focus on these compounds but another group, the prostaglandins, acting by different mechanisms, will also be described. The first group contains compounds of diverse structure (Table 11.5). They are all relatively simple molecules that elicit specific responses in different cell types. This specificity is generated by the presence or absence of individual receptors and by the genes whose transcription they regulate. The ligands include steroid hormones acting by endocrine and autocrine routes, thyroid hormone (endocrine) and derivatives of vitamin D (1,25-dihydroxy vitamin D3) and vitamin A (retinoic acids) obtained either through the diet (vitamins A and D) or by UV-induced reactions in the skin (vitamin D). To circumvent terminology problems, this disparate group are said to be nuclear receptor acting agents.

Nuclear receptor mediated events

There are no barriers to cell entry for such compounds and their physiological effects are mediated by intracellular, mainly nuclear, receptors. The ligand induces conformational changes in the receptor, resulting in dimerisation and exposure of DNA-binding sites which bind to DNA sequences (hormone response elements). Transcription from genes containing such elements is altered (Figure 11.20).

Ligands

The structures of three classes of ligand involved with cancers and the nature of this involvement are shown in Table 11.5. They act principally via endocrine routes, but autocrine effects may be important in older people (Figure 13.12); alteration of ligand types and concentrations are involved at several stages of cancer development. The sex steroids, oestrogens (female) and androgens (male) are produced endogenously as components of normal development but also find widespread use as exogenous agents that regulate contraception (oestrogens and progestins) or muscle development (anabolic androgens). Oestrogen overexposure from endogenous or exogenous sources increases the risk of endometrial and breast cancer and part of the protective effect of vegetable consumption may be due to antioestrogens in these plants (Chapter 4). There is speculation that environmental oestrogens (endocrine disrupters) produced as industrial by-products from oils, detergents and pesticides, might be responsible for the increased incidence of

Figure 11.20

Gene regulation by low molecular weight, hydrophobic molecules. Examples are steroid hormones, retinoic acid and thyroid hormone. The ligand and receptors can be altered in cancer cells.

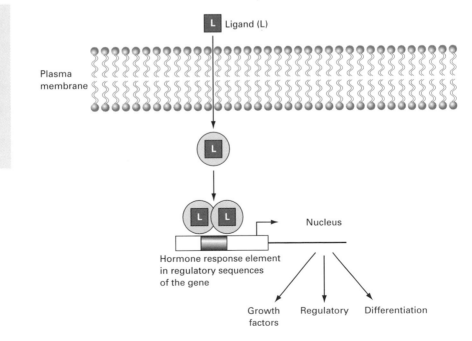

Table 11.5 Hydrophobic molecules involved in cancers and which act by nuclear receptors.

Compound	Involvement	Cancer	Example
Steroids			
Androgens	Tumour promotion, treatment	Prostate	
Oestrogens	Tumour promotion, treatment	Breast, uterus	
Glucocorticoids	Treatment	Leukaemia	
Progestins	Inhibit proliferation, treatment	Uterus, ovary	
			Oestradiol
Thyroid hormone	Hyperproliferation Differentiation	Chicken erythroblastosis	
			Triiodothyronine
Retinoic acids	Differentiation, treatment	Acute promyelocytic leukaemia	
			trans-Retinoic acid

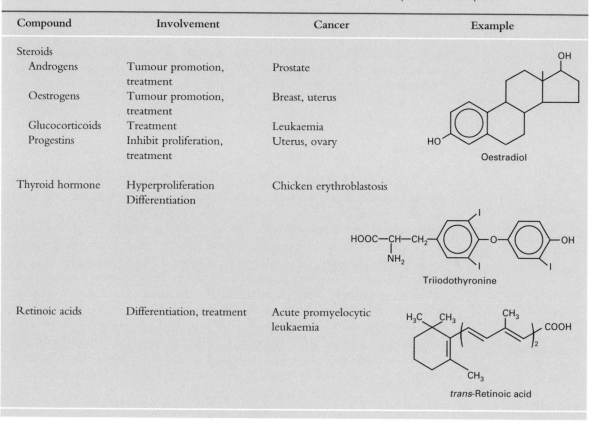

testicular cancer. Oestrogens are mitogens for cells such as those in endometrium and breast that contain oestrogen receptors; this accounts for the elevated risk of cancer at these sites associated with prolonged oestrogen exposure (Table 4.3).

Contraceptive pills contain progestins which, because of their antiproliferative effect, decrease endometrial and ovarian cancer risk (Chapters 4 and 14). Use of anabolic androgens for muscle building is associated with benign liver tumour development.

Manipulation of the sex hormone environment is used in the treatment of hormone-sensitive cancers either by removal of endogenous hormones or by giving antagonists. Glucocorticoids are also used in several treatments (Chapter 13).

Two isomers of retinoic acid exist with different functions. The *trans* isomer binds to both the **r**etinoic **a**cid **r**eceptor **a**lpha (RARA) and the **r**etinoic acid **X r**eceptor (RXR) whereas the *cis* isomer only binds to RXR. This specificity has consequences for normal development as RXR is needed for differentiation responses promoted by vitamin D and thyroid hormone (see below). Altered exposure to vitamin D, thyroid hormone or retinoic acids is not linked with cancer formation although nuclear accidents such as the Chernobyl incident (Chapter 7) increase thyroid cancers by a process involving thyroid hormones. These hormones contain iodine (Table 11.5), and the radioactive isotopes iodine-131 and iodine-125, released from the nuclear reaction, are incorporated into thyroid hormones and concentrated in the thyroid gland. These isotopes emit ionising γ radiation that causes mutational events (Chapter 7). Retinoic acids, vitamin D and thyroid hormones are all agents that induce differentiation and indirectly block proliferation (Chapter 10).

Receptors

Receptors are transcription factors whose function is blocked in the absence of ligand due to conformational restraints imposed by other proteins and hypophosphorylation. Details vary with different receptors but, in general, each receptor protein molecule has a number of overlapping domains, serving different functions (Figure 11.21). Ligand binding to a large C-terminal region dissociates associated proteins such as the **90 kDa h**eat **s**hock **p**rotein (HSP90), which allows dimerisation and exposure of the DNA-binding domain. With the steroid receptors, homodimers between similar receptors are usually formed, but retinoic acids, thyroid hormone and vitamin D act via heterodimers. These heterodimers comprise an RXR plus its *cis* retinoic acid and the relevant other monomer plus ligand (RARA–*trans*-retinoic acid, thyroid hormone receptor–triiodothyronine, vitamin D receptor–1,25-dihydroxy vitamin D3). Dimerisation also requires serine/threonine phosphorylations. The DNA-binding domain is made up of two separate amino acid sequences, each containing Zn^{2+}; these 'zinc fingers' recognise specific DNA base sequences (hormone response elements) in regulatory regions of sensitive genes. It is the amino acid sequence of these fingers plus the base sequence of the response elements that determines which genes are sensitive to which receptor. Other regions of the receptor, known as transactivation domains, bind additional nuclear proteins

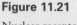

Figure 11.21

Nuclear receptor protein domains and gene transcription.

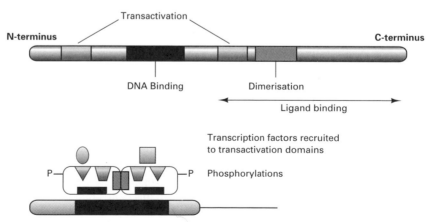

to form the active transcription complex. The coactivator proteins which form part of the transcription factor complex that activates gene transcription (Figure 6.1) can be needed for many genes regulated by pathways other than those discussed here. Furthermore, the coactivators can be present in rate-limiting concentrations so that activation of one gene inactivates others due to competition for coactivators. One such coactivator is **CREB-b**inding **p**rotein (CBP), needed for growth-related genes regulated by jun, fos (Figure 11.15), SMAD (Figure 11.9) and STAT (Figure 11.6). Retinoic acids and other differentiation-inducing ligands may inhibit proliferation by sequestering these rate-limiting coactivators for their own purposes and thus block transcription from the proliferation-related genes. Figure 6.1, which illustrates general transcriptional regulation, could also be used to describe the hormone-related events.

Hormone antagonists, such as the anti-oestrogen tamoxifen and the anti-androgen flutamide, act by binding to the relevant receptor and exposing the DNA-binding domain but not the transactivation domains (Figure 14.1). This means the complex will bind to DNA but not recruit all the other proteins necessary for initiation of transcription. Plant oestrogens (phyto-oestrogens) occur in seeds and vegetables (Chapter 4) and act as anti-oestrogens by this mechanism, but this generalisation should not be pushed too far as phyto-oestrogens can also have agonist properties. Compounds that have both agonist and antagonist effects in a tissue-specific manner are sometimes called selective oestrogen receptor modulators. A second oestrogen receptor, ER-β, has a different ligand specificity and tissue distribution to ER-α (the normal receptor in this book); ER-β may contribute to the selective actions of oestrogens.

Rats have a category of receptors called peroxisome proliferation activating receptors that have been implicated in carcinogenesis but peroxisome proliferation has not been detected in humans.

The presence or absence of receptors is a major determinant of whether or not a cell will respond to a ligand, and their concentrations determine the magnitude of response.

Genes influenced by hormone receptors

Proliferation events mediated by these ligands primarily act via the G_1 checkpoint of the cell cycle. Genes rapidly switched on include myc and fos, whilst those that are more slowly activated include growth factors and their receptors. Oestrogens increase TGF-α production and the number of IGF-I receptors, both events stimulating proliferation. Anti-oestrogens such as tamoxifen block these oestrogen effects but additionally activate genes coding for inhibitory growth factors such as TGF-β. Retinoic acids regulate differentiation-related genes such as osteopontin in bone osteoblasts and lung surfactant protein but the targets are uncertain in myeloid cells where defects occur. Retinoic acid activated receptors can block jun N-terminal kinase and thus antagonise genes containing AP1 regulatory sites (Figure 11.15); many of these are involved in cell proliferation.

Cancer

Changes in receptor type and magnitude occur in cancers. During breast and endometrial carcinogenesis, normal oestrogen receptor is upregulated at the transcriptional level but is then lost in some tumours as they dedifferentiate and become more aggressive. These changes decrease the likelihood of the tumour responding to endocrine treatment (Chapter 13). However, some oestrogen receptor positive breast cancers are resistant to endocrine treatment (Chapter 13); one possible reason is there are other pathways of receptor activation. MAP kinases can phosphorylate and dimerise the receptor in the absence of ligand so polypeptide growth factors produced by cancer cells could provoke hormone-independent growth. Changes in receptor type have been identified in acute promyelocytic leukaemia in which a t(15;17) chromosome translocation disrupts the retinoic acid receptor in its transactivation domain, thereby blocking differentiation (Figure 6.7). A rare type of acute myeloid leukaemia has a translocation between chromosomes 8 and 16 that disrupts CBP coactivator function. This prevents normal, retinoic acid induced differentiation of myeloid cells. In chickens the erythroblastosis virus carries the oncogene v-erbA, which codes for a thyroid receptor homologue and is responsible for generating erythroblastosis, a premalignant condition due to blocked differentiation. The v-erbA has deletions and substitutions in the ligand–binding domain such that the oncogene product blocks normal thyroid receptor binding to its response element.

Prostaglandins

This family of bioactive lipids, formed from a 20-carbon fatty acid, arachidonic acid (Figures 11.13 and 11.22), have multiple cellular effects with important clinical effects as judged from the fact that long-term inhibition of prostaglandin production halves the mortality from colon cancer. This serendipitous observation came to light from clinical trials on the use of **n**on-**s**teroidal **a**nti-**i**nflammatory **d**rugs (NSAIDs) such as aspirin to protect against heart problems and to treat arthritis. NSAIDs work by inhibiting two enzymes, **cycloox**ygenases (COX-1 and COX-2) required for the oxidation of arachidonic acid to produce prostaglandins. Aspirin acetylates a serine –OH at the active site of COX-1 and COX-2, thus preventing prostaglandin synthesis. More selective agents acting by different mechanisms have now been developed (Chapter 14).

COX-1 is constitutively expressed by many cells whereas COX-2 can be selectively induced by many mitogens. COX-2 is upregulated at early stages of colon carcinogenesis whereas COX-2 inhibitors block both adenoma and carcinoma formation in the colon. Prostaglandins have autocrine and paracrine effects on cell proliferation, apoptosis and angiogenesis via adenyl cyclase coupled receptors (Figure 11.10) and by nuclear receptors of the peroxisome proliferator family. The mechanisms involved are not well understood but they include stimulating the production of angiogenic growth factors by cancer cells and promoting proliferation of capillary endothelial cells. NSAIDs promote apoptosis by a ceramide pathway and block angiogenesis by inhibiting the COX enzymes (Figure 11.22). The COX enzymes may have additional functions relevant to

Figure 11.22

Prostaglandins: synthesis, function and NSAID inhibition.

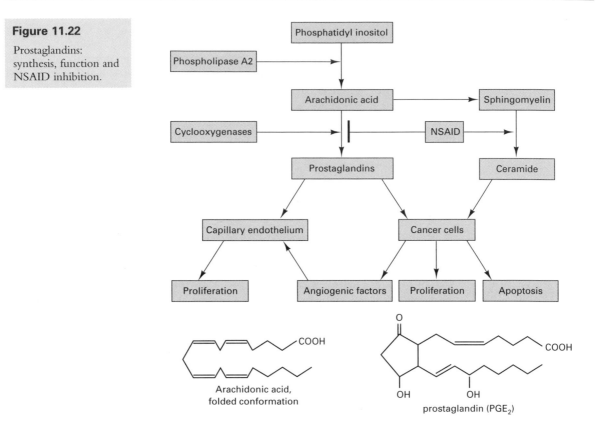

carcinogenesis. Aspirin inhibits acetylaminofluorene binding to DNA suggesting a role for the cyclooxygenases in carcinogen activation (Chapter 7). NSAIDs are being tested as agents for preventing or treating colon cancer but they may also be effective with breast and head/neck cancers (Chapter 14).

Crosstalk between signalling pathways

Normal cells have a network of cross-linked signalling pathways, but it is impossible to do this justice without losing the simple format used here. The interplay between tyrosine and serine/threonine kinase pathways is illustrated in Figure 11.11, and kinase signalling, phosphoinositol and CAMs are illustrated in Figure 11.14; the nuclear receptor and MAP kinase interaction was discussed above.

Under normal circumstances such cross-communications synergise to give fine control of the processes involved. In cancers it means that loss of control of one pathway can result in loss of other regulatory mechanisms to the detriment of the normal cells. It can also result in increased adaptability when it comes to cancer treatments based on manipulation of individual pathways; cancer cells are adept at circumventing the actions of inhibitory drugs by switching to alternative pathways (Chapter 13).

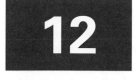

INVASION AND METASTASIS

Key points

- Metastasis is the escape of cancer cells from a primary site and their re-establishment at distant, secondary locations.
- Metastasis is inefficient in that most cells are destroyed in transit, but it is efficient in other ways as most human cancers successfully metastasise.
- Metastasis requires the disruption of local cell–cell interactions, invasion, penetration of blood or lymphatic vessels (intravasation), escape from those vessels (extravasation), migration and growth.
- Metastasis can occur via blood vessels, lymphatics or movement within the body cavities.
- The organ through which the transporting vessels first pass (first-pass organ) is a common site of new growth.
- Tumours metastasise to specific sites. This is determined by the anatomy of the transporting vessels, and by specific features of the cancer cells (the seed) and of the new environment in which they grow (the soil).
- Adhesion molecules help determine sites of metastasis. Local properties such as endothelial function, extracellular matrix composition and growth factor production also contribute.
- Metastases can be dormant for long periods.
- Individual metastases can be of clonal origin.
- Metastasis is a late event in the natural history of carcinogenesis, although early gene changes can influence later events.
- Oncogenes and repressor genes are important. Metastasis inhibitor genes have been identified.
- Invasion and migration require proteolytic enzymes and polypeptide motility factors.
- Two types of protease are required, both of which are generated from inactive proenzymes by the actions of other proteases. Activators and inhibitors of these events exist.
- Arrest of cancer cells within a vessel is a result of passive entrapment or requires the cooperation of lymphocytes, platelets and endothelial cells.
- Extravasation requires attachment to endothelium, dissolution of the basement membrane and migration.
- Growth at both the new primary and any new site requires the formation of new blood vessels (angiogenesis).
- Angiogenesis is activated by a change in the balance of inhibitory and stimulatory polypeptide factors in favour of stimulation. These factors are produced by cancers and normal cells. It can also be stimulated by hypoxia.

Introduction

The processes by which cancer cells escape from their local environment, invade their surroundings, become transported to remote sites and establish new foci of growth, represent the fundamental differences between a benign growth and a malignant growth (Chapter 3). Metastases also create the major clinical problems in handling cancer patients because treatments used for disease confined to the original site (local disease) are often ineffective against metastatic cancer.

At the time of first detection of cancer, about half of patients also have evidence of metastatic foci and it is likely that more patients have undetected, occult metastases. Many clinical oncologists think that cancer should be considered to have spread from the primary site at the time of first detection even if nothing can be detected at this time. Treatments should take note of this possibility.

Metastases can be detected where the primary cancer is small (less than 0.5 cm diameter) but, with most types of cancer, increasing primary size correlates with increased probability of metastasis. However, this is not true when comparisons are made between different types of cancer. Different cancers of similar sizes have variable rates of metastasis.

Although metastasis is an efficient process in the sense that most cancers will generate metastatic deposits, it is inefficient in terms of number of cells successfully moving to a new site. If melanoma cells are injected into an animal's bloodstream, over 99% are destroyed within 24 hours. Another indication of its inefficiency is that about 1 million cells a day are shed from a mammary cancer, less than 0.1% of which can be detected in the blood as they are rapidly destroyed by host defence mechanisms. The small number that do survive create the clinical problems, although that may take a long time to become apparent. Even 10 years after apparently successful breast surgery, some women still die from metastatic disease. Residual cancer cells can remain dormant for long periods. Metastases can themselves metastasise.

In terms of the natural history of cancer development, invasion and metastasis are considered as late stages of progression, which is not to say that contributory changes have not occurred earlier. Thus, ras mutations can increase metastatic potential but is an early gene change in colon carcinogenesis (Chapter 2). The first detected gene alteration in patients with familial adenomatous polyposis coli is in the APC gene that codes for a protein involved in cell–cell adhesion (Chapters 2 and 11), disruption of which is a prerequisite for escape from local control. Hence very early gene changes can contribute to late events in progression.

Both oncogene and repressor gene products are involved in metastatic spread. The ras and APC examples illustrate that point, although a specific metastasis gene has not been identified.

General features

Heterogeneity of metastatic potential

A striking feature of primary tumours is the heterogeneity of behaviour of their constituent cells. This is reflected in variability in expression of tissue antigens such as hormone receptors (breast and prostate cancers), melanin (melanomas) or more general features such as growth rates, drug sensitivity and response to radiation. This heterogeneity is also applicable to metastatic behaviour. There is debate as to whether all or a limited number of cells in a primary growth have metastatic potential but it is clear that, in at least some cases, individual metastases originate from a single cell (clonal origin) and that different metastases can arise from different parent cells. This heterogeneity can be due to either genetic differences of individual cells within a cancer or altered gene expression without observable gene mutations. Localised differences in gene regulation could be regulated by local factors, such as proximity to blood vessels or other cell types producing paracrine growth factors. This is referred to as phenotypic diversity, to convey differences in appearance of individual cells without implying a mutational cause. The definition also covers the fact that the behaviour of individual cells within a cancer can vary independently of nearby cells.

Escape from primary site and establishment at a new site

A formidable number of obstacles must be overcome for cells to grow at sites remote from their original one. That most cancers generate cells capable of achieving this objective points to the survival advantage cancer cells have over their normal counterparts. Only rarely can normal cells achieve growth away from their normal site. Apart from pregnancy, in which a fertilised egg invades the endometrium (lining of the uterus), the only common example is endometriosis, in which endometrial cells grow at sites such as the ovary and peritoneum, accessible from the endometrium via the fallopian tube.

The common cancers in humans arise from epithelial cells, which must break contacts with their neighbours, traverse the basement membrane and migrate through the stroma (invasion) in order to reach blood or lymphatic vessels that will carry them to other parts of the body (Figure 12.1). Invasion distinguishes *in situ* carcinoma from more advanced cancers and it is also one of the properties that differentiates benign and malignant lesions (Chapter 3). Progression to the invasive state also has clinical implications in that invasive cancers are more life-threatening. A breast cancer patient who has only *in situ* carcinoma can be cured by its excision, but this outcome is not as likely with invasive cancer. When the cells reach the vessels, they have to penetrate them (intravasation), avoid destruction during transit to remote sites and then repeat the process at the new site (extravasation). Having reached the metastatic site, the cancers must proliferate in the new environment. Again there are clinical implications regarding cells that successfully complete this series of events. About one-quarter of women whose breast cancer has metastasised to multiple lymph nodes will be alive 10 years after first diagnosis, compared to three-quarters of women with no nodal involvement.

Mesenchymal cancers, such as those arising from bone, have to accomplish a similar set of events with the exception that the cell–cell contacts are different to those seen in epithelia. Leukaemias are exceptional in that normal proliferation

Figure 12.1

Escape of cancer cells to a metastatic site. Within the capillary, cancer cells move as aggregates with other cells (not shown).

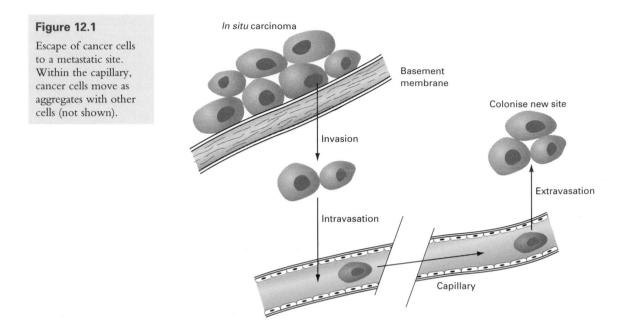

In situ carcinoma

Basement membrane

Invasion

Intravasation

Capillary

Colonise new site

Extravasation

occurs in the bone marrow or spleen, both of which have direct access to blood vessels.

Routes of transport

Three conduits are used for transfer to other sites: blood vessels, lymphatic vessels and movements within the body cavities (Figure 12.2)

Body cavities

The peritoneum and pleural cavities of the lungs (Figure 12.2) are the sites of main interest. Peritoneal spread is available to cancers of organs such as ovary and colon that lie within the peritoneal cavity. Cancer cells invading out from their primary site within such organs reach the surface, break away and are carried within the peritoneal fluid or by direct contact to other sites within the cavity. Secondary growths at the new site can also shed cells and establish multiple foci of disease. This creates two types of clinical problem: how to treat these disseminated growths and what to do about the attendant overproduction of ascitic fluid. Treatment features are dealt with in Chapter 13 but some comment is worthwhile about biological aspects of ascitic fluid. This is an exudate of plasma and as such contains proteins and growth factors that support growth. In effect, it provides a growth medium for cells capable of growing without anchorage (Chapter 2) as well as for foci of cancer cells on the surface of the peritoneum or the organs within it. Peritoneal metastases result in overproduction of ascitic fluid, causing abdominal swelling, so the excess fluid must be removed periodically.

A similar process can occur in the lungs, producing pleural effusions. Cancers in the lung, either primary lung cancers or, more commonly, metastases from other

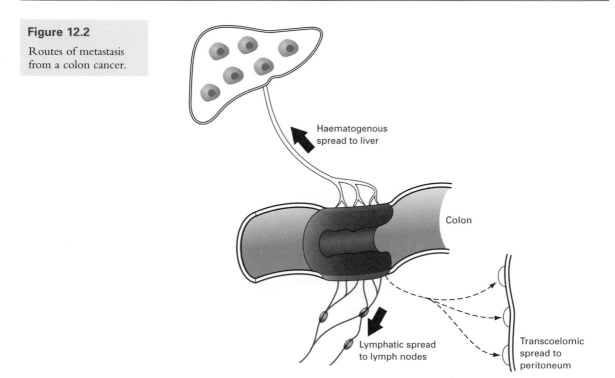

Figure 12.2

Routes of metastasis from a colon cancer.

sites, can colonise the space between the pleural membranes surrounding the lungs. This generates a cancer-containing, growth-supporting fluid (effusion), which must be removed to maintain lung function.

Blood vessels

Capillaries are at the start and finish of cancer cell redistribution within the body. They are constructed from a single layer of endothelial cells that forms the capillary lumen plus an external basement membrane of glycoproteins. They provide the least difficult barrier to entry and exit of cancer cells, as arteries have an additional smooth muscle layer to prevent intravasation and extravasation. Liver is exceptional in that the main afferent vessel, the hepatic portal vein, breaks down into sinusoids where the blood is not in vessels but in direct contact with the hepatocytes (Figure 12.3).

The anatomy of the blood circulation partly determines the sites of metastatic growth (see below). Blood from the gut collects in the hepatic portal vein, passes through the liver and is redistributed by the heart via the lungs (Figure 12.3). Blood from other parts of the lower body enters the inferior vena cava and blood from the head enters the superior vena cava. Liver and lung are therefore common sites for metastatic growth, but other factors also influence choice of sites (see below).

Lymphatic vessels

Lymphatic vessels provide less of a barrier than capillaries in that they do not have a basement membrane. Lymphatic vessels finally drain into the subclavian veins and

Figure 12.3

Transport routes of cancer cells around the body. Arrows indicate direction of flow.

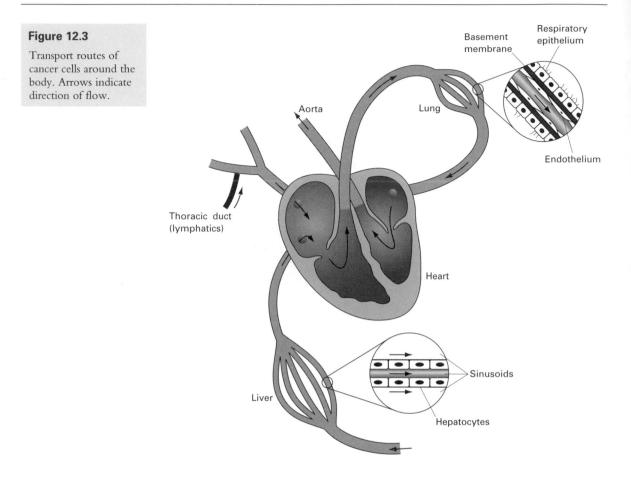

thence into the superior vena cava (Figure 12.3). Hence there is a route whereby cancer cells in lymphatic vessels can reach the general bloodstream.

Preferential sites of metastasis

Different cancers metastasise to different sites and two factors contribute to that variable distribution: the first-pass organ and selective growth of specific cells at different sites.

First-pass organ

The organ first encountered by vessels from a cancerous site frequently supports secondary growth. For blood-borne cells the liver is the main first-pass organ for cells reaching it via the hepatic portal vein (Figure 12.3). This accounts for liver being a common site of metastasis (Table 12.1). The absence of barriers between cancer cells in sinusoids and hepatocytes makes liver an accessible site in which to establish a focus of growth. Because liver function is essential for life and is destroyed during

Table 12.1 Metastatic sites for human cancers.

Primary	Metastatic site*	
	First-pass organ	Other sites
Colon	Liver	Lung
Prostate	Liver	Bone
Breast	Liver	Bone, brain
Melanoma	Liver	Brain, bowel
Head and neck	Lung	–

* Blood-borne. Lymph nodes are the first-pass organ for lymphatic spread.

cancer growth, metastases at this site are a cause of death. Venous drainage from the head enters the superior vena cava, missing the liver, so the first-pass organ is the heart. Attachment and extravasation are difficult in this organ so the cells pass on to the lung, which is the main metastatic site for head/neck tumours.

Lymphatic vessels drain into lymph nodes near the affected site. Thus, breast cancers are frequently detected in lymph nodes in the armpit and can be felt externally as enlargements. Their detection forms part of initial monitoring of patients and lymph node positivity or negativity is a major determinant of life expectancy in such patients (Chapter 13).

Final lymphatic drainage is via the lymphatic and thoracic ducts into the superior vena cava, which thus forms a connection with the blood system to allow wider dissemination of cancer cells.

Seed and soil

The sites of only about half of metastases can be predicted from anatomic features such as blood supply to the region. Thus lung cancers often metastasise to the brain whereas liver would be the anticipated organ based on blood-borne transport. There are additional homing mechanisms that attract certain cancers to specific sites. At the end of the nineteenth century Paget noted that successful metastasis required cancer cells (the seed) and the correct environment (soil) in which to grow. Few early concepts about cancer have withstood the test of time but his 'seed and soil' concept is an exception. In modern parlance the seed represents the cancer cells and the soil represents tissues in which the appropriate blend of growth factors whilst extracellular matrix (ECM) could be recognised by cancer cell receptors (Figure 12.4); the soil provides a homing mechanism by supporting growth.

Escape from local control and invasion

This first step in metastasis involves the breaking of links with, and control by, adjacent cells followed by migration through the stroma to blood/lymphatic vessels. The cells that have broken away from the tumour mass must also have the potential

219

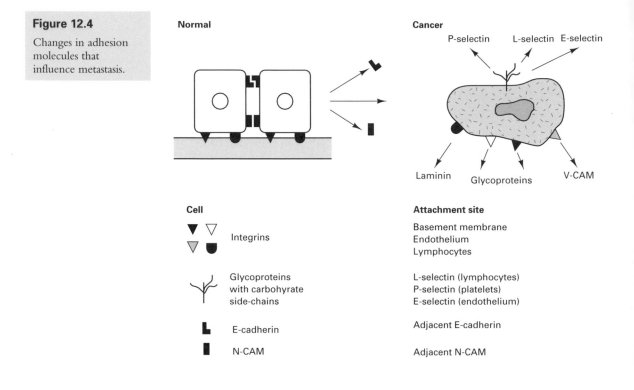

Figure 12.4

Changes in adhesion molecules that influence metastasis.

Normal

Cancer

P-selectin   L-selectin   E-selectin

Laminin   Glycoproteins   V-CAM

Cell

Integrins

Glycoproteins with carbohyrate side-chains

E-cadherin

N-CAM

Attachment site

Basement membrane
Endothelium
Lymphocytes

L-selectin (lymphocytes)
P-selectin (platelets)
E-selectin (endothelium)

Adjacent E-cadherin

Adjacent N-CAM

to invade those vessels (intravasation), form new associations with other cell types, evade destruction within the vessels, escape (extravasation) and invade their new surroundings. Many of the processes involved in extravasation are analogous to those required for local escape and intravasation, and as more information is available about extravasation, detailed discussion of the events involved in migration and invasion will be made in that section.

Molecules that mediate many of these interactions between cells and their immediate environment are called **c**ell **a**dhesion **m**olecules (CAMs) and they can be considered as receptors and ligands. An alternative nomenclature refers to receptors and counter-receptors because it is not always obvious which is the receptor and which is the ligand. The CAM terminology will be used here. The molecular characteristics of the molecules involved are described in Chapter 10, so only their biological functions are described here. Because this is an active area of current research, overlapping and confusing terminologies abound. For example, the general term CAM is also used to describe specific receptors with immunoglobulin-like sequences in their extracellular domains. When used in this context, CAM is prefixed by a capital letter to designate their original site of identification, even though this is inappropriate in some cases. Thus, the prefixes N and V refer to **n**erve and (blood) **v**essel, respectively, even though their expression is not confined to these cell types.

Three types of recognition process are important: (i) recognition of similar cells (homotypic); (ii) recognition of dissimilar cells (heterotypic); and (iii) cell–ECM interactions.

Cell–cell recognition

Normal cells

Homotypic interactions between normal epithelial cells are formed by morphological entities such as desmosomes, tight junctions and gap junctions. At the molecular level, cadherins and CAMs are involved through their interaction with similar molecules on the lateral faces of adjacent cells (Figure 12.4). Cadherins have cell-specific distributions, with E-cadherin being especially important in epithelial cells. N-CAM mediates homotypic interaction in colon epithelium, whilst V-CAM on activated endothelium binds integrins $(\alpha_4\beta_1)$ on lymphocytes (heterotypic interaction). The heterotypic interaction between endothelium and lymphocytes is required for the normal response to inflammation and tissue injury.

Cancer cells

Breaking of homotypic recognition and changes in heterotypic recognition are characteristic of invasive and metastatic cancers. Proteins like E-cadherin and N-CAM that promote homotypic recognition function as repressor proteins in that their loss facilitates escape from local control. This is seen in experimental and clinical settings. Experimentally, antibodies that block cadherin function increase metastatic potential, whereas overexpression of either E-cadherin or N-CAM has the opposite effect. E-cadherin is lost at an early stage of breast carcinogenesis; and loss of N-CAM in gliomas is associated with a high probability of metastasis.

Inactivating mutations in the extracellular domain of E-cadherin have been identified in epithelial cancers such as gastric and prostate carcinoma. In keeping with the general principle of cancer cells using multiple mechanisms to achieve the same objective, E-cadherin can also be functionally inactivated by the indirect route, i.e. mutation of the APC protein that mediates signal transduction from E-cadherin to the cytoskeleton.

Cell–ECM interactions

Normal cells

Integrins provide a major mechanism whereby cells recognise proteins in the extracellular matrix and basement membrane. This family of receptors are formed from a range of α and β subunits, the heterodimer of α and β chains forming the active receptor. Ligands include collagen IV, laminin and fibronectin (basement membrane), and collagen I, laminin and fibronectin (stroma). Specificity as to which ligand is recognised is determined by which α and β subunits make up the receptor (Table 11.4).

Interaction with the basement membrane provides an important mechanism for regulating cell function. Normal breast epithelium in culture will only express differentiated functions such as milk protein production if grown on an artificial basement membrane. The reason for this is that the gene for one such protein, casein, has regulatory sequences that respond to signals from adhesion molecules. In the absence of these signals, transcription of the gene does not occur. Given the inverse relationship between differentiation and proliferation, loss of basement membrane interaction in cancers would indirectly generate a more aggressive phenotype. Anchorage-independent growth of cultured cells is a laboratory index of that increased aggressiveness and reflects the altered link between substrate attachment and cell proliferation (Chapter 11).

Integrins transduce signals from the extracellular matrix and sometimes heterotypic cells to the cytoskeleton. Cells have specialised regions of their membrane called focal adhesions that link the extracellular matrix to the cytoskeleton and other intracellular functions (Box 11.1). Focal adhesions are sites of integrin accumulation and binding of these receptors to their matrix ligands activate cytoskeletal changes by interaction with a **f**ocal **a**dhesion **k**inase (FAK) capable of phosphorylating its own or other tyrosine residues. Such phosphorylations result from mitogenic signals such as growth factors and are required for the proliferative response (Figures 11.7 and 11.18).

The $\alpha_3\beta_1$ integrin is localised on the basal surface of normal epithelial cells, where it binds to laminin in the basement membrane (Figure 12.4).

Cancer cells

Integrin changes resulting from carcinogenesis cannot be defined in simple terms of increase or decrease, but cancers often have different types and membrane distributions of these receptors compared with their normal counterparts. In general, integrins involved in tissue organisation are decreased whereas those needed for migration are not. Several integrin changes relevant to carcinogenesis are listed in Table 11.4, and the increased expression of $\alpha_V\beta_3$ illustrates the influence integrins can have on invasion and metastasis. $\alpha_V\beta_3$ has a broad ligand specificity, is little expressed on normal cells but is increased on melanoma cells and normal endothelium participating in cancer-directed angiogenesis (see below). The ability of this integrin to recognise virtually any of the glycoproteins of the ECM means that cells expressing $\alpha_V\beta_3$ can migrate over whatever matrices they encounter on their route to distant parts. The integrin's ability to bind metalloproteinases also helps digest a path through the ECM. Upregulation of $\alpha_V\beta_3$ coincides with the appearance of a more aggressive growth pattern. Melanomas initially expand radially but invasion is heralded by a change in direction to vertical growth. Upregulation of $\alpha_V\beta_3$ integrin occurs at this stage. In contrast to these increased expressions, $\alpha_2\beta_1$ that recognises laminin and collagen, is decreased in colon and breast cancers.

Laminin receptors (integrins $\alpha_3\beta_1$ and $\alpha_6\beta_1$) are frequently upregulated in epithelial cancers such as those of endometrium and breast; their distribution is altered such that they are found throughout the cell membrane, not just in the basal region.

Upregulation of all types of protease (serine/threonine, cysteine, aspartate and metalloproteinases) is a common event in carcinogenesis, with increased secretion of plasminogen activator, a serine protease, preceding the acquisition of anchorage-independent growth in culture (Figure 2.6). Activation of these enzymes facilitates invasion, extra- and intravasation, and angiogenesis (see below).

Intravasation

Cancer cells attach to the stromal face of the blood vessel basement membrane, digest that membrane with proteases (see below) and migrate between the endothelial cells into the bloodstream. Entry into lymphatic vessels is easier because there is no basement membrane to circumvent.

Bloodstream transport

Cells are carried in the direction of blood flow; whilst they are in the bloodstream, cells must first avoid destruction and then have their movement arrested at potential sites of new growth. The bloodstream is a hostile environment with greater than 99% of injected cancer cells being destroyed by a combination of mechanical stresses, proteolytic destruction and surveillance by the host immune system. Immune surveillance can also occur outside the vessels; it involves cells of the immune system and **m**ajor **h**istocompatibilty **c**omplex (MHC) proteins on the cancer cells (Chapter 5).

The contribution of host immune surveillance to metastatic spread is a subject of debate because, other than viral cancers in which foreign proteins are expressed, cancer cells are composed of host proteins that are unlikely to activate the immune system. Strains of mice that are immunodeficient due to lack of T-cells do not develop increased numbers of metastases when injected with cancer cells, but they do have natural killer cells capable of destroying abnormal cells, so this does not rule out a host contribution. On the other hand, MHC changes are commonplace in cancer cells. MHC-I proteins are required for antigen presentation to cytotoxic T-cells, so loss of MHC proteins should give the cancer cell a survival advantage (Chapter 5). In experimental systems, overexpression of MHC-I proteins decreases metastatic potential, and metastatic potential is inversely correlated with MHC-I expression in a range of melanoma cell lines. Clinically, lymph node metastases from breast, colon and kidney cancers have lower expression of MHC-I proteins than the primaries from which they were derived.

Cancer cells are transported in the blood as single cells or as aggregates (emboli) of several cancer cells, lymphocytes and adhering platelets (Figure 12.5). Formation of emboli may provide protection from mechanical stress and immune attack. The formation of emboli also facilitates attachment to the endothelium and therefore helps arrest the cancer cells at potential metastatic sites.

Extravasation

Escape from the vessel involves three steps: (i) attachment to the endothelial lining; (ii) retraction of the endothelial cells followed by cancer cell attachment to, and destruction of, the basement membrane; and (iii) migration into the surrounding stroma (Figure 12.5).

223

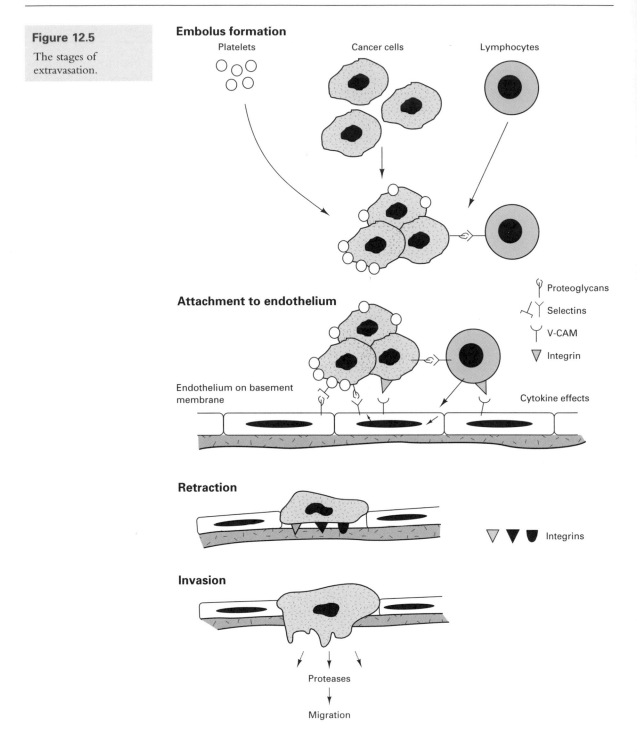

Figure 12.5

The stages of extravasation.

Embolus formation

Platelets

Cancer cells

Lymphocytes

Proteoglycans

Selectins

V-CAM

Integrin

Attachment to endothelium

Endothelium on basement membrane

Cytokine effects

Retraction

Integrins

Invasion

Proteases

Migration

Arrest within the blood vessel

Arrest within the blood vessel occurs by attachment of cancer cell aggregates, lymphocytes and platelets (emboli) to the capillary endothelial cells; each of the three cell types that constitute the embolus participate in this process. Platelets interact with fibrinogen on the endothelial surface, and via their P-selectin they interact with endothelial proteoglycans. Endothelia from different tissues vary in their properties and this contributes to the site specificity of metastases. Endothelial cells carry organ-specific cell membrane determinants, some of which have been identified as CAMs and selectins. Endothelial E-selectins bind to proteoglycans on the tumour cells, the proteoglycans being characterised by sialylated fucosylated lactosamine side chains. $\alpha_4\beta_1$ integrins on both the tumour cell and lymphocytes contribute to this initial braking of the embolus movement and its tethering to the endothelium. This weak, heterophylic cell interaction does not achieve complete arrest; stronger cell interactions between $\alpha_4\beta_1$ integrins and endothelial V-CAM (Table 11.4) are required to achieve that. Normal endothelium expresses low levels of V-CAM but cytokines (interleukin-1, tumour necrosis factor) from both lymphocytes and tumour cells upregulate V-CAM expression. Strong interaction between tumour cell, lymphocytes and endothelium results from clustering of the integrins (affinity modulation) that form multiple interactions with V-CAM (Chapter 11). This generates a localised 'stop' mechanism. Endothelia from many sites express V-CAM but L-CAM is present in lung; this provides a degree of selectivity as to which metastatic site is selected (soil). .

The process just described is a normal response to tissue injury, with T-cells accumulating at an inflammation site providing the cytokines. Cancers use this mechanism to stop their movement by interaction of endothelial V-CAM with integrins on the cancer cell. This heterotypic cell interaction is the first phase of extravasation.

An analogous process, involving endothelial selectins and carbohydrate side chains on cancer cell membrane proteins or attached platelets, contributes to arrest of movement. Cytokine induction of E- and P-selectins on the endothelial surface are capable of recognising carbohydrate side chains on the cancer cells (E-selectin) or platelets (P-selectin) that form the embolus. Many cancers have ill-defined, altered expression of surface glycoproteins that facilitate this heterotypic interaction.

Escape from the blood vessel

Retraction of the endothelial cells exposes the glycoproteins of the basement membrane, to which the cancer cells attach and then digest with proteases and glycosidases. The basement membrane proteins include laminin, collagen IV and fibronectin, which are ligands for the integrin family of receptors on the cancer cell surface (Figure 12.5). Different cancers display distinct patterns of integrins. Thus, bone cancers (osteosarcomas) have increased $\alpha_1\beta_1$ integrin whereas colon cancers possess $\alpha_6\beta_4$ forms. As $\alpha_1\beta_1$ recognises collagen and laminin whereas $\alpha_6\beta_4$ binds laminin, it follows that glycoprotein composition of basement membrane and extracellular matrix of a target site can contribute to 'soil' specificity. Differential expression of laminin receptor also influences 'soil' specificity. Epithelial cancers, such as those originating from colon, lung and breast, have high expression of this receptor whereas non-epithelial cancers like bone and brain do not.

Proteases involved in metastatic spread

Endopetidases involved in metastatic spread are used at three stages: (i) invasion of the primary growth site; (ii) digestion of the endothelial basement membrane; and (iii) invasion of the metastatic site. Two major types of protease are secreted by the cancers, categorised according to whether or not they require Zn^{2+} or Ca^{2+} (metalloproteinases): those that require the ions are collagenase types I and IV and stromolysin; those that do not require the ions have a serine residue at the active site (serine proteases) and plasminogen is an example.

A feature common to both categories is that these proteases are secreted as inactive proenzymes, which must be activated by other proteases (Figure 12.6). Tissue inhibitors of activation also exist such that invasion can be influenced by any of three components: the amount of proenzyme, the activator (a protease) and the inhibitor (a protease inhibitor). All these components can be produced by normal cells but their balance is altered in cancers in favour of proteolysis.

The serine protease precursor plasminogen is converted to the active protease plasmin by other proteases called plasminogen activators (Figure 12.7). These activators must themselves be proteolytically converted from inactive, proenzyme forms. Plasminogen activators are categorised as tissue-type (tPA) or urokinase-type (uPA). This nomenclature, based on their original characterisation, can be confusing because it is uPA that is most important in tissue proteolysis whereas the prime function of tPA is to dissolve blood clots. Antibodies directed against uPA inhibit invasion whereas overexpression has the opposite effect. Synthetic inhibitors of uPA such as amiloride also decrease the number of metastatic colonies in model systems. Cancer cells have membrane receptors for uPA, which concentrate that enzyme along with associated proteolytic activity at centres of active invasion.

Metalloproteinases fall into three categories as defined by their substrate specificity. Collagenses such as MMP1 digest collagens I, II, III, VII, VIII and X; gelatinases like

Figure 12.6

General features of extracellular protein digestion.

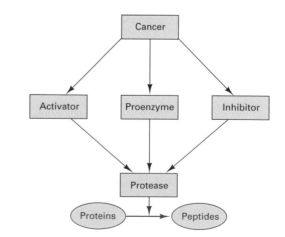

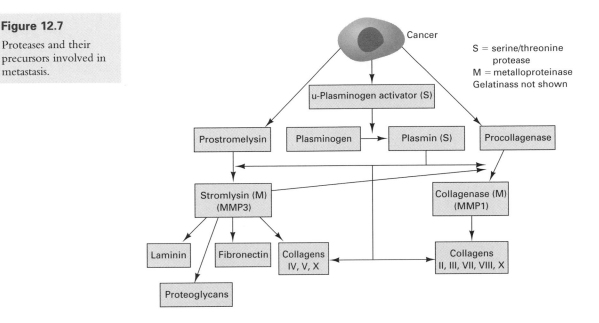

Figure 12.7

Proteases and their precursors involved in metastasis.

MMP2 digest gelatin, fibronectin, elastin and collagens I, IV, V, VII and X; and stromelysins (MMP3) hydrolyse fibronectin, laminin and collagens IV, V and IX. Thus, the MMPs can digest all the individual components of the ECM and remove physical barriers to metastasis. In addition to these secreted MMPs, a few transmembrane members of the family exist. MMPs are secreted as latent proenzymes that have their prodomains removed by the extracellular serine protease, plasmin or other MMPs (Figure 12.7). Plasmin can thus serve two functions, digestion of the ECM and activation of MMPs. The active site of MMPs contains a histidine.glutamate.any amino acid.glycine.histidine motif; the two histidines coordinate the Zn^{2+} that is essential for activity. Tissue inhibitors of metalloproteinases (TIMP) can also be secreted by cells, and if this occurs it is associated with decreased metastatic potential. TIMPs are broad-spectrum inhibitor proteins that form complexes with MMPs. They all contain cysteine residues arranged so that six intrachain —S—S— bonds are formed. Synthetic MMP inhibitors are currently being tested as potential antimetastatic drugs (Chapter 13).

Digestion products of ECM glycoproteins such as collagen XVIII and plasminogen can influence angiogenesis (see below).

Migration

After extravasation the cancer cells must migrate to their new site of growth. This requires continued production of proteases to digest the matrix but additional features are also important. Migration is achieved by alternate attachment of the leading edge of the cell to matrix proteins and detachment of the rear edge. Integrins in the cancer membrane mediate these events by transducing the external signals from the matrix to the actin cytoskeleton of the cell. Movement is achieved by contraction and relaxation of this cytoskeleton (Box 11.1).

Peptides released during proteolysis of matrix also act as chemotactic agents to attract additional cancer cells to the region. Proteolysis of matrix proteins does not always destroy the peptide sequences that form the binding site of the protein. Such peptides are capable of binding to integrins, thereby blocking cell attachment to the matrix and facilitating movement elsewhere.

Another class of polypeptides called motility factors are also important for migration as they stimulate movement by different mechanisms to those just mentioned. They can be produced by normal cells and act in a paracrine manner on cancer cells, or they can be produced by cancer cells themselves and have an autocrine action. The names of these factors, such as autocrine motility factor, scatter factor and migration-stimulating factor, reflect their original method of detection.

As with the related growth factors, surface receptors exist that can be altered in cancers. In the case of scatter factor, the receptor is a tyrosine kinase coded by the c-met oncogene. Little is known about post-receptor events.

Growth

Proliferation of the cancer cells at their new site is initially confined to a cuff of cells within 1 mm of the blood vessel. This growth occurs under the influence of locally produced growth factors and the distance is largely determined by the diffusion of oxygen from the blood. For further growth, new blood vessels must be formed (angiogenesis) to supply essential nutrients and oxygen.

Angiogenesis

Angiogenesis is the rate-limiting step that determines whether or not a metastasis remains dormant or grows to a size greater than about 1 mm. Although this section will discuss angiogenesis in the context of metastatic spread, remember that the same process is essential for the establishment of primary tumours at their initial site of genesis (Figure 2.3).

Capillaries form a web of vessels between the afferent, arterial blood supply and the efferent, venous conduits. They are composed of a single layer of endothelial cells attached to a basement membrane (Figure 12.8) across which nutrients and gases such as oxygen can diffuse. Cells within capillaries cannot usually escape into the stroma but normal events such as inflammation permeabilise the endothelium, so leucocytes can penetrate between adjacent cells to counteract the inflammation. Endothelial cells are normally quiescent, having low proliferation rates, and mitoses are rarely seen. Angiogenesis (neovascularisation) occurs in three phases. It is initiated by tumour-derived growth factors that, by paracrine routes, stimulate local endothelial proliferation as sprouts which penetrate towards the source (the cancer) of those growth factors. This invasive and proliferative phase requires extensive remodelling of the ECM through protease digestion of the existing glycoproteins, formation of a new ECM, altered cell–ECM contacts and directional chemotactic stimuli to promote the endothelial sprout towards the cancer (Figure 12.8). These events occur at numerous capillary sites such that individual sprouts fuse to form a new capillary bed in and around the cancer. This final phase involves maturation and differentiation of the endothelial cells, formation of

Figure 12.8

The phases of angiogenesis.

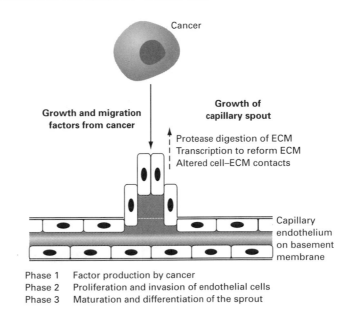

Phase 1 Factor production by cancer
Phase 2 Proliferation and invasion of endothelial cells
Phase 3 Maturation and differentiation of the sprout

the basement membrane and recruitment of ancillary cells. Only about 10% of metastatic cells become angiogenic, some die but others remain as dormant foci that can be reactivated. Initiation of angiogenesis is due to increased tumour secretion of mitogenic growth factors such as platelet-derived growth factor, **f**ibroblast **g**rowth **f**actor (FGF) and **v**ascular **e**ndothelial **g**rowth **f**actor (VEGF), of which FGF and VEGF are particularly important. Their production is low in normal cells but is upregulated in cancers and in normal cells existing in a low-oxygen environment (hypoxia). Thus, inadequate blood supply can generate hypoxia, promote angiogenesis and increase oxygen and nutrient availability. Oxygen can only diffuse short distances (< 1 mm) from the supplying capillaries, so the further they are from the capillary, the more hypoxic the cancer cells become. In small foci of cells, the hypoxia is not sufficient to kill the cells by necrosis but it does inhibit proliferation (Figure 2.3). Both normal and cancer cells have a mechanism for overcoming this adverse effect by increasing the local blood supply. The low oxygen tension activates a series of serine/threonine protein kinases, the **s**tress **a**ctivated **p**rotein **k**inases (SAPKs), which stimulates transcription from specific genes via **h**ypoxia-**i**nduced transcription **f**actors (HIFs); see Chapter 11. One such is the gene for VEGF, which has specific base sequences in its promoter (HIF response element) that bind HIFs. There is also a hypoxia-sensitive, HIF-independent mechanism for increasing VEGF; proteins bind to the 3′ untranslated region of the mRNA (Figure 6.1) and stabilise the mRNA. Transforming events such as ras activation also upregulate VEGF secretion, as do growth factors like EGF (Figure 12.9). The supressor gene VHL (**v**on **H**ippel–Landau), codes for a protein that inhibits functions which depend on hypoxia-inducible genes such as VEGF; this is due to destabilisation of the mRNA involved. Loss of this inhibitory function, as occurs in some kidney tumours, activates angiogenesis; cancers in which this occurs are hypervascularised. VEGF is secreted as a large glycoprotein that can be proteolytically cleaved to a smaller, but still active protein. Like FGF, VEGF can be stored as inactive

Figure 12.9

Influence of hypoxia on angiogenesis.

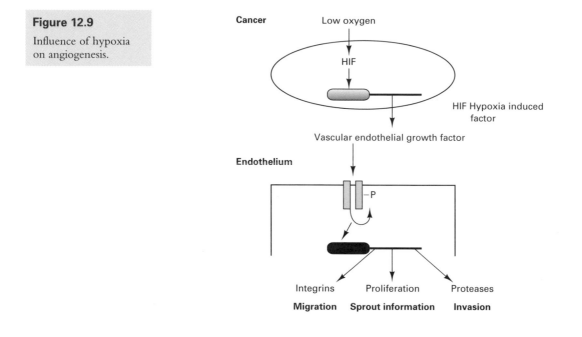

complexes with ECM proteoglycans like heparan; the active growth factor is released by ECM digestion (Figure 12.10).

The paracrine effect of VEGF is mediated via transmembrane receptors that are only present on endothelial cells, so VEGF is only mitogenic at this site; FGF receptors have a wider distribution. VEGF and FGF have synergistic effects on endothelial cells. VEGF receptors are typical tyrosine kinase receptors in that they require dimerisation, tyrosine phosphorylation of the cytoplasmic domain and recruitment of SH domain proteins (Chapter 11); recruited proteins include phospholipase C, GAP and phosphatidylinositol-3-kinase, each capable of transducing the proliferative signal to the endothelial cell nucleus (Figure 12.9 and Chapter 11). The VEGF receptor gene also contains an HIF response element and is activated by hypoxia. In addition to these proliferative effects, VEGF also promotes the secretion of serine proteinases and metalloproteinases as well as inducing integrins, VCAM and ICAM, all of which facilitate capillary sprout invasion of the ECM.

Several polypeptide inhibitors of angiogenesis have been identified, e.g. angiostatin, endostatin and thrombospondin. The thrombospondin gene is activated by p53 (Figure 6.13) and this helps to block angiogenesis; mutant p53 does not have this effect. Angiostatin and endostatin are partial proteolytic products of plasminogen and collagen XVIII respectively; they may act by binding to and blocking growth factor receptors needed for endothelial proliferation. In a normal cell mass the balance of inhibitors and activators favours inhibition; cancers shift this balance to favour activation (Figure 12.10).

Invasion of the ECM is mediated in part by serine proteases and metalloproteinases secreted at the leading edge of the sprout in response to VEGF. Migration towards the cancer also involves attachment to the remodelled ECM, helped by the altered profile of endothelial integrins. The upregulation of $\alpha_V\beta_3$ by

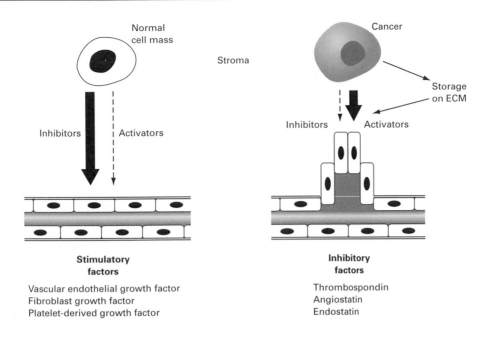

Figure 12.10

Activators and
inhibitors of
angiogenesis.

VEGF helps because the broad ligand specificity of this integrin enables interaction between endothelial sprout and diverse types of ECM (Chapter 11). As these interactions are needed for cell migration (Box 11.1), cell migration is enhanced by $\alpha_V\beta_3$ expression. And angiogenic growth factor FGF induces integrin, $\alpha_V\beta_5$.

Angiogenesis involves more than proliferation and proteolysis. Capillary sprouts extend out towards the source of angiogenic stimuli, such as a clump of tumour cells, so chemotaxis is also important. The molecules involved in its regulation must reflect this fact, so it is not surprising that fibroblast growth factor (FGF), a potent angiogenic factor, can stimulate all three of the required properties: proliferation, protease secretion and chemotaxis of endothelial cells.

The maturation and differentiation phase of angiogenesis includes processes that determine the direction of blood flow. Smooth muscle cells are recruited to capillaries destined to become afferent arterioles but not those destined to become efferent venules. Little is known about the underlying mechanisms involved in adult life, but in embryos the boundary between these two types of vessel is marked by differential expression of proteins. At the junction, the potential arterial endothelial cell expresses a transmembrane ligand (an ephrin) that interacts with an ephrin tyrosine kinase receptor (Tie) only present on the adjacent venous endothelial cell. These proteins may play an as yet indeterminate role in angiogenesis linked to metastatic spread of cancer.

Now that the basic features of angiogenesis are known, attention is being focused on their manipulation for therapeutic purposes. Avenues of investigation include blocking $\alpha_V\beta_3$ integrins with neutralising antibodies, inhibiting MMPs with synthetic peptides and increasing levels of inhibitors like endostatin (Chapter 13). Some of the components associated with angiogenesis can also help to determine subsequent behaviour of a cancer at the time it is first detected (prognostic use). Antibodies against several of the proteins can be used as histochemical stains to identify vessels in tissue sections. A high vessel density correlates with poor survival in breast and prostate cancers, and sometimes the angiogenic switch (appearance of new capillaries) can be seen microscopically before the invasive cancer is evident. Thus, in cervical carcinogenesis, angiogenesis begins in the preinvasive CIN II–III stages (Chapter 2) before invasion begins. This fits with the view that angiogenesis is a rate-limiting event in cancer formation at the primary stage as well as during metastasis (discussed here).

Gene changes involved in metastasis

Many gene products that influence metastatic spread have been mentioned in the preceding sections of this chapter. An important point to note is that different pathways are utilised by different cancers so there is no gene change that is common to all cancers. A caveat to this generalisation is that the gene products involved in angiogenesis are common to all cancers.

Both oncogenes and repressors are involved in metastasis, some of which have been implicated in other aspects of cancer biology. Thus, ras activation is associated with increased proliferation and is an early event in colon carcinogenesis. Ras-transfected cells have increased metastatic potential. Other oncogenes such as v–src and v–raf can also increase proliferation, tumorigenicity (transformation in culture) and invasiveness. Although properties such as transformation and proliferation are essential for metastasis, the following experiment shows how they can be separated. Experimentally, ras transforms some cells without affecting metastasis, whilst viruses such as adenovirus can block metastatic properties of ras but not its transforming effect. This indicates that transformation and metastasis can be divorced and metastasis is not simply a consequence of early events in carcinogenesis and proliferation. It is not clear how changes in a gene such as ras can influence transformation in some situations and metastasis in others. As ras is a focal point for multiple upstream and downstream signal pathways (Chapter 10), it is possible that different responses are modulated in different cells.

The additional gene changes required for metastasis are poorly defined. Genes involved in angiogenesis, protease production and cell adhesion molecules are clearly important but others have yet to be characterised. Fusion of metastatic mouse melanoma cells with normal cells can produce non-metastatic hybrids, which indicates that normal cells contain something that inhibits metastasis. Several putative metastasis-repressing genes have been identified. One such gene is nm23 (**non-m**etastatic protein **23**), which has clinical relevance in that its loss is correlated with increased metastasis in some tumours, e.g. liver tumours. However, nm23 changes do not occur in all tumours and it is actually increased in cancers such as ovary. The function of nm23 is obscure. It has nucleoside diphosphate kinase activity but this can be blocked without effect on its metastasis-inhibiting properties. The mammalian nm23 gene has a homologue in fruit flies, AWD, that is required for wing and eye development, so cell–cell interaction and differentiation may be involved.

The cell adhesion molecule CD44 may be linked to metastatic spread. Expression of normal CD44 is decreased in metastatic colon and breast cancers whereas variant CD44s present a confusing picture – increased in some cases and decreased in others (Chapter 11).

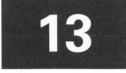

PRINCIPLES OF CANCER TREATMENT

Key points

- Treatment is required when a cancer is first detected and at later stages if it spreads to other parts of the body.
- Surgical removal of as much of the cancer as possible is important.
- If a cancer has metastasised, drugs or radiotherapy are used.
- The fewer cells there are when treatment begins, the greater the probability of achieving a cure.
- The objective of treatment is to prevent proliferation (cytostatic effect) and to kill the cancer cells (cytotoxic effect).
- Cell sensitivity to therapeutic agents varies at different times of the cell cycle.
- Future behaviour of a cancer can be predicted from its characteristics at the time of first treatment. The useful characteristics are tumour size, degree of spread from the original site, histological appearance and biochemical markers of growth and aggressiveness.
- Chemotherapy disrupts DNA synthesis and cell division by mechanisms common to all cells. This causes side effects.
- Optimal drug treatment reflects a compromise between effects on the cancer and toxicity to normal tissues.
- Drugs used in chemotherapy include alkylating agents that damage DNA, antimetabolites that inhibit nucleic acid synthesis and natural products that have several effects.
- Combinations of drugs are more effective than single agents.
- Chemotherapy is used as a primary (neoadjuvant) therapy or as an adjuvant to other types of treatment. It is the main method for treating advanced cancer.
- Cancers arising from hormone-sensitive cells regress if deprived of hormone. This receptor-mediated process is not common to all cells so hormone treatment has fewer side effects than chemotherapy.
- Radiotherapy generates DNA strand breaks through free radical formation.
- Photodynamic therapy involves laser activation of sensitive compounds that generate free radicals.
- Cells with DNA damaged by chemotherapy or radiotherapy die by the apoptotic pathway.
- New forms of treatment are being investigated based on interference with signal transduction, gene function, angiogenesis or cytokine action. Improved immunotherapy is also a goal.
- Cells within a cancer have heterogeneous sensitivities to drugs. This can be due

to properties of the cells, to their place in the cell cycle or their distance from blood vessels.

- Resistance to drugs is acquired as a result of treatment. This can be due to altered cell permeability, altered metabolism, increased number of targets or more efficient DNA repair.

Introduction

The options available when a cancer has been detected and needs treatment are illustrated in Figure 13.1. If it is localised, surgical removal of the primary cancer may be accompanied by additional (adjuvant) drug or radiation treatment to kill residual cancer. The period from first treatment for primary cancer to the appearance of first metastasis (relapse) is called the relapse-free or disease-free survival; the longer this period, the better the outlook for the patient. If the primary cancer has been detected at an early stage, the patient can be cured. If all the original cancer is not removed, a metastatic growth appears that is not amenable to surgery; additional forms of therapy are required. These are infrequently curative and death eventually results. The period from first detection to death is called the overall survival time.

The ideal treatment would be one that removed all the cancer cells without affecting normal cells; such a treatment does not exist and may be unattainable. Treatments are based on preventing growth; given that growth is such a general property of cells, methods designed to stop it will inevitably have side effects. Therefore, the objective of all current treatments is to maximise effects on the cancer

Figure 13.1

Detection and treatment: clinical events.

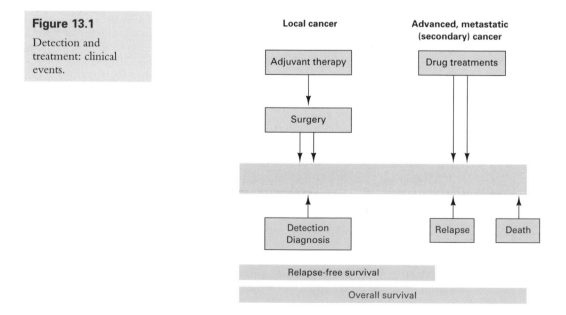

whilst minimising adverse side effects on normal tissues. For established cancers, surgical removal of a tumour mass is the best approach but it has limitations. Cancers of blood cells, leukaemias, are not amenable to surgery and the same is true for solid cancers that have metastasised to inaccessible sites like bone and brain.

Drug treatment is the most widely used alternative therapy to surgery; the majority of drug treatments are designed to disrupt cell proliferation. The term 'chemotherapy' is used to describe treatments based on drugs that have a broad cell specificity because they affect cell processes such as DNA synthesis and cell proliferation common to all cells: side effects inevitably ensue. On the other hand, major cancers such as those of the prostate, breast and endometrium can be susceptible to more specific treatments based on differentiation properties of the cells. Growth modulation of such cells is achieved by factors specific to these cell types, like the male (androgens) and female (oestrogens, progestogens) sex steroids. Hormone therapy therefore generates fewer side effects than chemotherapy. The term 'drug' will be used here where no distinction is made between chemotherapeutic agents and other chemicals used for growth control. DNA can be irreversibly damaged by ionising radiation such as X-rays, and X-rays are widely used in radiotherapy to kill cancer cells, often in conjunction with surgery.

Compounds used for treatment are described as being cytotoxic or cytostatic depending, respectively, on whether they kill the cells or only stop proliferation of the cells. Cytotoxic drugs have the potential to cure a patient whereas cytostatic drugs can prevent further growth but not always eliminate the cancer.

Newer methods of therapy are aimed at better targeting of drugs to cancer cells or at exploiting differences between normal and cancer cells. An example of better targeting would be the linkage of cytotoxic drugs to antibodies against a cancer cell membrane protein. Differences between cells are exploited by drugs that prevent metastatic growth. Metastasis is a process specific to cancers and has its own control mechanisms, which include angiogenesis (Chapter 12). Thus, anti-angiogenic drugs may have a promising future in reducing metastatic growth and with minimal effect on normal tissues.

Adjuvant drug treatments extend the relapse-free survival period and generate remissions in about half of patients with advanced cancers. Unfortunately, the duration of this remission is calculated in months rather than years. The main feature of cancer cells that contributes to this limited success with the common cancers is the heterogeneous sensitivity of the cell population. Furthermore, changes continue to occur within this population after treatment has begun. These changes include faster growth, more aggressive behaviour and the development of resistance to drugs that were originally effective. Of these properties, resistance to the treatment drugs presents major clinical problems because there are only a limited number of treatment options.

The likely future behaviour of a cancer is referred to as its prognosis, and the assessment of prognosis can be facilitated by prognostic factors. Prognostic factors can be clinical features such as tumour size or how far a cancer has spread, or they can be biochemical markers of tumour behaviour (tumour markers). Characterisation of the cells prior to treatment can be helpful because they can predict subsequent behaviour. A cancer with many proliferating cells is likely to recur sooner than a cancer with few such cells; the cancer with many proliferating-cells requires treatment more urgently than the cancer with few. If a recurrence occurs after surgery, it is important to ensure that the most effective type of therapy is chosen. Prognostic factors can help in these objectives.

The earlier a cancer is detected, the more likely it will be to achieve a cure; several important points follow from this simple principle. Screening programmes for early detection of cervical, breast and colon cancer exist but even small cancers detected by these methods have progressed a long way through their natural development. Thus, although good screening programmes save lives, they do not eliminate cancer deaths. That would best be achieved by preventing cancer cells from being generated in the first place. The smallest possible number of cancer cells is zero and the dictum that prevention is better than cure is now being applied in several prevention trials. Individuals can be identified who are at very high risk of developing cancer, and methods exist to prevent normal cells in such individuals becoming neoplastic. Antioestrogen treatment of women who have a greater than 50% chance of developing breast cancer because of inherited defects is one such approach; persuading people to change their diet is another.

This chapter will deal with the biological principles relevant to the various forms of cancer treatment and provide examples of the three major types of therapy: chemotherapy, radiotherapy and hormone therapy. Immunotherapy is described in Chapter 5.

Principles behind the treatment of cancer

Definition of response

It is important to have agreed criteria as to what constitutes a response so that effectiveness of regimens can be compared and patients informed as to the likely outcome of their treatments.

Relapse-free or overall survival times are good ways of covering both objectives. As people relapse at different rates, it is usual to plot a graph showing the proportion of patients with no detectable cancer or the proportion who are still alive at different times after treatment. Figure 13.2 shows such a graph of overall survival for breast cancer patients whose cancers had (node positive) or had not (node negative) metastasised to the lymph nodes at the time of initial surgery. In the node negative group, about one-quarter of the patients had died within 10 years with little change thereafter, whereas three-quarters of the node positive patients had died within the same time period and the group continued to do badly. It is bad news if cancer has spread at the time of first treatment. In order to compare different patient subgroups, treatments or cancer types, it is inconvenient to present many such graphs; however, information can be presented in a simpler format as the proportion of patients being relapse-free 5 years after treatment. Table 13.1 presents this data for different cancers. In all cases, metastasis is accompanied by worse outcome; pancreatic and liver cancer have a poorer prognosis than testicular cancer, with colon and breast cancer showing intermediate characteristics. The data for patients with non-metastatic testicular cancer indicates that they are cured by the primary treatment.

Another set of definitions applied to advanced cancers classifies responses

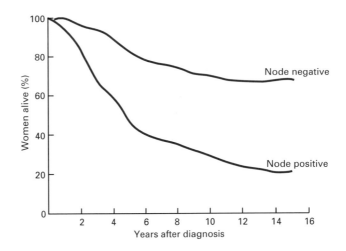

Figure 13.2

Overall survival for breast cancer patients. The node status was determined at the time of first treatment.

Table 13.1 Survival rates from first treatment for various cancers.

Cancer	Metastasis	Percentage alive at 5 years*
Colon	no	80
	yes	40
Breast	no	80
	yes	40
Pancreas	no	3
	yes	0
Testis	no	98
	yes	60
Liver	no	25
	yes	0

* Average value with wide variations.

according to whether a cancer disappears completely (complete response), partially (partial response), remains static (no change) or continues to grow (progressive disease). Partial and complete responses are often combined. A response period of 6 months is usually specified.

Using these criteria, chemotherapy can achieve response rates of 50%, although this figure covers wide variations depending on type of cancer and treatment used.

Patient criteria: Stage and Grade

When comparing different patients or treatments, like must be compared with like, such that the patients in the comparison groups begin with similar stages of cancer.

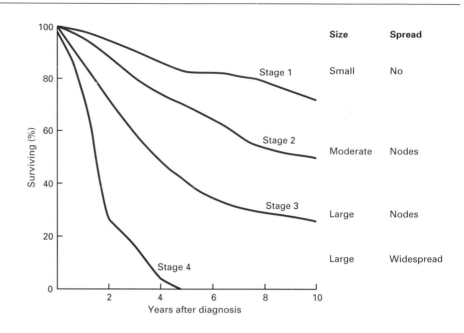

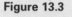

Figure 13.3

Overall survival for breast cancer patients. The stage of the cancer is the stage at diagnosis.

Two types of criteria are used for this: one based on tumour size and degree of spread, i.e. stage of disease, the other on the cellular characteristics of the cancer, i.e. grade. Thus, a large cancer that has invaded its surroundings and metastasised to other parts of the body is at an advanced stage compared to one that is confined to one site. Staging is done by the TNM system, based on the three criteria of **t**umour size, spread to the lymph **n**odes and **m**etastasis to distant sites. A stage 1 cancer is one of small size that has not progressed outside its original site whereas a stage 4 growth is large and has spread widely. Figure 13.3 shows the influence of tumour stage on overall survival of women with breast cancer; a quarter of stage 1 patients are alive at 10 years compared with none of the stage 4 group even at 5 years.

A low-grade tumour has a histological resemblance to the tissue of origin, whereas a high-grade cancer has undergone so many changes that it only marginally resembles the tissue of origin. Criteria for grading include number of mitoses, irregularities in nuclear shape (nuclear pleiomorphism) and architectural resemblance to normal tissue. Both stage and grade are important in that they measure different parameters of the cancer and can be used to predict the likely course of the cancer.

Early detection means better results

It was pointed out in Chapter 2 that, when a cancer can be physically detected, it has been developing for a long time, such that a 1 cm tumour has passed through three-quarters of its lifespan (Figure 2.8). As time equates with increased cellular change towards aggressiveness, it follows that the earlier a cancer can be detected, the fewer changes it will have undergone and the more likelihood there will be of getting a good response to treatment. Animal experiments have indicated the increased likelihood of

Table 13.2 Influence of cell number on response to a 5 log (99.999%) cell kill by a chemotherapeutic agent.

Cell number		Percentage of animals with tumours
Before treatment	After treatment	
10^4 (0.01 mg)	0	0
10^6 (1 mg)	10	50
10^9 (1 g)	10^4	100

achieving a cure when small numbers of cancer cells are present at the start of therapy (Table 13.2). If a drug treatment kills 99.999% of the cells, the fraction left alive is 0.001%. This is referred to as a 5 log kill because 1×10^{-5} of the starting cells remain. Injection of 10^4 cells followed by the same degree of kill would leave no cells alive and all the animals would be cured. Injection of 10^9 cells followed by a 5 log kill would leave 10^4 viable cells, which are capable of killing all the animals. An intermediate number of remaining cells would result in the cure of some but not all animals. Achieving a 5 log kill is just possible in animals but virtually unattainable in patients because of toxic side effects. To put this in perspective, a cancer comprising 10^9 cells is only just detectable by physical examination of patients (Figure 2.8), so it is problematic to achieve a cure by anything other than surgical removal of all the cells.

These types of data indicate that early detection of very small or premalignant growths should result in more cures. Screening large numbers of people for early signs of cancer should therefore be beneficial, provided a suitable test is available. Abnormal cells can be detected in smears taken from the cervix and this form of cervical screening does save lives (Figure 13.4). Cervical smear tests were widely introduced into Denmark and Finland in the late 1960s and death rates from

Figure 13.4

Effect of screening on deaths from cervical cancer. Widespread screening programmes were available in Denmark and Finland but not in Norway.

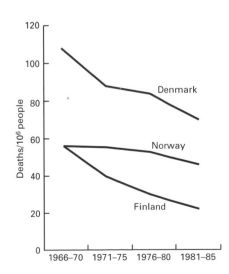

cervical cancer have fallen since then. In contrast, tests were not widely introduced into Norway until the 1980s and deaths did not fall there until after this date. Screening for breast cancer by photographing the internal features of the breast with weak X-rays (mammography) can also be beneficial. Deaths from breast cancer are falling in some countries, partly reflecting the widespread use of mammography and partly reflecting the added benefits of more efficient treatments.

Surgery

Surgical removal of cancer tissues can result in a cure, provided all the cells have been removed. Even if some remain, the debulking effect of cell removal means that subsequent drug treatment is more likely to be successful. It has been estimated that, at first detection, about 70% of cancers have spread elsewhere in the body and are not amenable to surgical removal. The treatment options for killing the remaining cancer cells are drugs and ionising radiations.

Drug treatment

Drug treatment can be divided into two categories depending on the degree of specificity involved. Chemotherapy is the term given to drugs that influence many cell types and whose actions are largely based on blocking cell proliferation. It is most effective against rapidly dividing cells and its efficacy depends on the concentration of drug reaching the tumour and the duration of this exposure. As chemotherapeutic drugs also affect normal cells, their side effects can be considerable. The gap between the minimum effective dose of drug and the maximum dose tolerated by the patient can be small. In trials of one effective anticancer drug, doxorubicin, several patients suffered heart attacks because that gap was crossed. The difference between the minimum effective dose and maximum tolerated dose is called the therapeutic index – the wider it is, the fewer the side effects. The problems of side effects can be minimised by using combinations of drugs with different toxicities (combination or polychemotherapy).

Combination chemotherapy also has the benefit of partially circumventing another problem, the development of drug-resistant cells that are no longer sensitive to the agent used. Cells become resistant by different mechanisms; in a heterogeneous population, some cells will be resistant to one drug, other cells to a different drug, whilst a third group will be insensitive to all reagents. Use of multiple drugs optimises the chances of hitting all the cells with at least one drug to which it is sensitive.

Chemotherapy is the most widely used type of drug treatment and can be used at different stages of cancer progression. Primary or neoadjuvant chemotherapy describes its use as a first line of treatment for local disease. For adjuvant chemotherapy, the agent is used in addition to other treatments such as surgery to kill undetected cancer cells. It can also be used for treating advanced disease where surgery is not an option. In this situation, chemotherapy will not cure a patient but it will improve the quality of life.

The DNA-damaging property of many chemotherapeutic agents means that they are mutagens and can actually cause cancers as well as cure them. Thus, patients who receive chemotherapy can have a tenfold increased risk of developing leukaemia. This is considered an acceptable risk in comparison with the certainty of dying from the existing cancer if it is left untreated.

With some cancers, specific properties of the cells can be exploited that have fewer side effects. Two major cancers, prostate and breast cancer, fall into this category because steroid hormones are required for their growth. Responsive cells must contain specific receptors for the hormone and, as most cells in the body do not have those receptors, they are unaffected by the hormone antagonists used.

Other forms of therapy are being developed based on recent discoveries about components involved in tumour biology, such as gene therapy, targeted delivery, signal transduction and angiogenesis.

Radiotherapy

Radiations such as X-rays damage DNA and, provided the damage is extensive, the cell dies by the apoptotic pathway (Chapter 7).

Cellular heterogeneity

By the time a cancer reaches the stage of requiring treatment, molecular changes associated with progression have taken place to a variable extent, so the constituent cells behave in a heterogeneous manner. This is reflected in some cells responding to treatment whilst others remain unresponsive. This heterogeneity is due to individual characteristics of the cells themselves and to their location within the cancer (Figure 13.5). Unfortunately, individual cells can develop resistance against drugs to which they are exposed (intrinsic resistance). The mechanisms underlying that resistance are discussed later on. Some potentially sensitive cells are resistant because of external factors (extrinsic resistance). This can be due to their stage in the cell cycle or their location relative to blood vessels. Cells that are in G_1 are refractory to most treatments as compared to those in S or M. Thus, if DNA synthesis takes up 1% of the cycle time, only 1% of cells will be in the S phase at any moment and only 1% of cells will be sensitive to S-phase-specific drugs. In cancers such as colon or skin where stem cells are present, a cure will not be achieved unless they are destroyed; killing the other cells will help but it will not eliminate the cancer.

Location of the cells within a cancer can also influence response because drugs must reach those cells from the general circulation. The further a cancer cell from a blood vessel, the less likely it is to receive enough drug to kill it. Likewise, radiotherapy relies on the generation of reactive oxygen species from molecular oxygen to damage the DNA (Chapter 7) and this oxygen is delivered by the blood.

Figure 13.5

Cells within a cancer have different sensitivities.

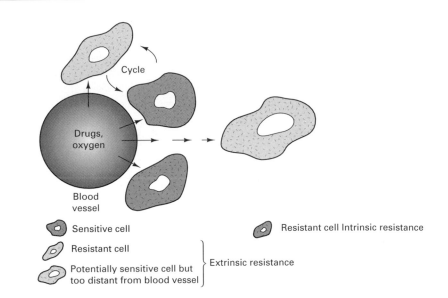

Hypoxia increases with distance from a blood vessel, so radiation sensitivity decreases. Some areas of a tumour are well vascularised whereas others are not; poorly vascularised cells will be hardly affected by drugs. For example, it would take an antibody several months to travel from the outside to the centre of a 1 cm tumour by diffusion alone. Blood vessels within the cancer are essential if this time period is to be reduced.

Cytostatic and cytotoxic effects: cell death and proliferation

The best results are obtained if cancer cells are killed (cytotoxic effect) rather than growth arrested but viable (cytostatic effect). This is not to suggest that cytostatic effects are not beneficial. Definitions of whether or not a response has occurred include a 'no change' category, which is considered to be a partial success rather than a partial failure because cancer expansion has been stopped. It is also worth remembering that growth is a balance of proliferation and death, and that relatively small changes in either property can tip the balance in favour of increased or decreased size (Table 13.3). During active growth, it has been estimated that for every 100 cells that divide to give 200 daughter cells, 80 die leaving 120 to continue the expansion process. The dying cells do not necessarily come from the proliferating pool; however, if the number dying can be increased to more than 100, there would be a net cell loss and the tumour would shrink. This type of argument is used in favour of maximising the doses of chemotherapeutic drugs a patient can stand in order to optimise cell kill at a time of low tumour cell burden.

With the realisation that cell death can be actively induced via the apoptosis pathway, attention is being directed at its manipulation as a form of treatment. Indeed, DNA damage, be it drug or radiation induced, activates the apoptosis pathway (Chapters 7 and 10). The other form of cell death, necrosis, can also be

Table 13.3 Influence of cell death and proliferation on tumour growth.

Cell death $\overset{\text{Regression}}{\leftarrow}$ Stasis $\overset{\text{Growth}}{\rightleftharpoons}$ Proliferation		
Number of cells dying per 100 proliferating*	Net change	Result
80	+120	Growth
100	0	Stasis
120	−20	Regression

* To generate 200 daughter cells.

increased by preventing angiogenesis. In the absence of new blood vessel formation, oxygen and essential nutrients are not available to maintain cell functions and necrotic death ensues. Death sets in at about 150 μm distance either side of a blood vessel, which limits tumour size to 300 μm around individual vessels.

Cell cycle-specific effects

The majority of drugs used for treating cancer are based on preventing DNA synthesis or mitosis. Actions of individual drugs are discussed later but some general points will be described here.

Most of the agents mentioned in Figure 13.6 act at specific phases (phase–specific drugs) of the cell cycle whereas others, such as cyclophosphamide, function at several phases and are referred to as cycle-specific. This distinction is a relative one in that most drugs act at several phases of the cycle but are especially effective at certain points. Thus, cultured cells are four times more sensitive to ionising radiation during mitosis than during DNA synthesis, with intermediate effects being seen in G_1. Likewise, vincristine blocks cells in mitosis but the effective interaction between it and its target, tubulin, occurs earlier.

It is also evident from Figure 13.6 that treatment regimens are targeted at several molecules although effects on DNA predominate. Again these specificities should only be taken as guidelines because **5–fluorouracil (5FU)** inhibits DNA synthesis as well as RNA transcription (see below).

Many biological processes are more active at certain times of the day (circadian rhythms) causing changes in drug metabolism and elimination that may have a profound effect on therapeutic index. Cell proliferation is also subject to circadian rhythms, so it has been shown that giving drugs at specific times of the day can generate greater levels of cell kill with fewer toxicities than when given haphazardly.

Two of the agents mentioned in Figure 13.6, hormones and retinoic acid, are more specific because they only affect cells that contain specific intracellular receptors for these ligands. Retinoic acid induces differentiation in one form of leukaemia, acute promyelocytic leukaemia (Chapter 6), and thus blocks their proliferation, whereas steroid hormone antagonists block receptor–positive cells in G_1 (Chapter 11).

243

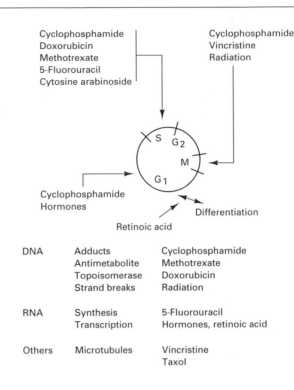

Figure 13.6

Drug effects related to the cell cycle.

Apoptosis as a conduit for cell killing

Cells damaged during therapy must be removed and apoptotic death can achieve that objective. Ionising radiations and genotoxic drugs, which include many used in chemotherapy, switch on the repressor gene p53 that stops proliferation and activates apoptosis (Chapters 7 and 10). Cells with defective p53 are resistant to some chemotherapeutic agents and to radiation damage. An attractive hypothesis is that resistance to apoptosis may contribute to drug resistance. Oncogene-transformed mouse cells are sensitive to apoptosis induced by 5FU, doxorubicin or radiation only if normal p53 is present; loss of its function results in resistance to each of these agents.

Side effects

Minimising side effects of treatments is a major consideration in deciding treatment options. In breast cancer, hormone therapy has fewer side effects than chemotherapy and is the preferred method for certain patients (see below). Agents that are relatively non-specific because they modulate general functions such as proliferation present special problems. Because cancer cells can have increased levels of signal transduction molecules such as growth factor receptors, they can respond to lower doses of some drugs but side effects still occur. Treatments under development are directed at increasing specificity by targeting drugs preferentially to cancer cells (see below).

Normal haemopoietic cells in the bone marrow are particularly sensitive to many chemotherapeutic agents, although protection can be achieved by removing bone marrow and returning it after treatment is finished (autologous bone marrow transplants). Alternatively, patients can be kept in sterile surroundings during chemotherapy to minimise complications due to destruction of immune cells in the bone marrow and elsewhere. Repopulation from remaining normal cells occurs after treatment is completed.

Germ cells in the ovary and testis are also chemosensitive, so young patients can become sterile as a result of treatment, which illustrates one of the many difficult decisions that must be taken with life-threatening conditions such as metastatic cancer. Hair loss also commonly accompanies chemotherapy because the rapidly dividing hair follicles are destroyed. Hair loss can be minimised by wearing a refrigerated cap that lowers skin temperature, thus decreasing follicle proliferation and reducing local cytotoxic effects.

Nausea and vomiting are frequent side effects of chemotherapy because the drugs activate vomiting centres in the brain stem; dopamine and 5-hydroxytryptamine receptor antagonists alleviate some of these symptoms.

Radiation damage is minimised by giving the radiation in fractionated doses and by focusing the radiation on the target area from multiple directions.

Drug resistance

Some cells have an intrinsic resistance to chemotherapeutic agents but virtually all cells have mechanisms whereby they can acquire resistance when exposed to a drug. The multiple ways in which this resistance can be acquired are listed in Table 13.4 together with the drugs involved. Development of resistance is the main cause of treatment failures following an initial good response. Mechanisms will be described here; additional points about specific drugs will be given in later sections dealing with those drugs.

Table 13.4 Mechanisms of resistance to chemotherapeutic drugs.

Process	Cause	Drugs affected
Decreased influx	Folate transporters	Methotrexate
Increased efflux	P-glycoprotein	Vincristine, doxorubicin
Increased inactivation	Glutathione S-transferase	Alkylating agents
Decreased activation	Kinases	5-Fluorouracil, cytosine arabinoside
	Polyglutamation	Methotrexate
Increased targets	Dihdrofolate reductase	Methotrexate
Increased DNA repair	Repair proteins	Doxorubicin, alkylating agents
Poor blood supply	Inadequate drug	All drugs
Sanctuary sites	Blood–brain barrier	All drugs

Membrane transport and the P-glycoprotein

When cells are exposed to a single drug such as vincristine, they develop cross-resistance to other drugs derived from natural products that are of dissimilar structure and function such as doxorubicin and etoposide, as well as to vincristine itself. Their only common feature is that they are lipophilic. This insensitivity is caused by an approximately thousandfold increase in the level of P-glycoprotein, a 170 kDa transmembrane protein that functions as an ATP-dependent efflux pump for the drugs. Increased expression can result from either gene amplification or increased transcription from the normal gene. This is called the **m**ulti**d**rug **r**esistance (MDR) phenotype and the responsible genes are the MDR genes. Compared with cells that have normal levels of P-glycoprotein, MDR cells can be one hundred times more resistant to drugs such as adriamycin. The normal function of P-glycoprotein is as a Cl^- ion efflux pump and its ability to pump out such diverse chemicals is due to multiple binding sites on its cytoplasmic face. The drug can reach the internal plasma membrane but it is then transferred to the exterior before reaching the cytoplasm. Ca^{2+} ion channel blockers such as verapamil will compete with vincristine for binding sites; thus verapamil can reduce the degree of resistance to vincristine.

The cross-resistance does not apply to all drugs, as alkylating agents and antimetabolites are unaffected by levels of P-glycoprotein. There is a good general correlation between P-glycoprotein expression and degree of drug insensitivity.

Resistance mechanisms for alkylating agents and antimetabolites are more specific than MDR, causing cross-resistance to other drugs only if they use the same enzyme transport mechanisms or are subject to the same repair mechanisms. Cells can become resistant to methotrexate by loss of reduced folate carrier, the membrane protein required to transport it into the cell. These cells would be cross-resistant to other antifolates, such as Tomadex, which use the same transporter.

Drug metabolism

All drugs are inactivated by metabolism but some require a metabolic activation step before they are active. Changes to both processes can result in resistance. Alkylating agents are conjugated to glutathione by glutathione S-transferase and upregulation of this enzyme increases the rate of drug inactivation. Antimetabolites like 5FU or cytosine arabinoside are activated by phosphorylations, and the kinases involved (see below) are downregulated by prolonged drug exposure. A different type of drug-induced change to an activation step occurs with methotrexate. It inactivates its target protein, dihydrofolate reductase, on its own but that activity is enhanced once it penetrates the cell by addition of four to six glutamate residues (see below). This process does not alter its ability to inactivate dihydrofolate reductase but it does reduce efflux and methotrexate remains active for a longer period. Loss of the polyglutamation process reduces this activity.

Altered targets

Prolonged exposure to methotrexate also causes amplification of the gene for its target protein, dihydrofolate reductase. The amplified genes are expressed so that insufficient drug is available to inhibit all the dihydrofolate reductase. The same end result, increased enzyme activity, can also be achieved by gene mutations.

DNA repair

Cells contain efficient mechanisms for repairing damaged DNA (Chapter 8). Increased activity of this complex series of processes therefore minimises the biological effect of DNA damage caused by alkylating agents and natural products like doxorubicin.

Blood supply and sanctuary sites

Poor blood supply results in inadequate drug delivery (see above) whilst the blood–brain permeability barrier prevents drugs carried in the blood from reaching cancer cells growing in the brain. These are called sanctuary sites.

Tumour markers

An ability to predict how a cancer might behave is useful in deciding what treatment to give or in monitoring whether it is working. This can be achieved by looking at the physical characteristics of the cancer plus tissue and serum from the patient. Patient characteristics such as nodal status or TNM stage are used to decide whether adjuvant therapy is required at first diagnosis (see above); serum or tissue analysis can refine decision making by providing additional information. The main questions that can be answered in this way are: How fast is the cancer growing? Is it likely to metastasise? Which is the best drug to use and is the drug effective? The majority of chemicals that provide such information are proteins detected by specific antibodies, so the term 'antigen' will be used to describe them. They are known as tumour markers. The term 'prognostic factor' is sometimes used but this can include features such as nodal status and histological tumour grade. The availability of polymerase chain reaction (PCR) kits to amplify and detect altered DNA base sequences in minute samples of cells has identified additional uses for tumour markers. They include the detection of tumour cells in blood or lymph nodes and the diagnosis of cancer types that are difficult to categorise by conventional pathology. Indeed this methodology, plus the ability to detect antigens in tissue sections by immunohistochemical means, makes the dividing line between chemical pathology and histopathology (Chapter 3) somewhat artificial.

Blood

Some cancers produce antigens that enter the general circulation and can then be assayed in a serum sample after removal of blood cells by clotting. Their detection can be useful in two settings: screening for undetected cancer and monitoring the behaviour of an established cancer because the amount of antigen is related to the number of cancer cells present. The useful antigens are glycoproteins identified by antibodies, although the terminology is confusingly related to the antibody used. Thus, one marker used for ovarian cancers is CA-125, a 200 kDa glycoprotein of unknown function. It can be used to indicate how much cancer may be present in a patient (tumour burden) and also for monitoring how much of that tumour is being destroyed by chemotherapy. CA-125 is most frequently present in serum from ovarian cancer patients but it can be detected in smaller proportions of people with cancers of the pancreas, colon and breast. Therefore, it cannot be used to identify the type of cancer a patient might have.

Prostate-**s**pecific **a**ntigen (PSA) is another marker that is useful for monitoring response to treatment. Increased levels can be detected months before clinical evidence of tumour regrowth is available. This antigen has also been used to screen healthy men for signs of early prostate cancer. The test can partially achieve this objective in that a high serum PSA is indicative of something that warrants further investigation but it is also increased in some men without cancer. This false-positive rate is matched by false-negatives in which some men with early prostate cancer do not have detectable PSA in their blood. For these reasons it has not been recommended for large-scale screening of healthy populations.

In healthy people the only nucleated (DNA-containing) cells in the blood are leucocytes; patients with cancer have additional blood-borne metastatic cells. These cells are too sparse to be detected by conventional means but they can be identified through the remarkable sensitivity of the PCR. Amplification of specific DNA sequences by this method means they can be assayed in samples containing less than 10 nucleated cells. All cells in an individual contain essentially the same DNA, so directly detecting specific sequences would not achieve the desired objective of distinguishing cancer cells from normal leucocytes. However, expression of those sequences in the form of mRNA is relatively cell-specific, so specificity can be achieved by first converting the mRNA sequences to their DNA homologues with a **r**everse **t**ranscriptase enzyme followed by PCR (RTPCR). The choice of which mRNA to monitor depends on the cell of interest, but cytokeratins are particularly useful for detecting epithelial cancer cells; epithelia express different cytokeratins to those in leucocytes (Box 11.1).

Tissue

Tissue is available at the time of surgery or as a result of a biopsy at other times. Expression of a wide range of antigens can be assayed either biochemically or immunohistochemically. Cell-sorting devices can identify the number of proliferating cells or ploidy status of the nuclear DNA.

The biological properties of a cancer for which assays are useful are cell proliferation, aggressiveness and treatment sensitivity. A rapidly growing, aggressive tumour will recur rapidly and requires treatment immediately. Proliferation can be assayed by incorporation of bromodeoxyuridine into DNA followed by its quantitation with an antibody raised against the nucleoside. A simpler assay is immunohistochemical detection of nuclear antigens related to DNA synthesis. Two antigens of proven use are **p**roliferating **c**ell **n**uclear **a**ntigen (PCNA) and Ki-67. PCNA is required for DNA polymerase function (Chapter 10) but the action of Ki-67 is less clear. Flow cytometry can also be used to assess the proportion of S-phase cells in a population. DNA in tumour nuclei is stained with a fluorescent dye and fractionated according to the DNA content per nucleus. The number of cells with double DNA content indicates the cells in $S+G_2$ of the cell cycle prior to mitosis.

Aggressiveness is a vague term covering many functions, and a multitude of antigens have been proposed for its prognosis. Two groups are worth mentioning, adhesion molecules and growth factor receptors. Invasion and metastasis require loss and gain of various cell adhesion molecules (Chapter 12). E-cadherin is lost in many metastatic epithelial cells whereas integrins can increase or decrease depending on the type of integrin and the type of cell. Growth factor receptors such as epidermal growth factor or erbB2 (Chapter 11) are elevated in malignant tumours, and increased expression of either of these antigens indicates a poor prognosis. An aneuploid DNA profile detected by flow cytometry also points to an aggressive cancer.

To predict responses to treatment, there are few antigens available. And there is no totally reliable marker for response to chemotherapy. However, the presence of oestrogen and progestogen receptors in endometrial and breast cancers indicates a high probability of response to hormone therapy.

Chemotherapy

Chemotherapy remains the main form of drug treatment at all stages of cancer development. The chemicals involved are directed at disrupting the cell cycle: RNA, DNA and protein molecules are the targets (Figure 13.6). The information contained in this figure can be presented in an alternative manner as the type of chemical related to the process it affects (Table 13.5). Synthetic chemotherapeutic agents in current use can be categorised according to whether they alkylate DNA (alkylating agents) or antagonise metabolites needed for DNA synthesis (antimetabolites). A third group are natural products from plants and fungi.

Single agents can be effective, as exemplified by the curative effect of methotrexate on early choriocarcinoma (cancer of the placenta), but it is more usual to use a combination of drugs. The beneficial effect of this approach is illustrated in Figure 13.7, which shows that with increasing numbers of drugs in a combination the remission rate is improved in patients with Hodgkin's lymphoma. Different drug combinations are used for different cancers but a common combination is the CMF regimen containing

Table 13.5 Processes affected by chemotherapeutic drugs.

Type of agent	Process affected	Cancers treated
Alkylating agents		
Cyclophosphamide	DNA synthesis	Breast, leukaemia
Cisplatin	DNA synthesis	Ovary, testis
Antimetabolites		
Methotrexate	Dihydrofolate reductase	Breast, placenta
5-Fluorouracil	Thymidylate synthase, RNA synthesis	Stomach, breast, colon
Cytosine arabinoside	DNA polymerase	Leukaemia, lymphoma
Natural products		
Doxorubicin	DNA and RNA synthesis	Lung, breast, leukaemia
Vincristine	Tubulin polymerisation	Lymphoma, testis
Taxol	Tubulin depolymerisation	Ovary, breast

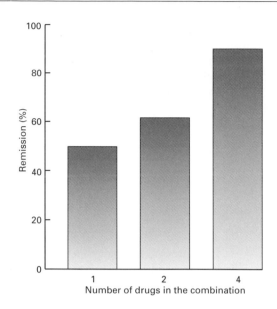

Figure 13.7

Number of drugs in a combination. The graph shows remission of Hodgkin's lymphoma for drug combinations containing 1, 2 and 4 drugs.

cyclophosphamide, methotrexate and 5FU. Cyclophosphamide is an alkylating agent whereas the other two are antimetabolites. Cells develop different types of resistance to each of these compounds (see above), so the combination increases the likelihood that one of the drugs will be effective on all the cells. Each drug has its own toxicity profile, thus a combination means that individual toxicities can be minimised without diminishing the cell-killing effect. Because many of the drugs are themselves carcinogenic (Chapter 7), secondary cancers can appear about 5 years after successful chemotherapy (e.g. leukaemia, lymphoma).

The potential benefits of primary (neoadjuvant) chemotherapy are being investigated but its worth in both the adjuvant and metastatic settings is established. Adjuvant chemotherapy after surgery plus radiotherapy for Wilms' tumour (kidney) in children can double the survival rate. Beneficial, but less dramatic, effects are seen with adult tumours. Chemotherapy is often the only treatment option for metastatic cancers.

Most chemotherapeutic agents in current use were discovered years ago but treatment responses have improved because they can now be delivered to the cancer more efficiently. Maintaining an effective concentration of the drug over a long period of time is more effective than giving one large dose; it also produces fewer side effects. For cycle-specific drugs, prolonged delivery also has the benefit of targeting cells at different cycle phases because the cells eventually reach a phase at which the drug is most effective.

Drugs can sometimes be perfused through the affected area without entering the general circulation.

Alkylating agents

Alkylating agents form adducts with DNA bases that disrupt DNA synthesis (Chapter 7). Most alkylating agents have two functional groups, each of which can react with a DNA base and form interstrand and intrastrand cross-links within the DNA double helix. These links can be formed at any stage of the cell cycle, so alkylating agents are not phase-specific.

Cyclophosphamide

The structure of cyclophosphamide is shown in Figure 13.8 together with the guanine adducts resulting from its metabolic activation and through which its effects are mediated. Cyclophosphamide metabolites block proliferation at several stages of the cycle (Figure 13.6) and are used in combination with methotrexate and 5FU for treatment of many cancers, such as those of the breast. Its side effects include immunosuppression, hair loss and sterility. Resistance to its actions occurs through changes in cellular transport and increased DNA repair. Alkylating agents such as nitrosoureas methylate DNA guanines (Figure 7.7) which are repaired by alkyl transferase (Figure 8.4). There is increased activity of alkyl transferase in brain tumours, which renders them less sensitive to methylating drugs.

A related compound, ifosfamide, is as effective as cyclophosphamide but it has a different toxicity profile.

Cisplatin

Cisplatin and its analogue carboplatin are converted to alkylating species in the body (Figure 13.8), preferentially forming adducts at the N-7 position of guanine and

Figure 13.8

Alkylating agents that cross-link DNA guanines.

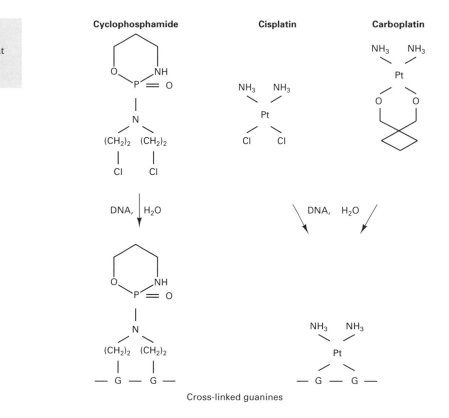

Cross-linked guanines

Figure 13.9

Cisplatin resistance
may be due to
glutathione
S-transferase.

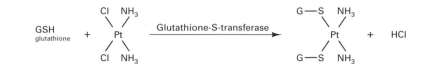

adenine. These adducts can interact with adjacent bases on the same strand
(intrastrand adducts) or on separate strands (interstrand adducts). The order of
preference for adduct formation is $G:G > A:G >$ others. Intrastrand adducts distort
the DNA helix whilst interstrand links prevent strand separation so that replication
is inhibited or abnormal.

Cisplatin is particularly effective against ovarian and testicular cancers and has the
advantage over other chemotherapeutic agents in that it has minimal effect on the
bone marrow. Its main toxicities are nausea, renal dysfunction (nephrotoxicity) and
neural effects. Carboplatin has a similar anti-tumour profile to cisplatin but it has
greatly reduced side effects, especially nephrotoxicity.

Resistance to cisplatin can result from its altered cellular transport, enhanced
repair of damaged DNA or inactivating reactions of the cisplatin with sulphydryl
groups in proteins and glutathione. Cisplatin derivatives are not influenced by
MDR mechanisms but they are substrates for glutathione-*S*-tranferase, the
detoxifying enzyme which conjugates the drug with reduced glutathione (Figure
13.9); cisplatin-resistant cancers can overexpress the enzyme. This drug also
upregulates metallothionine, whose sulphydryl groups interact with the drug by a
reaction analogous to that of glutathione. Decreased efficiency of apoptosis may play
a role in cisplatin resistance. In experimental systems, increased expression of the
antiapoptosis protein Bcl2 (Chapter 10) correlates with decreased drug sensitivity of
ovarian and breast cancers but the correlation is not good enough to use Bcl2 as a
predictive test for chemoresistance in patients.

Antimetabolites

Antimetabolites inhibit nucleic acid synthesis; the actual mechanism depends on the
compound.

Methotrexate

Methotrexate is one of the few drugs capable of curing a cancer, choriocarcinoma,
on its own although it is more commonly used in combination with other agents.
Methotrexate is a derivative of folic acid and competitively inhibits the enzyme
dihydro**f**olate **r**eductase (DHFR), essential for purine and pyrimidine production
and therefore DNA synthesis (Figure 13.10). Folic acid is reduced to tetrahydrofolic
acid (FH_4), which accepts a one-carbon fragment from serine to form either
N^5,N^{10}-methylene-FH_4 or N^{10}-formyl-FH_4. The methylene group in N^5,N^{10}-
methylene-FH_4 can be donated to phosphoribosyl glycinamide in the purine
biosynthetic pathway, whilst the formyl group of N^{10}-formyl-FH_4 methylates

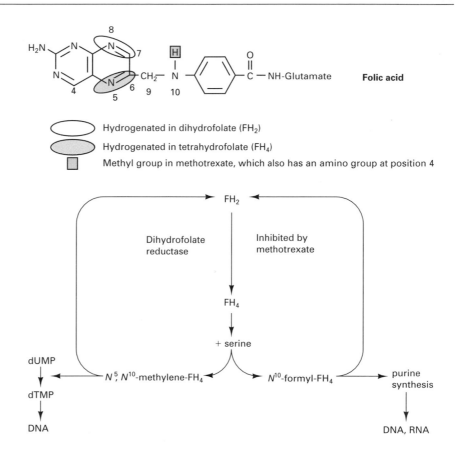

Figure 13.10

Folic acid: structure and derivatives. Methotrexate inhibition of nucleic acid synthesis.

dUMP under the action of thymidylate synthase, thus forming dTMP. In the process of carbon donation, FH_4 is converted to FH_2 and must be reconverted to FH_4 by DHFR. Methotrexate, which has a methyl group on the N-10 position of folic acid plus a 4-amino group, inhibits this hydrogenation and this depletes the pool of reduced folate.

If high doses of methotrexate are used, its toxic effect on the bone marrow cells can be considerable but this can be counteracted by providing reduced folate in the form of leucovorin (folinic acid, N^5-formyl-FH_4).

Methotrexate enters the cell by active transport, and drug resistance can result from decreased activity of this transport process. Two other types of resistance are encountered: amplification of the DHFR gene and decreased polyglutamate formation within the cell. Exposure to methotrexate can generate a several thousandfold amplification of the DHFR gene plus DNA regions on either side, to the extent that the changes can be seen in stained chromosomes. This can take the form of homogeneous staining regions within the chromosome due to the amplified DNA or it can take the form of double minute chromosomes which are separate from the standard chromosome. Amplification of the DHFR gene results in overexpression of the enzyme, and methotrexate will not inhibit all the available enzyme. Folic acid can have four to six glutamate residues added within the cell and this biologically active derivative is retained within the cell to a

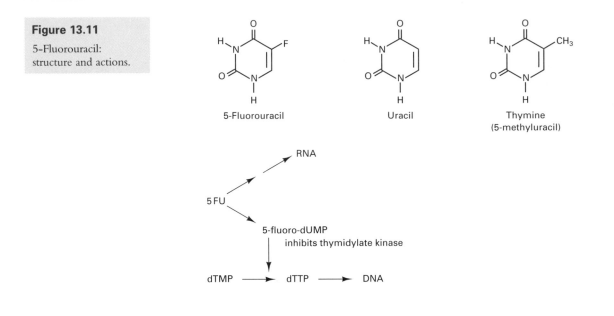

Figure 13.11

5-Fluorouracil:
structure and actions.

greater extent than the parent compound. The enzymes involved in glutamate addition become less active in cancers, so the inhibitory activity of the methotrexate is diminished.

5-Fluorouracil

5-Fluorouracil (5FU) is a derivative of uracil that can be phosphorylated and incorporated into RNA, which is thus not functional (Figure 13.11). Additionally, it produces 5-fluoro-dUMP that forms an inactive ternary complex with the N^5, N^{10}-methylene-FH_4 and thymidylate synthase, thereby inhibiting DNA synthesis. It is used to treat breast and stomach cancers, and its main toxicity is to bone marrow cells. Resistance results from increased catabolism and downregulation of its activating enzymes.

Cytosine arabinoside (Ara-C)

When deoxyribose in cytidine is replaced by arabinose, another 5-carbon sugar, the product is Ara-C; this can be phosphorylated to form Ara-CTP, which is an inhibitor of DNA polymerase α. Some Ara-C is also incorporated into DNA. Both processes block DNA synthesis so Ara-C is an S-phase inhibitor. It is effective against leukaemia and its main toxicity is on bone marrow. Resistance results from loss of activating kinases and increased catabolism.

Natural products

Doxorubicin (adriamycin)

Doxorubicin is a multi-ring fungal anthracycline and a related compound is epirubicin. Both doxorubicin and epirubicin have several effects on DNA. They intercalate and cause partial unwinding of the double helix but they also generate single- and double-strand breaks as well as binding to the enzyme topoisomerase II. This enzyme is needed for the cleavage, unwinding and rejoining of DNA strands during DNA synthesis. Doxorubicin blocks the religation step but it can also generate free radicals, which may contribute to its strand-breaking action. All the effects of doxorubicin on DNA contribute to the drug being an S-phase-specific agent.

Doxorubicin is widely used in the treatment of leukaemias and solid cancers such as those of breast, lung and ovary. Its main side effect is on heart function and this is dose limiting. Drug resistance results from overproduction of the multidrug resistance, P-glycoprotein (see above) and decreased efficiency in repairing DNA strand breaks (Figures 8.7 and 8.8). Topoisomerase II mutations have been detected in experimentally induced doxorubicin-resistant cell lines but the clinical relevance of this observation is uncertain.

Vinca alkaloids and Taxol

Vincristine and vinblastine are plant alkaloids that bind to tubulin and prevent its polymerisation. As polymerised tubulin forms the spindles that retract chromosomes into daughter cells at mitosis, its disruption results in blocked mitosis. Although the effects are seen at this time, the actual vincristine–tubulin interaction occurs during interphase. Although chemically unrelated, the terpene taxol (from yew trees) acts at the same locus but prevents tubulin depolymerisation.

These compounds are effective against a broad spectrum of cancers such as leukaemia, ovarian cancer and testicular cancer. They have bone marrow and neural toxicities, and development of drug resistance is via overproduction of P-glycoprotein.

Hormone therapy

Breast cancer is the most common cancer in women in the West and prostate cancer has that dubious honour in men (Figure 1.3). The normal progenitor cells require oestrogens (women) or androgens (men) for their proliferation. This mitogenic effect of the sex steroids is mediated by specific, intracellular receptors that are gene transcription factors (Chapter 11) which overcome a block in the G_1 phase of the cycle. Antagonising this effect generates a cytostatic response, although additional cytotoxic effects may occur. Because relatively few cell types contain these receptors, drugs aimed at their disruption have a degree of specificity missing with chemotherapeutic agents. As breast and prostate cancers occur predominantly in older people, disruption of reproductive function, the main side effect of hormone therapy, is not a problem. This is not true for younger people, in whom the menstrual cycle can be disrupted.

Treatment of hormone-sensitive cancers is based on the principle of depriving them of the mitogenic hormone, which can be achieved by either preventing steroid synthesis or blocking their effects at the target cell level via the receptor machinery (Figure 13.12).

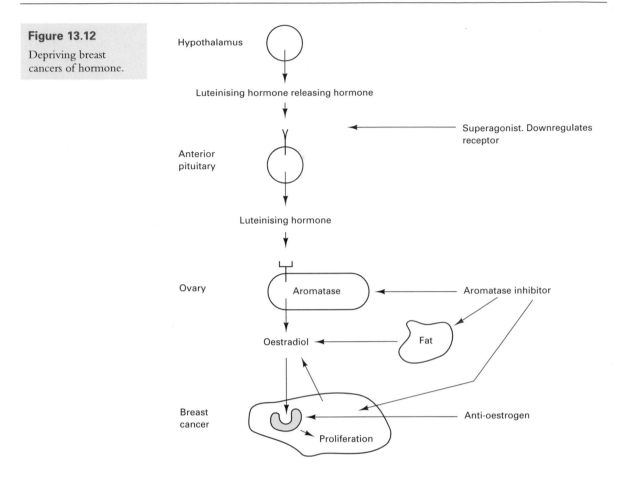

Figure 13.12

Depriving breast cancers of hormone.

Disruption of steroid synthesis

Disruption of steroid synthesis was originally achieved by removing the relevant glands – ovary, testis, adrenal or pituitary. Medical rather than surgical ablation is now the method of choice, except for ovarian destruction by radiotherapy without recourse to surgery. Inactivation of ovarian function is only effective in premenopausal women, as the postmenopausal ovary has already stopped producing oestradiol. As far as breast cancer is concerned, oestradiol (Figure 13.12) is the main oestrogen in humans and is mostly synthesised in the ovary, so the function of this gland is central to treatments based on removing oestradiol. Ovarian function is regulated by polypeptide hormones produced by the anterior pituitary gland – luteinising **h**ormone (**LH**) and **f**ollicle-**s**timulating **h**ormone (**FSH**). These hormones are collectively known as gonadotrophins. LH and FSH have their release modulated by polypeptides synthesised in hypothalamic centres of the brain. **LH-r**eleasing **h**ormone (**LHRH**), synthesised in the hypothalamus, is especially important because its effect can be blocked by antagonists. In postmenopausal women the ovary becomes refractory to pituitary hormones, and ovarian oestradiol synthesis stops, but synthesis continues at a low level in extraglandular sites such as fat cells and breast cancer cells, if present. This represents a change from an endocrine effect (premenopausal women) to an autocrine response (postmenopausal women) of oestradiol.

LHRH superagonists

The hypothalamic decapeptide LHRH stimulates membrane receptors in the pituitary gland to release LH. Synthetic analogues of LHRH bind so avidly to the LHRH receptors that they downregulate them. These LHRH superagonists thus desensitise the pituitary gland, causing decreased oestradiol production in the ovary. These agonists are also effective against prostate cancer because the same hypothalamic–pituitary regulation process occurs in both sexes. Additionally, the LHRH agonists may have direct antiproliferative effects on the cancer cells.

Inhibitors of steroid synthesis

Another way to decrease oestradiol production is via drugs that block steroid biosynthesis. The last step in this pathway requires an aromatase enzyme that converts testosterone to oestradiol. Aromatase inhibitors such as Formestane and 4-hydroxy-androstenedione are clinically effective, with the advantage over LHRH agonists that aromatase inhibitors also block extraglandular oestrogen synthesis. These steroidal aromatase inhibitors irreversibly inactivate the enzyme (type I or suicide inhibitors). Non-steroidal triazols such as Anastrozole (type II inhibitors) are reversible.

Steroid receptor antagonists

Anti-oestrogens bind to the oestrogen receptor but do not activate gene transcription (Chapter 11). Receptor binding by the antagonist prevents oestradiol binding and blocks its mitogenic effect (Figures 13.12 and A.1). A few oestrogen-sensitive genes, such as the gene for TGF-β, act in reverse in that they are activated by anti-oestrogens and inactivated by oestrogens. Anti-oestrogen blockade of oestradiol binding to its receptor synergises with the induction of growth inhibitory polypeptides to stop proliferation.

The most widely used anti-oestrogen is tamoxifen, a derivative of the non-steroidal oestrogen diethylstilboesterol (Figure 13.13). Interference with the action of other classes of steroid hormone, such as progestogens, glucocorticoids or androgens, is also effective in treating advanced breast cancer. Interestingly, male breast cancer responds to the same hormone treatments as the female disease. An analogous situation occurs with prostate cancer in men; its growth is driven by androgens from the testis. Anti-androgens such as flutamide induce remission.

The main toxic effect of hormone therapy is interference with sexual functions such as ovulation, but it also causes secondary cancers of the endometrium. Resistance can result from loss of receptors but many receptor-positive breast cancers are hormone insensitive, so other mechanisms must exist. One possibility is

Figure 13.13

Structure of oestradiol and its antagonist tamoxifen.

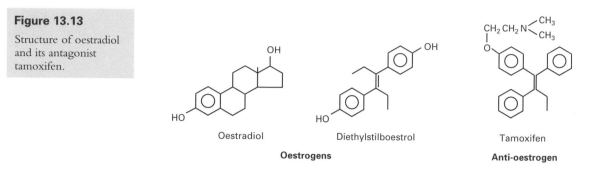

Oestradiol   Diethylstilboestrol   Tamoxifen

Oestrogens   **Anti-oestrogen**

hormone-independent upregulation of locally produced growth factors. And another route to hormone insensitivity is ligand-independent activation of steroid receptors via the MAP kinase signalling pathway (Chapter 11).

Radiotherapy

Ionising radiations generate reactive oxygen species which in turn produce DNA strand breaks that can result in cell death (Chapter 7). Because the oxygen is derived from the air, it follows that air composition influences radiation response. Fortunately, the responses are near maximal at the oxygen concentration in air and trials of higher oxygen (hyperbaric oxygen) levels have not yielded convincing benefits. The same conclusion applies to the use of electrophilic chemicals such as misonidazole that can sensitise cultured cells to the killing effect of ionising radiations but are mostly ineffective in patients. Nevertheless, all tumours have regions of hypoxia related to poor blood supply and cells in these regions are radioresistant.

Cells differ in their inherent sensitivity to radiotherapy and this influences the responses obtained. Thus, 99% of normal bone marrow cells are killed by a radiation dose (4 Gy) that must be increased fourfold to kill the same proportion of thyroid cells.

Doses of radiation that can be used on patients are limited by the damage done to normal tissues. The adverse effects on normal tissues can be minimised by focusing multiple radiation beams from different angles onto the cancer and also by dividing the total dose into fractions given over several weeks. Typically, daily doses of 2 Gy are given which, in total, are appreciably greater than those shown to cause cancer (Chapter 7). Hence the overall DNA damage is sufficient to kill the cells rather than just generate changes that can be repaired.

Immunotherapy

This is dealt with in Chapter 5.

Photodynamic therapy

Visible light on its own does not damage cells but it can have deleterious effects in the presence of light-sensitive (photosensitive) chemicals such as porphyrins plus oxygen. Naturally occuring porphyrins like haemoglobin bind and transport oxygen (O_2). In the laboratory, haemoglobin can be modified with acid so that light in the 630 nm (red) region of the spectrum provides energy to transfer an electron from the photosensitive porphyrin to oxygen and generate the reactive superoxide radical, $O_2^\bullet$; the porphyrin is a prodrug. This free radical has a short half-life ($<0.04\,\mu s$) and therefore will only damage molecules less than $0.02\,\mu m$ from the site of O_2 formation. Given a cell diameter of about $10\,\mu m$, this means that only cells containing porphyrin are directly destroyed, although there are secondary effects such as an inflammatory response with accumulation of leucocytes and an immune reaction. Photodynamic therapy has been adapted so the porphyrin is given systemically and the target cancer is illuminated with 630 nm light focused on the cancer and not the surrounding tissues.

Multiple processes are activated such as vascular shutdown, an inflammatory reaction, stress-activated kinase increase (Chapter 11) and apoptosis. All of them contribute to treatment effectiveness but apoptosis is particularly relevant. The basis for the selective uptake of the porphyrin by the cancer cells is unclear but it involves both the high blood vessel density in cancers and the presence of mitochondrial membrane binding sites for porphyrins. Formation of $O_2^\bullet$ radicals in the mitochondrial membrane activates the apoptosis pathway downstream from the processes requiring RNA and protein synthesis such as p53 formation (Figure 10.14). Cell death is thus independent of p53 status and stage in the cell cycle, so the potential causes of intrinsic and extrinsic resistance are circumvented.

The original prodrug was a complex mixture of acid-treated porphyrins, partially purified to remove inactive components and give a mixture called Photofrin; nowadays there are single compounds which are more selective and which have more precise actions. Photodynamic therapy has been successfully used to treat cancers of the bladder, head/neck and oesophagus. Side effects include skin photosensitivity and renal problems; local heating occurs due to the activating light.

New forms of treatment

We now have a reasonable idea of the molecular events driving the major processes linked to carcinogenesis and new therapies are being developed based on this information. Most currently used drugs prevent either nucleic acid synthesis or mitosis, so there is scope for widening the molecular targets; this is important for several reasons. A consequence of chemotherapy is that resistant cells appear (see above). Generation of cancer cells with intrinsic resistance results from the inherent genetic instability of those cells (Chapter 8). This problem will apply to all treatments aimed at the cancer cell but it should not arise if normal cells are the targets; blood vessels (angiogenesis) are one such target. Nevertheless, targeting cancer cells continues to be important; resistance to one drug does not always mean resistance to another, so the broader the available drug

Table 13.6 New types of cancer treatment.

Type	Targets	Drugs
Signal transduction: cancers more active than normal cells		
Ras	Block membrane binding	Inhibit prenylation
Tyrosine kinases	Inhibit tyrosine phosphorylation	Inhibit ATP binding
Growth factors	Block ligand binding	Receptor antibodies
Angiogenesis: prevent new blood vessel formation		
Growth factor	Inactivate by binding to other molecules	Pentosan polysulphate
Metalloproteinases	Prevent invasion	Marimastat
Endothelial proliferation	Prevent vessel formation	Integrin antibody
		Endostatin
Influence specific genes: counteract growth related products		
Antisense oligodeoxyribonucleotides	Destroy mRNA	Bcl2
Gene therapy	Introduce repressor gene	p53
	Increase immunotoxicity	Interleukins
Immunotherapy		
Tumour antigens	Increase immune attack	Immunodominant peptides

armamentarium, the longer beneficial treatments can be provided. Side effects are often related to drug type so widening the number of cellular pathways that can be targeted may minimise side effects and increase the therapeutic index of a multidrug regime. Some of the more interesting developments are described below; they have been chosen because of their relevance to the topic of this book but also because they illustrate general points about drug development. The potential treatments are at various stages of development but most have shown potential in cell culture or animal experiments; there is only limited information on their clinical use. Table 13.6 lists the types of treatment that fall into this category.

Signal transduction

Cancer cells upregulate signal transduction pathways that convey messages from outside the cell to its interior. Features of these pathways that are being tested as avenues of therapy are the ras protein, protein kinases and growth factor availability. Growth factor availability is discussed in the section dealing with anti-angiogenic agents.

Ras

The ras oncogene is at the hub of several signalling pathways (Chapter 11) and is activated in more than 80% of cancers. If its function could be blocked, beneficial effects would theoretically occur with a range of cancers. Most attention has been directed at inhibiting ras prenylation thereby preventing membrane attachment and biological function. The theory has been validated in that inhibitors of prenylation will reverse the classical transformation characteristics of cultured cells (morphology, anchorage dependence, uncontrolled growth) and block the growth of human cancers transplanted into immunodeficient mice (xenografts). Clinical trials are under way but laboratory work has highlighted some of the difficulties encountered when theory is translated into practice.

The major type of prenylation involves enzymic attachment of a farnesyl group to the cysteine (C) of the C-terminal CAAX amino acid motif (A = aliphatic amino acid, X = any amino acid, commonly methionine, serine or glutamine). This requires farnesyl diphosphate and farnesyl transferase (FTase). Synthetic CAAX tetrapeptides are substrates for FTase, but if the aliphatic amino acid preceding X is replaced by an aromatic one, the peptide is a competitive inhibitor of the enzyme (Figure 13.14). Several peptidomimetic inhibitors are available that work on cultured cells but they are of limited use *in vivo* because their –CO–NH– peptide bonds are attacked by serum proteases and therefore have limited half-lives. And the negatively charged terminal methionine –COO⁻ carboxyl group limits cell entry. Replacing the peptide bonds with protease-resistant –C–N– or –C–O– linkages and methylating the carboxyl group are two ways to overcome these problems (Figure 13.14); intracellular demethylation releases the active inhibitor. Alternatively, prenylation can be blocked with competitive inhibitors of farnesyl diphosphate binding; α-hydroxyfarnesyl diphosphate and manumycin will achieve this effect.

Despite the encouraging effects obtained in laboratory studies, there are still some problems. In normal human cells there are three ras genes, H-ras, K-ras and N-ras, each with slightly different base sequences. The majority of mutations in solid

Figure 13.14

Prenylation of ras: a target for therapeutic drugs.

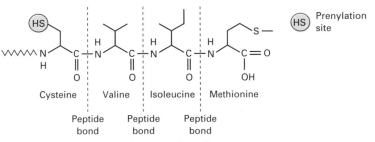

Natural C-terminal substrate for farnesyl transferase

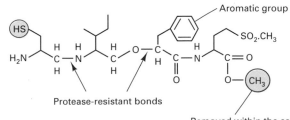

Competitive inhibitor L739, 749

tumours occur in K-ras but H-ras changes predominate in bladder and head/neck cancers. The CAAX motifs are different in these two oncogenes such that X is a serine in H-ras and a methionine in K-ras, which alters the prenylation characteristics of the preceding cysteine. Farnesyl transfer is the only option with H-ras, so FTase inhibition blocks function; but this is not true for K-ras. When FTase is blocked, the enzyme geranygeranyl protein transferase prenylates the cysteine with an alternative 20-carbon lipid; K-ras remains active albeit at a decreased level. The implication of this observation is that some tumours may be susceptible to FTase inhibitors and others less so. Predicting which are the susceptible cancers is further confused by the fact that the drug effect can be independent of the mutational status of ras; even normal ras must be membrane-bound to be active.

Two other features of prenylation inhibitors have to be considered. The biological outcome of inhibition depends on external factors such as the extracellular matrix. Under anchorage-dependent culture conditions (Figure 2.5), FTase inhibition has a cytostatic effect by inhibiting proliferation, whereas anchorage-independent culture generates a cytotoxic response by activating apoptosis; the mechanistic bases for these different responses are described in Chapter 11. Clinically, a cytotoxic response is more beneficial than a cytostatic response but it is not immediately apparent how the culture conditions relate to cancers growing *in vivo*. Also the ras protein is not the only substrate for prenylation. Other substances are also activated by this route and they may generate unwanted side effects; two of them are rho, a GTP-binding protein (Chapter 11), and PRL, a protein tyrosine phosphatase.

Overall the theoretical attractiveness of this approach to disrupting signal transduction is tempered by practical realities but it is well worth pursuing. Given the many problems encountered, it is not suprising that it takes £20 million to bring a drug to the market!

Protein kinases

Drugs are available that will inhibit either serine or tyrosine kinases with varying degrees of specificity. The microbiological product staurosporin blocks cyclin-dependent serine kinases (Chapter 10) at concentrations 100 times lower than required for the EGF receptor tyrosine kinase, and the synthetic flavopiridol exhibits a sixtyfold preference for serine kinases. However, it is the tyrosine kinases that are receiving most attention with drugs that exhibit a remarkable specificity for individual members of the family. Design of these compounds is based on inhibiting ATP binding to the kinase. Specificity is determined by adding peptide side chains to the drug so it will bind more strongly to one kinase protein but less strongly to another. Presumably this specificity is determined by amino acids in the vicinity of the ATP binding site. Compounds are available that inhibit EGF receptor autophosphorylation but with virtually no effect (<1000-fold) on kinase receptors for PDGF, FGF or IGF; intracellular kinases like src and abl are also unaffected.

The EGF family of receptor tyrosine kinases are particularly attractive targets as their activity is increased in many cancers and they are associated with aggressive tumours that have poor prognosis (Chapter 11). Figure 13.15 illustrates the type of structure used for anti-EGF receptor kinase drugs in comparison to ATP, the natural substrate. Known up to now only by their in-house names, e.g. PD165557

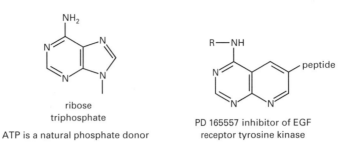

Figure 13.15

Competitive inhibitors of ATP binding to tyrosine kinases.

ribose
triphosphate

ATP is a natural phosphate donor

PD 165557 inhibitor of EGF
receptor tyrosine kinase

and ZD1839, in culture these drugs inhibit all the downstream events associated with EGF action such as receptor autophosphorylation, proliferation and anchorage-independent growth. They also block EGF-dependent growth of human tumour xenografts in immunodeficient mice. Interestingly, they antagonise effects mediated by other members of the EGF receptor family like erbB2. This could be important as the erbB2 proteins are poorly expressed by normal adult cells but are upregulated in many cancers (Chapter 11); this property might limit side effects in patients.

Related compounds exist that specifically target either PDGF or FGF receptors associated with angiogenesis (Chapter 12). There is a feeling that high specificity should be linked to fewer side effects but this remains to be proven. Given the multiple signalling pathways involved in cell proliferation with their ability to cross-communicate, broader spectrum kinase inhibitors may be more effective. As these agents block proliferation, they are cytostatic rather than cytotoxic and in the animal models tested so far, tumours reappear when treatment is stopped.

Growth factor receptors

A different approach to blocking EGF receptors is via neutralising **monoclonal antibodies** (mAb) and clinical trials with such reagents are under way. The mouse mAb225 blocks EGF binding without itself activating the receptor. This property is important because antibodies are bivalent and therefore have the potential to react with two receptor proteins thereby dimerising and activating them. mAb225 will localise to cancers such as breast, lung and ovary, and in laboratory studies it will inhibit EGF effects. The main problem is that mAbs are usually generated in mice, and when given to humans they will produce inactivating, antimouse antibodies. By genetic engineering it is possible to generate human–mouse chimeric antibodies in which the antigenic mouse determinants have been replaced with human homologues without losing the antireceptor activity. Humanised forms of mAb225 and another monoclonal antibody against erbB2 (Herceptin) are currently in trials; preliminary results indicate responses in breast cancer patients with no accompanying antimouse antibody problem.

Angiogenesis

Tumours will not grow in the absence of new blood vessel formation (Chapter 12). Angiogenesis requires proliferation of capillary endothelial cells and penetration of the surrounding tissue by the new vessels. Proliferation can be blocked by interference with growth factors, and tissue penetration is inhibited by antagonising protease action. Both endothelial proliferation and invasion are treatment targets. The use of antagonising proteases will also disrupt the tumour cell's invasion of its surroundings.

Attacking angiogenesis should create a cytotoxic environment with benefits over the mainly cytostatic responses seen with most of the other novel treatments described above. Additionally, targeting genetically stable, normal endothelial cells means less likelihood of resistant cells appearing than with cancer cells. Current trials are aimed at three different components of the angiogenesis mechanism: blocking endothelial proliferation via growth factor sequestration, interfering with endothelial invasion with anti-integrin antibodies and disrupting both endothelial and cancer cell invasion with metalloproteinase inhibitors. A fourth route, increasing tissue concentrations of angiogenesis inhibitors like endostatin, is also yielding promising results in animal tests. Endostatin caused regression of established tumours which regrew when treatment was stopped. However, after prolonged endostatin exposure, the tumours did not regrow, although residual cancer cells were present in a dormant state.

Growth factors

Angiogenic growth factors such as VEGF and FGF, produced by cancers, bind to and are inactivated by negatively charged proteoglycans (Chapter 12). Infusion of sulphated polysaccharides such as pentosan polysulphate or tegogalan polysulphate achieves the same objective; these compounds are active in animal experiments.

Integrin antibodies

Vitaxin (LM609), a humanised monoclonal antibody against integrin $\alpha_V\beta_3$, reduces tumour-associated angiogenesis without affecting normal blood vessels. This reflects $\alpha_V\beta_3$ expression in the growing sprout of new capillaries but not on mature capillaries; prevention of cell–ECM interaction in this way induces apoptosis (Chapter 12). Vitaxin inhibits growth of human xenografts in mice and is being tested against a variety of advanced cancers in patients. The same integrin is downregulated by TNF and IFN, indicating another potential antiangiogenic therapy.

Metalloproteinase (MMP) inhibitors

MMPs are required for invasion by capillary sprouts and by cancer cells themselves (Chapter 12), so antagonising these enzymes should have a dual effect; this appears to be the case and several clinical trials are nearing successful completion. Two types of inhibitor are being studied, polypeptide tissue inhibitors (TIMPs) and synthetic drugs that chelate the Zn^{2+} required for MMP activity. The majority of these drugs use a hydroxamate group for this purpose, linked to hydrophobic peptide-like structures to improve inhibitor binding to the active site of the MMP (Figure 13.16). Marimastat, an example of this formulation, illustrates the potential of these compounds. The original compound, Batimastat, was poorly absorbed after oral ingestion and Marimastat evolved as the compound that resolved the problem. It is a broad-spectrum inhibitor of all the metalloproteinases, albeit with varying

Figure 13.16

Inhibition of metalloproteinases by Zn^{2+}-chelating peptides.

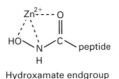

Hydroxamate endgroup

efficiencies, and in all the laboratory tests it exhibited the required properties. It inhibited capillary sprout formation and blocked tumour growth in various animal models, including models assaying metastatic spread. Clinically, Marimastat has mainly been tested as an antimetastatic against ovarian, gastric, lung and pancreatic cancers. It effectively reduces serum markers secreted by the cancers, e.g. CA125 in ovarian cancer patients, and it decreases the proportion of cancer cells in relation to stroma in gastric cancers. Other drugs of this type are being tested against primary cancers.

The development of Marimastat illustrates a problem common to all new drugs: How do you test them in humans? This must be done to ascertain clinical effectiveness. For ethical reasons, the usual procedure is to test the drug on patients with advanced cancers who have failed all other treatments – not the best group of patients for identifying responses. Marimastat is not effective against advanced pancreatic cancer that, even in its early stages, has a very poor prognosis (Table 13.1). A negative result against such advanced, aggressive cancers does not imply the drug will be ineffective against other cancers.

Genes coding for TIMPs have been cloned and incorporated into expression vectors so that adequate quantities of TIMPs will be available. They have the requisite properties in laboratory experiments and clinical studies have now begun.

'Gene' therapy

The coding sequences of DNA are transcribed into mRNA before synthesis of the protein specified by the DNA coding sequence (Box 6.1); synthetic oligodeoxynucleotides with bases complementary to those in the mRNA (antisense oligonucleotides) will hybridise with the mRNA (Figure 13.17). This heteroduplex of mRNA (ribonucleotides) and deoxyribonucleotides is a substrate for ribonuclease H, which preferentially hydrolyses the mRNA strand to release the antisense oligonucleotide; the antisense oligonucleotide then hybridises with another mRNA molecule. This catalytic effect has the potential to selectively destroy specific target mRNAs and the proteins translated therefrom. The concept worked with cultured cells and short (7–30) oligomers were an acceptable compromise between cell permeability (shorter = better) and hybridisation specificity (longer = better). There were problems of hybridisation to other sequences, along with problems of toxicity and drug delivery, but clinical trials have now been started.

The original oligonucleotides had the natural phosphodiester linkages between deoxynucleotides, and this made them susceptible to destruction by phosphodiesterases. Substitution of the phosphate with a phosphothiorate overcame this

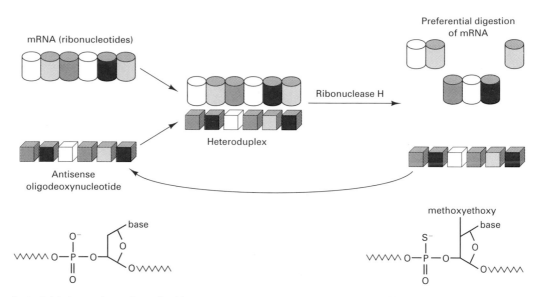

Phosphodiester link between deoxyribonucleotides

Phosphothiorate link

Figure 13.17

Antisense oligodeoxynucleotides can destroy specific mRNAs.

problem, and modification of the 2′ position of the deoxyribose (Figure 13.17) increased the plasma half-life of the drug. Choice of which mRNA to target depends on the protein to be eliminated; trials have begun targeting raf, ras, protein kinase C (signal transduction, Chapter 11), the human papilloma virus E6 and E7 proteins (proliferation and DNA repair, Chapter 6) and Bcl2 (apoptosis, Chapter 10).

The Bcl2 gene is upregulated in about half of advanced cancers and, as the Bcl2 protein blocks apoptosis, this produces resistance to chemotherapy and radiation treatment. Bcl2 is overexpressed in some non-Hodgkin's lymphomas and a small trial with these patients elicited hopeful results. That trial followed the usual intuitive method of designing the antisense oligonucleotides against base sequences at the start site of mRNA synthesis. Laboratory studies have now shown that a more effective region to target lies further into the coding region. The different efficacies reflect the fact that mRNAs have a secondary structure, so certain regions are more accessible to antisense oligonucleotides than others. Thus far, rules to identify accessible regions have not been formulated, so trial and error methods must be used.

The alternative approach of inserting a gene that will downregulate growth-promoting products has also been achieved in animals. This can take the form of introducing a repressor gene such as p53 or a gene coding for a cytokine that activates immune attack on the cancer cell. The cytokine method is being tested in clinical trials on melanoma and colon cancers. Tumour or bone marrow is taken from a patient, lymphocytes isolated and transfected with a cytokine gene such as interleukin-2 or tumour necrosis factor. The cells are then returned to the patient where the cytokines recruit cytotoxic lymphocytes to the tumour.

Gene delivery is a major problem in applying gene therapy to inaccessible cancers and it still remains unsolved. Nevertheless, there are some promising results from accessible head/neck and lung cancers which were directly injected with constructs of the normal p53 gene linked to a viral vector.

Immunotherapy

Manipulation of the immune system to kill cancer cells has been tested in various settings with limited success (Chapter 5). A better understanding of the processes involved in antigen presentation to immune cells (Figure 5.4) has indicated a number of potential improvements to the way immunotherapy is used. Tumour antigens, usually proteins, are proteolytically cleaved to short peptides (about 10 amino acids) within the **a**ntigen **p**resenting **c**ell (APC) that are presented to lymphocytes via the MHC complex: MHC-I for T-cells and MHC-II for macrophage interaction. The two exploitable advances are (i) the identification of specific tumour antigens that efficiently activate the system, and (ii) determination of amino acid sequences of the immunodominant peptides that generate the link between MHC and immune cells. Identification of proteins and peptides has opened up the possibility of priming the immune system with these reagents. Coating APCs with peptides before their reinjection into the patient can improve active immunisation protocols against the parent antigen. Alternatively, coated APCs will activate lymphocytes (tumour or blood derived) *in vitro* and their numbers can be amplified in culture with interleukins and before they are returned to the patient (passive immunisation).

Tumour antigens   Previous work in this area used trial and error methods, but a systematic approach to the identification of tumour antigens has been developed with the acronym of SEREX (**ser**ological analysis of recombinant DNA **ex**pression library) (Figure 13.18). APCs are constructed in the laboratory from cells that have MHC-I but which do not produce peptides capable of activating T-cells; breast cancer cell lines have been used for this purpose. The cells are transfected with recombinant DNA expression libraries constructed from melanomas known to activate T-cells; the breast cells then express proteins determined by the transfected melanoma DNA. Most such cells produce new proteins that do not activate their

Figure 13.18

Identification of tumour antigens and their immunodominant peptides.

1. Transfect recombinant melanoma DNA to express proteins (expression library)

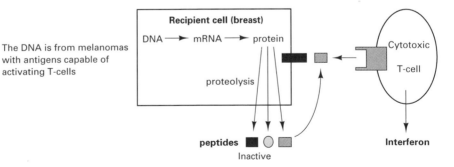

2. Isolate recipient cells that promote interferon production
3. Isolate its melanoma DNA coding for protein/peptides
4. Repeat stages 1, 2 and 3 with fragments of DNA from 3
5. Sequence DNA to identify responsible genes. Predict amino acid sequence of protein/peptides
6. Synthesise immunodominant peptide. Test for biological effect (interferon production, lysis of recipient cell)

MHC-I but some express tumour antigens and immunodominant peptides formed therefrom. Co-culture with autologous T-cells (serology) will detect the active breast cells by the interferon produced by the T-cells in response to MHC interaction. DNA is isolated from positive breast clones; DNA can be isolated after using electrophoresis to distinguish it from breast DNA. Part of the DNA must code for the activating antigen. This cycle of transfection, interferon production and DNA isolation is repeated with fragments of the melanoma DNA isolated during the first round of experiments. The melanoma DNA is sequenced to determine the codons responsible for producing the tumour antigen or immunodominant peptide. The protein or peptide predicted to be formed from the DNA sequence can be identified; peptides are chemically synthesised and tested for biological activity.

An alternative route to defining immunodominant peptides is to purify the MHC together with its bound peptide; subsequent separation and sequencing of the peptide provides the required information. This method has been used to identify families of melanoma tumour antigens (Table 5.3) and to analyse normal expression by other types of cancer. All these antigens elicit a cytotoxic T-cell response *in vitro* but they do this with varying efficiencies; characterising which antigens evoke the best response for different tumour types should improve clinical response rates.

The information obtained about tumour antigens and their peptides can be used to improve both active and passive methods of therapy by bolstering antigen presentation to T-cells. One active immunotherapy trial with malignant melanoma patients involves incubating APCs with a cocktail of peptides based on the melanoma antigen series gp100 and then injecting the cells directly into the patient's lymph nodes. This route was chosen to improve targeting of the APCs to T-cells; good remission was seen in some patients. The APC used in this trial was also novel in that it was not a melanoma cell but a rare type of dendritic cell. This cell type has proved to be very efficient as an APC, and although present in small numbers in a patient's blood, the population can be expanded by culture with mitogenic interleukins. Interleukin-2 is also used for this purpose *in vivo* as an adjuvant to the other components of the immunotherapy regime. In fact, *in vivo* injection of interleukin-2 was required to get a clinical response in the dendritic cell trial. An additional technical advance was tested in that trial; the amino acid sequence of the immunodominant gp100 peptide was engineered so it would be anchored more efficiently to the MHC. The second amino acid of the octapeptide was changed from a threonine to a methionine.

In animal models, the interleukin-2 gene has been incorporated into the commonly used adjuvant bacillus BCG (Chapter 5) so that endogenous interleukin-2 is produced; it improves the immunogenicity of tumour antigens in experimental models. An analogous approach is being tested in which the inserted 'gene' codes for immunodominant peptides of the Mart and gp100 series.

Passive immunotherapy trials have used the principles just described but in which the APC is co-cultured with lymphocytes from a patient's blood or tumour. The cytotoxic potency of TLIs can be improved by a factor of 50–100 through repeated stimulation using dendritic cells coated with immunodominant peptides from the Mart tumour antigen.

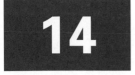

APPROACHES TO CANCER PREVENTION

Key points

- Some cancers can potentially be prevented.
- Chemoprevention of breast cancer has been achieved with the anti-oestrogen tamoxifen.
- Ovarian and endometrial cancer risk is decreased by combined oral contraceptive pills.
- Non-steroidal anti-inflammatory drugs reduce the risk of developing colon cancer.
- Side effects occur with drug use by normal people.
- Increasing fruit and vegetable intake has the potential to reduce the risk of getting several cancers.
- Dietary supplements such as β-carotene are not effective and they may be harmful to smokers.

Introduction

Cancers arise as a consequence of chemical reactions within the cell; it follows that blocking those reactions might prevent cancer. It is an index of our greater understanding of cancer biology that we can now use practical rather than theoretical approaches to chemoprevention. The principle that preventing contact with carcinogens decreases cancer risk is well established; stopping young children climbing soot-encrusted chimneys, preventing atom bomb use and banning smoking diminishes cancer risk in exposed people. There are now legal requirements for carcinogen testing (Chapter 6) which minimises hazards associated with industrial products such that industrial carcinogens cause less than 1% of cancers in developed countries (Table 4.9). However, cancer is still the second biggest cause of death in the Western world (Figure 1.4), so there is much more to be achieved. Antismoking measures would have a major impact (Chapter 3) but, as they are political rather than biological, they will not be discussed here. Likewise the impact of important public health measures such as screening for early detection of cervical (Figure 13.4), breast, prostate and colon cancer are outside the scope of this book. Manipulation of biological processes in normal people with the aim of preventing the appearance of clinical cancers is the objective of several current investigations and will form the basis of this chapter. The 'manipulations' involve giving drugs to healthy people, although in some cases the drugs are called health foods or dietary supplements. The ethical considerations of giving drugs to healthy people are different to those operating in ill people especially in relation to side effects. Chemoprevention trials have to pay great attention to side effects so that a good cost–benefit calculation can be made. An extreme example would be the elimination of breast and prostate cancer by removing the ovaries from young women or the testes from young men, but the consequence would be the extinction of the human race.

Breast cancer and tamoxifen

The major risk factor for breast cancer is oestrogen overexposure (Chapter 4). Hence, opposing that oestrogen should be beneficial; there are good data to support that notion, although all the problems of side effects have not been resolved. Oestrogen deprivation can be achieved by removing the ovaries or giving an anti-oestrogen. For practical reasons, the latter approach is the only feasible one, and the anti-oestrogen tamoxifen has been widely used (Chapter 13). Tamoxifen, a derivative of the synthetic oestrogen diethylstilboestrol (Figure 13.12), binds to the oestrogen receptor, and promotes dimerisation and DNA binding of the receptor (Chapter 11 and Figure 14.1). However, the conformation of the DNA-bound receptor is different to the conformation with an oestrogen; one of the transactivation domains is occluded by the C-terminal sequences, recruitment of essential transcription factors does not occur and gene transcription is not activated. Non-functional binding of tamoxifen to the oestrogen receptor blocks the effects of oestrogen. In fact, the situation is not as simple as this because some genes can be switched on by tamoxifen in a cell-specific manner. In pharmacological parlance, tamoxifen is a partial oestrogen agonist with different cell types exhibiting different proportions of agonist and antagonist activity. Endocrinologists have taken to calling

Figure 14.1

Oestradiol and tamoxifen binding to the oestrogen receptor. Other proteins are involved but they are not illustrated.

Domain structure of the oestradiol receptor

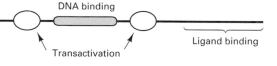

Inactive receptor in absence of ligand: DNA-binding domain occluded

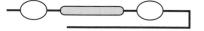

Oestradiol binding: DNA-binding and both transactivation domains exposed

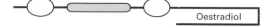

Tamoxifen binding: DNA-binding and one transactivation domain exposed

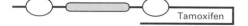

such drugs selective oestrogen receptor modulators. The selective action of tamoxifen can be beneficial in that one of the genes switched on in breast cancer cells is the gene for the antiproliferative cytokine TGF-β (Chapter 11). In other cells, such as those of the endometrium, growth-promoting genes are activated that generate adverse side effects (see below).

Induction of breast cancers in rats with carcinogens such as dimethylbenz(o)anthracene or N-methylnitrosurea (Chapter 8) is blocked by tamoxifen, as is growth of established breast cancers. This suggests that tamoxifen can inhibit both early and late events in carcinogenesis. Clinical data amply support the laboratory experiments that tamoxifen has beneficial effects on established breast cancer. The clinical data come from three main sources. (1) Tamoxifen induces good remission in about one-quarter of patients who have metastatic breast cancer and there are only limited side effects; better response rates (two-thirds) are seen with breast cancers that have retained the oestrogen response mechanism (oestrogen receptor positive cancers). (2) Women who have had a cancer removed from one breast are at risk of getting a subsequent cancer in their other breast; tamoxifen given after the first operation reduces that risk by one-third. (3) Pre- or postmenopausal women given adjuvant tamoxifen for primary breast cancer are less likely to get a recurrence than those who did not get the drug.

These data pointed to the potential of tamoxifen as a chemoprotective agent and trials were begun with normal women who were at high risk of developing breast cancer. The women were identified by the known risk factors (Chapter 4) of age, reproductive history and relatives with breast cancer. Having relatives with breast cancer is a surrogate indicator for families who carry a defect in one of the breast cancer genes (Chapter 9). Women in some families who carry such gene defects have an 80% probability that they will get breast cancer some time in their life; these women would especially benefit from a chemopreventive therapy. One trial in the USA was stopped early because it was so successful that it was considered unethical not to offer tamoxifen to the control group who had not been given the drug. There were half the number of cancers in the tamoxifen-treated group; the number of non-invasive carcinomas *in situ* was also reduced, suggesting that tamoxifen could act at a relatively early stage of carcinogenesis. In contrast, two European trials indicate no such benefits. It remains to be established whether this conflict of data reflects differences in characteristics of the participating women or something more fundamental.

Both beneficial and adverse side effects were noted in these trials consequential to the partial agonist nature of tamoxifen. Beneficial, agonist (oestrogen) effects on high-density lipoproteins and calcium deposition occurred with liver and bone respectively, but the endometrium showed an adverse hyperproliferation. Oestrogens induce high-density lipoprotein synthesis in liver that is associated with increased clearance of cholesterol and decreased risk of heart attacks. Oestrogen-induced calcium deposition in bone decreases the risk of osteoporosis (weak bones due to calcium loss). Tamoxifen is mitogenic for endometrial cells and the tamoxifen group in the US trial had twice as many endometrial cancers as the control group. The tamoxifen group also had a higher than expected incidence of problems linked to blood vessel dysfunction (pulmonary embolus and deep vein thrombosis). Many problems have to be resolved before wider use of tamoxifen as a chemopreventive agent can be recommended, but women might consider the risks worthwhile if they are almost certain to get breast cancer because they have an inherited gene defect. More selective anti-oestrogens with potentially fewer side effects are currently being tested. Despite these problems associated with tamoxifen, much poorly substantiated hyperbole is currently directed at potential benefits of dietary components, photooestrogens (see below) with similar properties to tamoxifen.

Ovarian/endometrial cancer and the contraceptive pill

Oral contraceptive (OC) pills were developed to suppress ovulation; the most effective agents contained two categories of female sex steroid, oestrogens and progestins, hence they were called combined oral contraceptive pills. Via their separate receptors (Chapter 11), these steroids suppress pituitary gonadotrophins and hence ovulation (Figure 13.12). Oral conraceptives have proved effective at controlling ovulation and they are extremely safe; a beneficial side effect has been a dramatic protective effect against endometrial and ovarian cancer (Figure 14.2). The protective effect is long-lasting and continues after stopping their use.

Ovarian cancer is the fifth most common cause of cancer deaths in women (Table 1.1) so it is especially gratifying that OCs have halved the risk of developing it, given that oral contraception is used by 100 million women worldwide. Oral contraceptives are also protective against familial types of ovarian cancer (Chapter 9). The mechanism behind this protective effect is clear for endometrium but less so for ovary. In endometrium, oestrogens are mitogenic and progestins counteract that effect. Acting via the progestin receptor, progestins downregulate the oestrogen receptor, making the cells refractory to oestrogens; but progestins also activate genes involved in differentiated functions (secretory proteins, glycogen synthesis). The events involved in ovarian carcinogenesis are poorly understood. The prevailing hypothesis is that tissue damage, consequent to egg release, generates DNA damage via free radical formation (Chapter 8). If this model is correct, OCs indirectly prevent this damage by inhibiting ovulation.

Figure 14.2

Women taking oral contraceptives: cancer risk for ovary and endometrium.

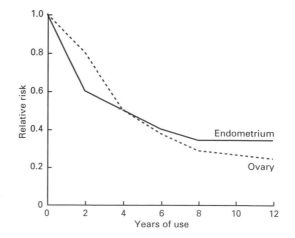

Adverse side effects of OC use are mainly limited to altered blood lipid profiles and damage to blood vessels in a minority of women. There is also a small (15%) increased risk of developing breast cancer, presumably via receptor-mediated events, but it disappears within 5 years of stopping OC use. Pill users are also at an increased risk of developing cervical cancer (Table 4.2). It is not clear whether this is due to a direct effect of OCs on the cervical epithelium or is an indirect consequence linked to increased sexual activity and exposure to the carcinogenic human papilloma virus (Chapter 4).

Colon cancer and aspirin

Colon cancer is the third most important cause of cancer-related deaths in both men and women (Table 1.1). The serendipitous observation that **n**on-**s**teroidal **a**nti-**i**nflammatory **d**rugs (NSAIDs) such as aspirin, taken for diseases like arthritis, decreased mortality from colon cancer by half (Figure 14.3), indicates a practical route whereby the incidence of colon cancers in the general population might be reduced. Arachidonic acid is a substrate for the **cyclooxy**genase enzymes COX-1 and COX-2 that produce a series of prostaglandins and thromboxanes (Figure 11.21); production of prostaglandin E2 is especially important in colon carcinogenesis. NSAIDs inhibit the COX enzymes and prostaglandin production. Prostaglandins stimulate angiogenesis and cell proliferation whilst blocking their synthesis increases apoptosis (Chapter 11); inhibiting prostaglandin production would influence all of these functions in a way that would antagonise cancer formation. Laboratory studies have demonstrated the relevance of these effects to colon carcinogenesis. The Min mouse, which lacks the APC gene (Chapter 2), develops colon polyps; deleting the COX-2 gene decreases both the size and number of those polyps. COX inhibitors have a similar effect on chemically

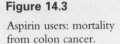

Figure 14.3

Aspirin users: mortality from colon cancer.

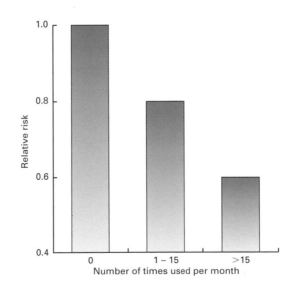

induced colon cancers. In cultured colon cancer cells, transfection of a COX-2 gene increases prostaglandin synthesis, increases cell adhesion and decreases apoptosis; these effects are blocked by COX inhibitors. Hence there is a good mechanistic explanation for how NSAIDs such as aspirin can prevent colon carcinogenesis.

Aspirin has been available for a hundred years so its side effects are well known; gastrointestinal ulceration and renal toxicity are such that long-term use as a chemopreventive agent would create problems. However, more selective NSAIDs that only inhibit COX-2 may not have these side effects. COX-1 enzyme is constitutively expressed in many cell types whilst COX-2 is usually low but can be induced by early events in colon carcinogenesis. The classical NSAIDs like aspirin, Sulindac and ibuprofen inhibit both COX-1 and COX-2, thus blocking cancer genesis (COX-2) but also generating the unwanted side effects (COX-1). Selective COX-2 inhibitors such as Celecoxib or NS-398 have all the anticancer effects of aspirin but none of its side effects in laboratory studies. They may be even more efficient than aspirin, as one animal study indicated a greater than 90% inhibition of invasive and non-invasive colon cancer formation. Selective COX-2 inhibitors have a promising future as chemopreventive drugs.

Diet

According to prestigious international bodies, '30–40% of cancers are preventable by dietary means'. This statement encapsulates the potential benefit of dietary manipulation but it is a best-case scenario; actually achieving changes of that magnitude is an improbable objective. Table 14.1 Indicates that potential benefits would accrue for a range of cancers and it points to the major food components involved. When considering these estimates of preventable cancers, remember that the data on which they are based were mainly obtained from observational epidemiological investigations in countries with different dietary habits (China versus USA) or groups with different lifestyles (vegetarians versus meat-eaters) within one country (Chapter 4). This type of study provides substantial evidence that food intake is an important factor but it overestimates the magnitude of change

Table 14.1 Diet and the five major (global) cancers: overall 3–4 million cancers are preventable.

Site	Incidence (millions)	Prevent by diet (estimate)	Dietary factor	
			Good	Bad
Lung	1.3	25%*	Fruit and vegetables	
Stomach	1.0	70%	Fruit and vegetables	Salt, salt foods
Breast	0.9	40%†	Fruit and vegetables	Fat, alcohol
Colon	0.9	70%	Fruit and vegetables	Meat, alcohol
Mouth, pharynx, nasopharynx	0.6	40%	Fruit and vegetables	Alcohol, salt fish

* Both smokers and non-smokers.
† If started before puberty; 15% if started in adult life

that could be achieved in practice. Although they indicate the food items involved, they do not reveal which components in those foods are the active agents. Nevertheless, any decrease in cancer incidence has to be a good objective.

Food contains both good and bad components (Table 14.1) with the good items consistently including fruit and vegetables. Based on this type of evidence, national and international bodies have recommended an increased intake of fruit and vegetables to include five portions per day (American Cancer Society, UK government), at least 400 g/day (World Cancer Research Fund, WCRF) or increase current consumption by 50% (UK government). This good advice is worth following, but based on previous experience with coronary heart disease, it is unlikely to achieve maximum response because people prefer hamburgers to lettuce. The 400 g/day of fruit and vegetables is almost twice the average UK consumption of these items. It would be more practical to adopt the 'pop-a-pill' approach of dietary supplementation provided one knew which pills to pop. Despite many subjective claims, there is no hard evidence that any dietary supplement is beneficial against cancer in humans. Micronutrients such as vitamins, selenium and antioxidants have received much attention and may have beneficial effects on general health of people with poor nutrition, but for a well-fed population the current conclusion from all the expert committees would be 'good hypothesis but no supportive data'. An exception to that conclusion might be β-carotene.

Found in vegetables, β-carotene is an antioxidant which can also be metabolised to vitamin A, and vitamin A induces differentiation in some epithelia. Observational studies indicate that a high vegetable intake correlates with a decreased risk of developing lung cancer (Figure 4.9); as vegetables contain β-carotene, serum levels of β-carotene indicate a similar risk pattern. Participants in these observational studies ate their normal diet so β-carotene supplements were not involved. The correlation between fruit and vegetable intake and lung cancer was stronger than that for β-carotene. It could be that the causal agent was something other than β-carotene and that the β-carotene was only a surrogate marker of the active ingredient. This is a real possibility because the observational results conflict with data from intervention trials in which β-carotene was given to people for several years; the incidence (Figure 14.4) and mortality from lung cancer increased by about one-fifth rather than decreased. One of the trials was stopped prematurely because the dietary supplements were harmful not beneficial. A caveat should be noted that the trial participants were mostly smokers. Cigarette smoke is such a strong carcinogen that data obtained from smokers may not be relevant to non-smokers.

Nevertheless, the current recommendation by bodies such as the UK government is to avoid β-carotene supplements. It remains to be seen whether the lung cancer data is relevant to cancers at other sites. This discrepancy between results from observational and intervention trials carries a warning against making conclusions for other dietary ingredients from a plausible hypothesis plus observational data; better data are required before a causal link can be established. Other β-carotene supplementation trials for effects on skin, oesophagus and stomach cancers have shown neither beneficial nor detrimental effects. The only dietary supplement trial that has shown a beneficial effect (incidence decreased by one-quarter) involves vitamin A (retinol) and squamous cell carcinomas. It has been emphasised that taking a pill is not a substitute for a varied diet.

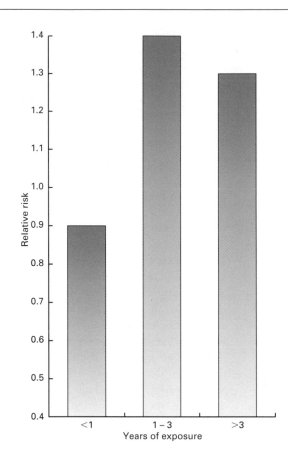

Figure 14.4

Smokers taking
β-carotene: risk of
developing lung
cancer.

Due to uncertain mechanisms (Chapter 4), dietary fibre (non-starch polysaccharides) may be protective against cancers of the gastrointestinal tract and both the UK government and the World Cancer Research Fund (WCRF) recommend an increased intake. The WCRF also concluded that insufficient data were available to make any recommendations on vitamins A, C or E consumption or fat intake. The WCRF suggested that fat and oil consumption should provide less than one-quarter of calorific intake and that less than 80 g of red meat should be eaten per day. No recommendations were made about selenium because current data are too sparse. Selenium was incorporated with tocopherol or carotenoids in several ineffective trials. Meat intake and cancer is an emotive topic; it generated disagreement within the UK government committee and the original report was withdrawn within days of its publication. The committee eventually concluded that red meat intake should not rise. Consumption of salt-cured or smoked foods should be minimised.

APPENDIX A
FEATURES OF SELECTED CANCERS

The cancers in this appendix are those whose incidence and mortality are listed in Table 1.1. Figure A.1 presents that data in a different format. Data for these cancers relates to European and North American populations. Unless stated otherwise, the factors mentioned increase risk. Multiple changes in gene structure and function have been identified in every cancer studied; a comprehensive list would not distinguish between genes that play a causative role in carcinogenesis and those that have ancillary effects such as changes relevant to progression. Furthermore, for any one type of cancer, specific gene changes often occur in only a proportion, commonly about one-third, of those cancers; there are multiple routes to a common endpoint, cancer. Rather than provide a catalogue of genes, I mention only those genes that are *probably* involved in early rather than late responses. This is a subjective exercise that may contain errors as good data is not available for many of the cancers mentioned. Hesketh's *Oncogene and Tumour Repressor Gene Fact Book*, 2nd edn (Academic Press, 1997) has a good table (Table IV) that lists genes identified in various human cancers. Where possible, I have cross-referenced the genes mentioned here to relevant parts of this book. In some cases it is not possible to identify causative changes for specific cancers.

Figure A.1

New cases and deaths from the main cancers. USA, 1995, % of all cancers at stated site.

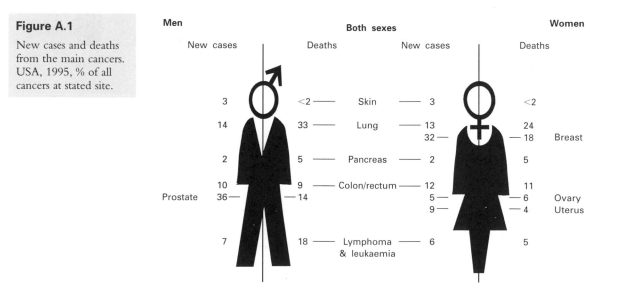

277

Breast (Figure A.2)

1. Adenocarcinomas: mostly of ductal (80%) or lobular (10%) epithelium.

2. Lifetime risk of getting breast cancer: 1:11 (women), 1:1000 (men).

3. Five-year survival rates: 80% but see Table 13.1 and Figures 4.3, 13.2 and 13.3 for subgroup data.

4. Risk factors: age of first pregnancy (<30, lower risk), early menarche, late menopause, family history, breastfeeding (premenopause, lower risk), diet (Chapter 4).

5. Metastasis: lymph nodes, bone and locally in the breast.

6. Inherited gene changes: BRCA1 and BRCA2, p53 (Figures 4.6 and 9.2, Tables 9.3 to 9.5).

7. Sporadic gene changes: oestrogen receptor (Table 11.5), cyclin D (Figure 10.9), EGF/ErbB family (Tzahar, E., and Yarden, Y., 1998, *Biochimica Biophysica Acta*, **1377**, M25–M37).

Comments   Breast cancer is the most common cancer in women. Men get breast cancer but the probability is about one hundred times less than for women. There are marked geographical differences in risk (Figure 4.2). Mortality is decreasing in developed countries due to the introduction of breast screening to detect early cancers and due to improved treatment regimes.

Figure A.2

Breast. Epithelial cells give rise to cancers. See also Figure 3.3. Blue type indicates cells that give rise to cancers.

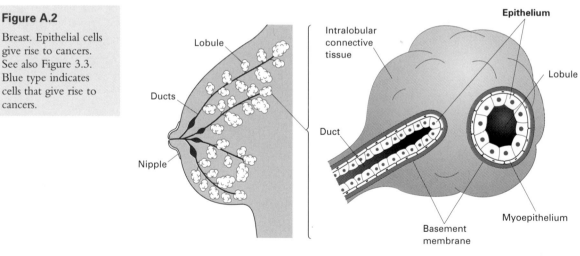

Colon (Figure A.3)

1. Adenocarcinoma: (90%) or mucinous adenocarcinoma (10%).
2. Lifetime risk of getting colon cancer: 1:20 (men and women).
3. Five-year survival rate: 59% but see Table 13.1.
4. Risk factors: family history, inflammatory bowel disease, diet (Table 4.1).

Figure A.3

Colon. Epithelial cells give rise to cancers. The endocrine cells secrete peptides and can form tumours (APUDomas); they are not described in this book. See also Figures 3.2 and 12.2.

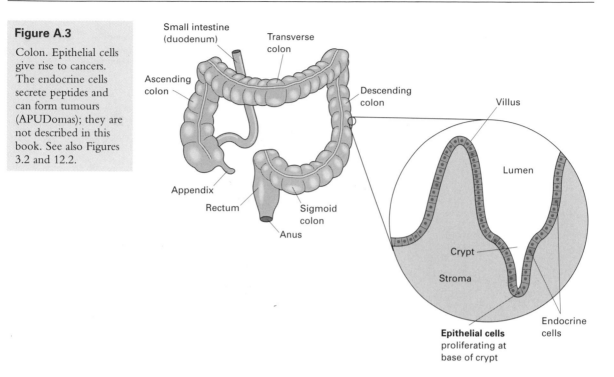

5. Metastasis: locally and to liver and lymph nodes.
6. Inherited gene changes: APC, MLH1, MSH2 (Tables 9.3 to 9.5).
7. Sporadic gene changes: APC, ras, p53, MLH1 (Figure 2.11 and Table 2.1).
    p53 (Figures 6.11 and 7.12, Table 7.9.)

Comments   The figures include rectal cancer (colorectal cancer); see Chapter 2 for additional information.

Leukaemia (Figure A.4)

Results from blocked haemopoietic cell differentiation; the type of leukaemia is determined by the stage at which differentiation is blocked. See Figure 10.18 and accompanying text. Each type of leukaemia has its own characteristics and the information given below contains major generalisations. Leukaemias constitute a third of childhood cancers. Gene changes in leukaemias vary with the type of leukaemia but chromosome translocations are common. Hesketh's book (Hesketh, R., 2nd edn, 1997, Academic Press) has a good table (Table III) that lists translocations and the genes involved that have been identified in various leukaemias. Chronic myeloid leukaemia (abl oncogene) and acute promyelocytic leukaemia (retinoic acid alpha receptor) are described in Figures 11.8 and 6.7, respectively. Inheritance of the ataxia telangiectasia gene defect (Table 9.3) predisposes individuals to a risk of developing leukaemia. The lifetime risk of getting leukaemia is 1:400.

Figure A.4

Leukaemia. Only the major types are shown.

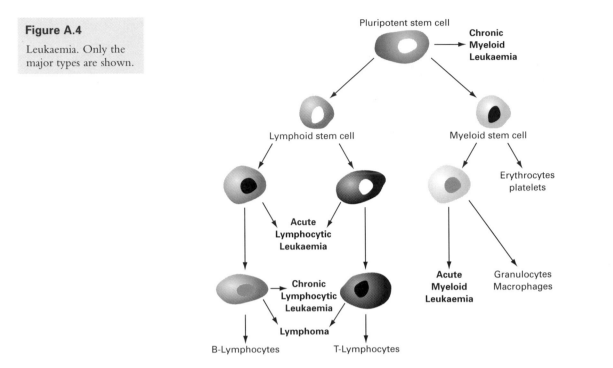

Chronic leukaemia.

1. Mostly B–cell (95%) but some T–cell (5%) leukaemias. Variants include chronic myeloid leukaemia (Chapter 2).
2. Five-year survival rate: 80%.
3. Risk factors: uncertain; not increased by radiation.
4. Abnormal cells accumulate in blood, bone marrow and spleen.
5. Gene changes: see above.

Comments Chronic leukaemia is the most common form; it is twice as common in men as in women. Efficient chemotherapy has greatly improved survival rates.

Acute leukaemia

1. Acute myeloid leukaemia (acute non-lymphocytic leukaemia) is five times more common than acute lymphocytic leukaemia. Variants include acute promyelocytic leukaemia (Figure 6.7).

2. Aggressive condition with 90% mortality within one year of diagnosis.

3. Risk factors: Down's syndrome, Bloom's syndrome (Chapter 9), radiation (Figure 4.4), T-cell leukaemia virus, previous chemotherapy for other cancers.

4. Accumulation of abnormal cells in bone marrow and other organs.

5. Gene changes: see above.

Comments Men are marginally more susceptible than women; acute leukaemia is ten times more common in adults than children but it accounts for 75% of childhood leukaemias (Figure 1.1). Chemotherapy has improved survival of childhood acute leukaemias.

Lung (Figure A.5)

1. Non-small-cell (90%) and small-cell (10%) variants of bronchial epithelial cancers exist. Small-cell carcinomas are derived from epithelial cells with features of neuroendocrine origin as they secrete neuropeptides such as vasopressin and ACTH. Non-small-cell carcinomas have squamous (35%), glandular (adenocarcinoma 40%) or large (10%) cell features. They may all derive from a common stem cell. Cancers of the mesothelial lining of the lungs (mesothelioma) are closely associated with asbestos exposure. There are epithelial and sarcomatous variants.

2. Lifetime risk of getting lung cancer: 1:12 (men), 1:23 (women).

3. Five-year survival rate: 13%.

4. Risk factors: smoking (Chapter 4), asbestos (mesothelioma), radon gas from building materials (Chapter 8).

5. Metastasis: lung, bone, liver.

Figure A.5

Lung. Respiratory epithelium and mesothelial lining give rise to cancers.

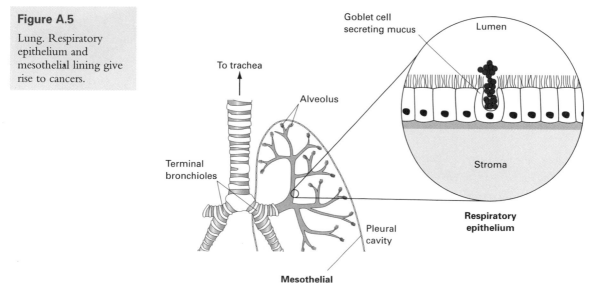

6. Gene changes: see Sekido, Y. *et al.* (1998) *Biochimica Biophysica Acta*, **1378**, F21–F59.
   - Small-cell variant: Bcl2, Rb, myc, telomerase, p53.
   - Non-small-cell variant: ras, Bcl2, p53, Rb, p16^{INK}, telomerase.
   - Mesothelioma: p16^{INK} (see Hall, M. and Peters, G. 1996. *Advances in Cancer Research*, **68**, 67–108).
   - p53 changes in lung cancers are described in Figures 4.6, 6.11, 7.12 and Table 7.9.

Comments   A 35-year-old man smoking 25 cigarettes per day has a 1:8 chance of dying from lung cancer before age 75 (Chapter 4). Men are more likely to get lung cancer than women but the difference between the sexes is getting smaller as women increase their smoking habit. Lung cancer has a poor response to chemotherapy.

Lymphoma (Figure A.6)

1. Two categories, Hodgkin's lymphoma and non–Hodgkin's (lymphocytic or malignant) lymphoma. Non-Hodgkin's lymphomas are mainly of B-cell origin,

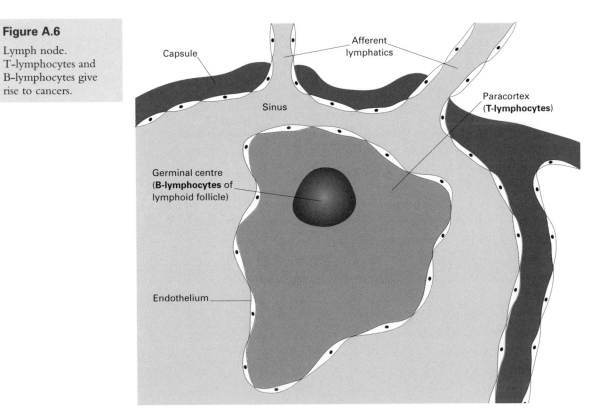

Figure A.6

Lymph node. T-lymphocytes and B-lymphocytes give rise to cancers.

including Burkitt's lymphoma (Figure 6.5); Hodgkin's lymphoma possibly has a multi-lineage aetiology. The nodular form of Hodgkin's lymphoma is a B-cell tumour.

2. Lifetime risk of getting lymphoma: 1:300 (Hodgkin's), 1:40 (non-Hodgkins).

3. Five-year survival rate: 79% (Hodgkin's), 52% (non-Hodgkins).

4. Risk factors: Epstein–Barr virus (Chapter 6), organ transplants (immunosuppression), AIDS virus, radiation, chemotherapy for previous cancer.

5. Metastasis: lymph nodes, spleen and viscera.

6. Chromosome translocations are common. Hesketh's book (see reference on p. 279) has a good table (Table III) that lists the major translocations and the genes involved. Burkitt's lymphoma involving the myc oncogene is detailed in Figure 6.5. Inheritance of the ataxia telangiectasia gene defect (Table 9.3) predisposes individuals to a risk of developing lymphoma.

Comments   Hodgkin's lymphoma has a bimodal age distribution with peaks at ages 20–30 and >50. The incidence of non-Hodgkin's lymphoma peaks at ages 40–50 but 10% occur in children less than 16 years of age. The childhood form of non-Hodgkin's lymphoma has different characteristics than the adult form. The childhood form derives mainly (40%) from T-cells; it is more diffuse; and under the age of 10 it is three times more common in boys than in girls.

Mouth

1. Mostly squamous carcinomas.
2. Lifetime risk of getting cancer of the mouth: 1:70.
3. Five-year survival: 52%.
4. Risk factors: smoking, alcohol.
5. Metastasis: lymph nodes and bone.
6. Gene changes: cyclin D (Figure 10.9), p53 (Figure 4.6).

Comments   Men are twice as likely as women to get mouth cancer, but this reflects tobacco use rather than a sex difference. Mouth cancer is usually included in a collective group of head/neck cancers. The histological picture is similar to squamous cell carcinoma of the cervix (Figure A.11).

Ovary (Figure A.7)

1. Over 90% arise in the epithelial layer surrounding the ovary. The cancers appear as mucinous cystadenocarcinoma (12%), serous cystadenocarcinoma (42%) or endometrioid carcinoma (15%) with a further fraction being undifferentiated carcinomas (17%).

Figure A.7

Ovary. Coelomic epithelial cells give rise to cancers. Granulosa cells can also give rise to cancers but they are not described in this book.

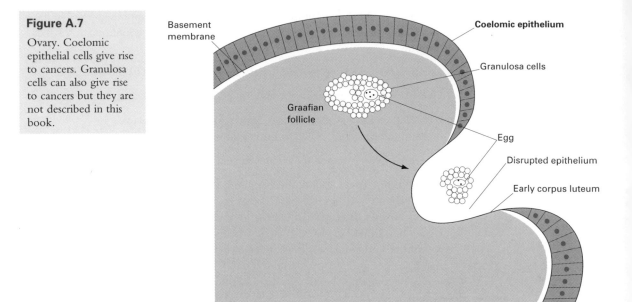

2. Lifetime risk of getting ovarian cancer: 1:56 (women).

3. Five-year survival: 42% (Table 4.3).

4. Risk factors: family history, ovulation, fertility treatment, pregnancy (decreased risk), combined oral contraceptive use (decreased risk, Figure 14.12).

5. Metastasis: surface shedding into the peritoneum; regrowth on viscera, including the other ovary.

6. Inherited gene changes: BRCA1 and BRCA2 (Table 9.5).

7. Sporadic gene changes: p53 see Steele, M. Gene aberrations. In *Ovarian Cancer*, Vol. 4, 1 Sharp, F., Mason, W.P. and Leake, R.E. (eds), Chapman Hall, London, pp. 61–75.

Comments   Poor prognosis is due to late initial detection.

Pancreas (Figure A.8)

1. Mostly (80%) ductal adenocarcinoma of the exocrine pancreas.
2. Lifetime risk of getting pancreatic cancer: 1:60 (men and women).
3. Five-year survival: 3% (Table 13.1).
4. Risk factors: smoking, pancreatitis.
5. Metastasis: intraperitoneal spread to viscera, lung, bone.
6. Gene changes: p16^{INK} (see Hall, M. and Peters, G., 1996, *Advances in Cancer Research*, **68**, 67–108).

Comments   Treatments ineffective.

Figure A.8

Exocrine pancreas. Glandular epithelial cells give rise to cancers.

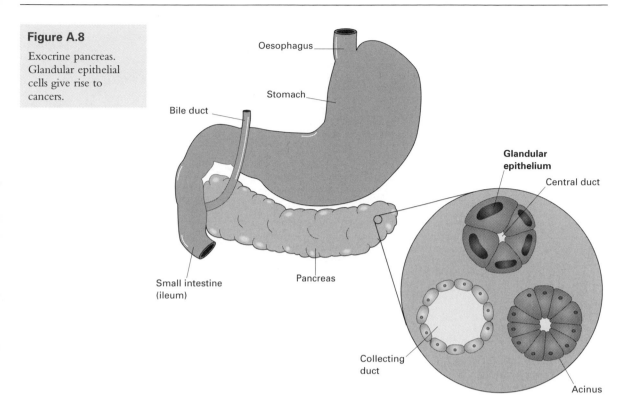

Oesophagus

Stomach

Bile duct

Glandular epithelium

Central duct

Small intestine (ileum)

Pancreas

Collecting duct

Acinus

Prostate (Figure A.9)

1. Adenocarcinomas of luminal epithelium.

2. Lifetime risk of getting prostate cancer: 1:14 (men).

3. Five-year survival rate: 80%

4. Risk factors: uncertain but include diet (Chapter 4) and family history of prostate cancer.

5. Metastasis: lymph nodes and bone.

6. Inherited gene changes: BRCA2 (Table 9.5), HPC1.

7. Sporadic gene changes: androgen receptor (Table 11.5), β-catenin (Figure 11.19), telomerase, DNA methylation, p53, CD44, E-cadherin, Rb, ras (see Ruijter, E., van de Kaa, C., Miller, G., Ruiter, D., DeBryne, F. and Schalken, J., (1999) Molecular genetics and epidemiology of prostate carcinoma. *Endocrine Reviews*, **20**, 22–45).

Comments   Prostate cancer is the most common cancer in men and its incidence is increasing. The reasons are unclear but they include improved diagnostic efficiency. Autopsy analysis indicates that most men have occult cancers of the prostate. There are marked geographical variations (Table 4.1 and Figure 4.2).

Figure A.9

Prostate gland. Glandular epithelial cells give rise to cancers.

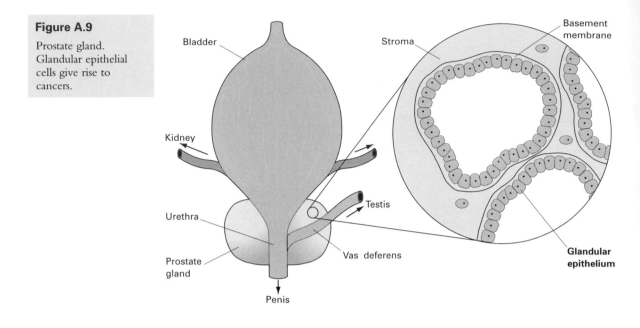

Skin (Figure A.10)

1. Three cell types can develop into cancers. Basal cell carcinoma (basal epithelium) accounts for 75% of all skin cancers with squamous cell carcinoma (keratinocytes) contributing another 20% to that total. Malignant melanoma (melanocytes) contributes only 5% of the total. Melanoma can also occur in the eye and vulva.

2. Lifetime risk of getting skin cancer: 1:60 (melanoma), 1:3 (other).

3. Basal cell cancers are curable as they rarely metastasise; squamous cell carcinomas are curable if detected early. Five-year survival rate for malignant melanoma: 85%.

4. Risk factors for all types of skin cancer: ultraviolet light, fair skin (White people are ten times more likely to get melanoma than Black people).

5. Melanoma metastasises to lymph nodes, skin and lung.

6. Gene changes: individuals who have inherited one of the xeroderma pigmentosum gene defects (Table 9.3) are at increased risk of getting skin cancers. p16^{INK} is involved in the formation of familial and sporadic melanoma (Table 9.3); see also Hall, M. and Peters, G. (1996) *Advances in Cancer Research*, **68**, 67–108). p53 is connected with basal cell carcinoma.

Comments Incidence of skin cancer is the same for men and women. Incidence figures for melanoma are increasing at a rate of 4% per year; this is due to increased exposure of skin to sunlight.

Figure A.10

Skin. Melanocytes, keratinocytes and basal epithelium give rise to cancers.

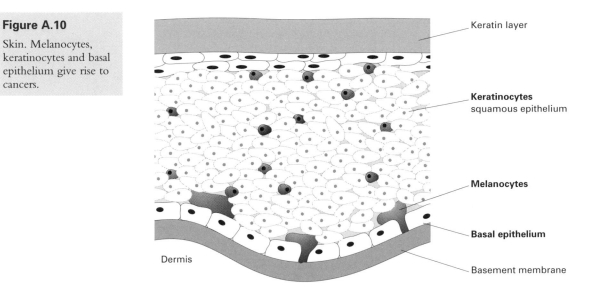

Keratin layer

Keratinocytes
squamous epithelium

Melanocytes

Basal epithelium

Dermis

Basement membrane

Uterus (Figure A.11)

Cervix

1. Most occur as squamous carcinomas (95%); the rest occur in the endocervical columnar cells as adenosquamous carcinoma (5%).
2. Lifetime risk of getting cancer: 1:100 (cervical), 1:77 (all uterine).
3. Five-year survival: 67%.
4. Risk factors: early age of first intercourse, multiple partners, smoking, exposure to human papilloma virus (Table 4.2).
5. Metastasis: lymph nodes, distant metastases are rare.
6. Gene changes: human papilloma virus contributing the E6 and E7 genes (Figure 6.7).

Comments   Cervical cancer is a sexually transmitted disease (Table 4.2). There are wide geographical variations in incidence (Table 4.1). Where screening programmes have been introduced, mortality has fallen (Figure 13.4).

Endometrium

1. Mostly adenocarcinomas (95%) of the epithelial cells, sarcomas (5%).
2. Lifetime risk of getting endometrial cancer: 1:120.
3. Five-year survival: 83%

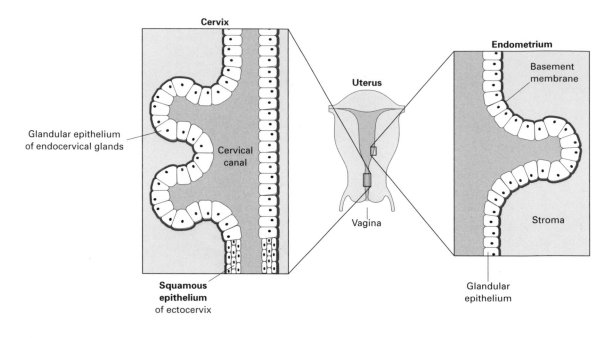

Figure A.11

Uterus. Glandular and squamous epithelia give rise to cancers.

4. Risk factors: oestrogen unopposed by progestins (oestrogen replacement therapy), obesity, history of infertility, early menarche, late menopause, combined oral contraceptive pill (reduces risk, Figure 14.2).

5. Metastasis: myometrial and cervical invasion.

Comments Good prognosis as detected early because of associated menstrual problems.

GLOSSARY

Acquired resistance: drug resistance resulting from drug exposure.

Adjuvant chemotherapy: chemotherapy given at the time of surgery or radiotherapy.

Alkylating agent: electrophilic chemical that alkylates nucleic acids; carcinogenic and used in chemotherapy.

Allele: gene on one chromosome that has a homologue on the other chromosome of a diploid cell.

Anaplasia: lack of differentiated features.

Anchorage dependence: cells that require a substrate on which to grow. Anchorage independent if substrate not necessary (suspension growth).

Aneuploid: inexact multiple of normal DNA (chromosome) content.

Angiogenesis: growth of new blood vessels.

Antigen: molecule capable of generating an immune response.

Antimetabolite: chemotherapeutic drug that blocks metabolic pathways.

Antioncogene: poor alternative term for a repressor gene. See Chapter 6.

Apoptosis: active cell death that requires nucleic acid and protein synthesis.

Apoptosome: protein complex containing protease responsible for final stage of apoptosis

Ascitic fluid: peritoneal fluid; can contain cells.

Athymic mouse: *see* Nude mouse.

Autocrine: secretion of regulatory molecules that function on the producing cell.

Autosome: chromosome that is not one of the sex chromosomes.

B-cell: lymphocyte capable of being activated to produce antibodies. See Chapter 5.

Benign: confined growth that is not malignant. See Table 3.2.

Biological response modifiers: heterogeneous group of chemicals that influence cells of the immune system. Also affect other cells. Include interferons, interleukins and tumour necrosis factor.

Cachexia: body wasting associated with advanced cancer.

Cancer: unregulated growth that is invasive and capable of spreading elsewhere (metastasis).

Carcinogen: agent capable of causing cancer.

Carcinogenesis: processes involved in the production of a cancer.

Carcinoma: epithelial cell cancer. See Table 3.3.

Carcinoma in situ: early stage of cancer that has not invaded its surroundings.

Case–control study: epidemiological method in which people with one characteristic are compared retrospectively with those without that feature.

Cell cycle: cycle of events required for cell multiplication.

cDNA: DNA sequence complementary to an mRNA.

Chimera: mixed function/cell type.

Chromatin: nuclear DNA plus its attached proteins.

Chromosome: structural unit that contains genetic material.

Clone: single cell that can produce identical cells. Also applied to the isolation of a single gene.

Coding region: part of a gene that is transcribed into mRNA. It codes for amino acids.

Codon: three-base sequence in DNA that codes for one amino acid.

Cohort study: prospective epidemiological study in which the characteristics of a group of people are followed over a period of time.

Contact inhibition: *see* Density regulation.

Cytostatic: agent that stops the growth of cells.

Cytotoxic: agent that kills cells.

Density regulation: cells that stop proliferating when they contact adjacent cells (contact inhibition).

Differentiation: development of specialist function by a cell.

Diploid: normal DNA content of cells with a double complement of each chromosome.

Domain: region of a protein serving one specific function.

Dominant: mutation that overcomes the influence of the other allele in a diploid cell. Change that results in a gain of function. See Table 6.1.

Dominant–negative: dominant mutation that has a negative effect on function. See Table 6.1.

Endocrine: chemical signals carried to the target cells by the bloodstream.

Enhancer: DNA sequence in regulatory region of a gene that is activated by appropriate DNA-binding proteins (transcription factors). See Figure 6.1.

Epigenetic: regulation of gene activity by means other than altering gene structure.

Epitope: region of an antigen that is recognised by an antibody.

Extravasation: escape of cancer cells from blood vessels and lymphatics during metastasis.

Exons: transcribed regions of a gene that are translated into protein. See Chapter 6.

Gatekeeper gene: gene in which a functional change is essential for carcinogenesis.

G_0, G_1, G_2: phases of the cell cycle. See Chapter 10.

Gene: DNA containing regulatory and coding sequences for one protein. See Chapter 6.

Genotoxic: agent that damages DNA.

Genotype: genetic (DNA) make-up of a cell.

Germ cell: sperm or egg whose genetic complement can be passed to children.

Grade: histological classification of a cancer based on mitoses, nuclear shape and differentiation. See Chapter 13.

Growth factor: secreted polypeptide that regulates growth. Usually stimulatory but can be inhibitory.

Haploid: half the normal DNA content. Single complement of chromosomes.
Heterodimer: dimer (protein) composed of dissimilar subunits. See Chapter 6.
Heterozygous: two alleles of a gene are different; heterozygosity.
Histogenesis: original cell type from which a cancer was derived.
Homodimer: dimer (protein) composed of similar subunits. See Chapter 6.
Homologous recombination: recombination between similar regions of DNA base sequence on each allele.
Homozygous: two alleles of a gene are the same; homozygosity.
Hyperplasia: increased cell number.
Hypertrophy: increased cell size.
Hypoxia: low oxygen level.

Immune surveillance: processes by which the immune system monitors the body for foreign antigens such as cancer cells.
Incidence: number of new cancers developing in a defined population over a defined time.
Initiation: initial stage of carcinogenesis.
Interphase: period between mitoses.
Intravasation: cancer cell entry into the bloodstream and lymphatics.
Intrinsic resistance: basic level of drug resistance of a cell.
Intron: gene sequences that are transcribed into RNA but removed before translation.
Invasion: spread into adjacent tissue.

Karyotype: the chromosome content of a cell.
Knock-out mice: mice in which both alleles of a gene have been inactivated. Also called nul/nul or −/− mice.

Ligand: agent that binds to a receptor.
Linkage: proximity of two genes on a chromosome.
Loss of heterozygosity: loss of the second allele of a gene. See Table 6.1.

Malignant: property of cancer cells to invade and metastasise.
Mesenchyme: bone, fat, connective tissue, blood vessels derived from embryonic mesoderm.
Metaplasia: reversible replacement of one normal cell type with another.
Metastasis: process by which cancers escape to other parts of the body.
Mitosis: phase of the cell cycle at which a cell divides to produce two daughter cells.
Mitotic index: percentage of cells in mitosis.
Mutation: a change in one or more bases in DNA.

Necrosis: cell death due to membrane disruption and release of lytic enzymes. Does not require RNA and protein synthesis.

Neoadjuvant therapy: chemotherapy given as a primary treatment.

Neoplasia: new growth of any type. Includes cancers and benign growths.

Non-genotoxic carcinogen: carcinogen that does not damage DNA.

Nude mouse: mouse with no thymus and therefore no T-cells. This inactivates the immune system. Has no hair.

Oligomers: multiple subunits.

Oncogene: a gene whose protein product contributes to carcinogenesis. Mutations relevant to carcinogenesis are dominant. Normal cellular oncogene is abbreviated to c-onc and viral oncogene is v-onc. See Chapter 6.

Overall survival: period from first diagnosis to death.

Paracrine: secretion of growth factors by one cell type that influences a nearby cell of a different type.

Phenotype: characteristics of a cell.

Pleural effusion: liquid plus cells in the space between the pleural membranes of the lung.

Ploidy: DNA (chromosome) content of a cell.

Primary cancer: site of first formation of a cancer.

Prognosis: future outlook for a patient with a cancer.

Prognostic factor: factor that helps define prognosis.

Progression: changes that result in increased aggressiveness (dedifferentiation) of a cancer.

Promotion: stage of carcinogenesis after initiation.

Promotor: (1) agent that promotes carcinogenesis; (2) regulatory region of a gene that initiates transcription.

Proteasome: ubiquitin-containing complex responsible for selective degradation of individual proteins.

Proto-oncogene: a gene that, as a result of mutation, can become an oncogene. See Chapter 6.

Provirus: viral DNA in host genome that can be transcribed into an RNA virus.

Purine: adenine or guanine base or derivative thereof.

Pyrimidine: cytosine, uracil or thymine base or derivative thereof.

Recessive: gene whose function is lost as a result of mutation. See Table 6.1.

Relapse: reappearance of a cancer.

Relapse-free survival: period between first diagnosis and appearance of secondary growths.

Relative risk: risk of developing a cancer in one group compared to that in a control group.

Remission: decline in cancer size as a result of treatment.

Replisome: complex responsible for DNA synthesis.

Repressor gene: gene whose protein product inhibits a cell function. See Chapter 6.

Restriction fragment length polymorphism (RFLP): DNA sequences cut with restriction nucleases that are different lengths in different individuals.

Retrovirus: RNA virus.

Sarcoma: mesenchymal cell cancer.

Secondary growth: a metastasis or local recurrence.

Silencer: regulatory DNA sequences that bind appropriate proteins to produce gene inactivation. See Chapter 6.

Somatic cell: not a germ cell so genetic complement cannot be passed to children.

S phase: phase of the cell cycle in which DNA is synthesised.

Stage: tumour classification based on size, nodal status and metastasis. See Chapter 13.

Stem cell: cell capable of an unlimited number of divisions.

Suppressor gene: *see* Repressor gene.

T-cell: class of lymphocytes with various subtypes. See Chapter 5.

Telomere: repeated DNA sequences at the end of a chromosome. See Chapter 9.

Telomerase: enzyme that extends telomere length. See Chapter 10.

Therapeutic index: ratio of maximal tolerated dose to minimal effective anticancer dose.

Totipotent cell: cell that has not differentiated and is capable of developing along several, alternative pathways.

Transcription: RNA synthesis from DNA. See Figure 6.1.

Transcription factor: protein that regulates transcription. See Chapter 6.

Transfection: experimental insertion of DNA sequences into cells.

Transformation: cell characteristics change from normal to more like those of a cancer.

Transgenic mouse: mouse in which every cell contains a 'foreign' gene (a transgene).

Transition: mutation that changes a purine to another purine (adenine/guanine) or a pyrimidine to another pyrimidine (cytidine/thymine).

Translation: protein synthesis from RNA. See Figure 6.1.

Transversion: mutation that changes a purine to a pyrimidine or vice versa.

Tumour: a growth that can be benign or malignant.

Tumour antigen: tumour cell antigen capable of eliciting an immune response.

Tumour marker: antigen that provides prognostic information about a cancer.

Tumour repressor (suppressor) gene: *see* Repressor gene.

FURTHER READING

General books

De Vita, V.T., Hellman, S. and Rosenburg, S.A. (eds) (1997) *Cancer: principles and practice of oncology*, 5th edn. J.B. Lippincott, Philadelphia PA. Multiauthor book containing chapters on basic science and detailed information on different cancer types, including treatments.

Franks, L.M. and Teich, N.M. (eds) (1997) *Introduction to the cellular and molecular biology of human cancer,* 3rd edn. Oxford University Press, Oxford. Multiauthor book containing chapters on various aspects of cancer biology. Does not deal with individual cancer types.

Meisenburg, G. and Simmons, W.H. (1998) *Principles of medical biochemistry.* Mosby, St Louis MO. Biochemistry text book dealing with all the pathways described here including a chapter on cellular growth control and cancer (pp. 603–36).

Alberts, B., Bray, D., Lewis, J., Raff, M., Roberts, K. and Watson, J.D. (1994) *Molecular biology of the cell*, 3rd edn. Garland Publishing, New York. Chapters on all the cell biology described in this book including one on cancer biology (pp. 1255–94).

Chapter 2

Kinzler, K. W. and Vogelstein, B. (1996) Lessons from hereditary colorectal cancer. *Cell*, **87**, 159–170.

Kinzler, K. W. and Vogelstein, B. (1997) Cancer-susceptibility genes; gatekeepers and caretakers. *Nature*, **386**, 761–62.

Sekido, Y., Fong, K.M. and Minna, J.D. (1998) Progress in understanding the molecular pathogenesis of human lung cancer. *Biochimica Biophysica Acta*, **1378**, F21–F59.

White, R. I. (1998) Tumour suppressing pathways. *Cell*, **92**, 591–92. Evidence that DCC is a SMAD.

Chapter 3

Underwood, J.C.E. (1992) *General and systematic pathology*. Churchill Livingstone, Edinburgh.

Chapter 4

American Cancer Society (1995) *Cancer facts and figures*. American Cancer Society, Atlanta GA. Concise data on incidence of and deaths from individual cancers in the USA.

Doll, R. and Crofton, J. (eds) (1996) Tobacco and health. *British Medical Bulletin*, **52**(1). This issue contains a series of articles covering all aspects of tobacco and health.

American Institute for Cancer Research (1997) *Food, nutrition and the prevention of cancer: a global perspective*. World Cancer Research Fund/American Institute for Cancer Research, Washington DC. Detailed review and conclusions of current data on all foodstuffs implicated in specific cancers.

Greenblatt, M.S., Bennett, W.P., Hollstein, M. and Harris, C.C. (1994) Mutations in the p53 suppressor gene: clues to cancer aetiology and molecular pathogenesis. *Cancer Research*, **54**, 4855–78.

Hussain, S.P. and Harris, C.C. (1998) Molecular epidemiology of human cancer. *Recent Results in Cancer Research (molecular epidemiology of human cancer)*, **154**, 22–36.

Nutritional aspects of the development of cancer (1998) *Report on Health and Social Subjects*, Vol. 48 (COMA report). Stationery Office, London. Detailed review and conclusions of current data on all foodstuffs implicated in specific cancers.

Parkin, D.M. (1998) The global burden of cancer. *Seminars in Cancer Biology*, **8**, 219–35.

Villa, L.L. (1997) Human papillomaviruses and cervical cancer. *Advances in Cancer Research*, **71**, 321–41.

Chapter 5

Brooks, C. (1998) NK cells, a class I act. *Immunology News*, **5**, 249–50.

Kuly, J. (1997) *Immunology*, 3rd edn. W.H. Freeman, New York. General book on the topic that includes a section on tumour immunology.

Nestle, F.O., Burg, G. and Dummer, R. (1999) New prospects on immunobiology and immunotherapy of melanoma. *Immunology Today*, **20**, 5–7.

Rosenberg, S. A., Kawakami, Y., Robbins, P.F. and Wang, R.-F. (1996) Identification of the genes encoding cancer antigens: implications for cancer immunotherapy. *Advances in Cancer Research*, **70**, 143–77.

Scott, A.M. and Welt, S. (1997) Antibody-based immunological therapies. *Current Opinion in Immunology*, **9**, 717–22.

Van den Eynde, B.J. and van der Bruggen, P. (1997) T cell defined tumor antigens. *Current Opinion in Immunology*, **9**, 684–93.

Yee, C., Ridell, S.R. and Greenberg, P.D. (1997) Prospects for T cell adoptive immunotherapy. *Current Opinion in Immunology*, **9**, 702–8.

Chapter 6

Brehm, A. and Kouzarides, T. (1999) Retinoblastoma protein meets chromatin. *Trends in Biochemical Science*, **24**, 142–45.

Grimwade, D. and Solomon, E. (1997) Characterisation of the PML/RAR alpha rearrangement associated with t(15:17) acute promyelocytic leukaemia. *Current Topics in Microbiology and Immunology*, **220**, 81–112.

Hesketh, R. (1997) *The oncogene and tumour suppressor gene facts book*, 2nd edn. Academic Press, London. Contains molecular details of major oncogenes and repressor genes plus a short introduction to their biological functions.

Ko, L.J. and Prives, C. (1996) p53: puzzle and paradigm. *Genes and Development*, **10**, 1054–72.

Lavia, P. and Jansen-Durr, P. (1999) E2F target genes and cell-cycle checkpoint control. *Bioessays*, **21**, 221–30.

Prives, C. (1998) Signalling to p53: breaking the MDM2–p53 circuit. *Cell*, **95**, 5–8.

Selivanova, G., Kawasaki, T., Ryabchenko, L. and Wiman, K.G. (1998) Reactivation of mutant p53: a new strategy for cancer therapy. *Seminars in Cancer Biology*, **8**, 369–78.

Slack, J.L. (1999) The biology and treatment of acute progranulocytic leukemia. *Current Opinion in Oncology*, **11**, 9–13.

Taya, Y. (1997) Rb kinases and Rb-binding proteins: new points of view. *Trends in Biochemical Sciences*, **22**, 14–17.

Villa, L.L. (1997) Human papillomaviruses and cervical cancer. *Advances in Cancer Research*, **71**, 321–41.

Chapter 7

Blancher, C. and Harris, A.L. (1998) The molecular basis of the hypoxia response pathway: tumour hypoxia as a therapy target. *Cancer and Metastasis Reviews*, **17**, 187–194.

Collins, A.R. (1999) Oxidative DNA damage, antioxidants, and cancer. *Bioessays*, **21**, 238–46.

Dogliotti, E., Hainaut, P., Hernandez, T., D'Errico, M. and DeMarini, D.M. (1998) Mutation spectra resulting from carcinogen exposure: from model systems to cancer-related genes. *Recent Results in Cancer Research (molecular epidemiology of human cancer)*, **154**, 97–124. Gives specific examples of mutations generated by tobacco smoke, UV light, aflatoxin and vinyl chloride.

Finkel, T. (1998) Oxygen radicals and signalling. *Current Opinion in Cell Biology*, **10**, 248–53.

Neckers, L.M. (1999) aHIF: the missing link between HIF-1 and VHL? *Journal of the National Cancer Institute*, **91**, 106–7.

McGregor, D.B., Rice, J.M. and Venitt, S. (eds) (1999) The use of short- and medium-term tests for carcinogens and data on genetic effects in carcinogenic hazard evaluation. *IARC Scientific Publication* 146. IARC Press, Lyon. Series of articles on the topic.

Mercurio, F. and Manning, A.M. (1999) Multiple signals converging on NF-kB. *Current Opinion in Cell Biology*, **11**, 226–32.

Chapter 8

Biggs, P.J. and Bradley, A. (1998) A step towards genotype-based therapeutic regimens for breast cancer in patients with BRCA2 mutations. *Journal of the National Cancer Institute*, **90**, 951–53.

Genetic instability and cancer (1996) *Cancer Surveys*, **28**. Series of articles.

Greenblatt, M.S., Grollman, A.P. and Harris, C.C. (1996) Deletions and insertions in the p53 tumor suppressor gene in human cancers: confirmation of the DNA polymerase slippage/misalignment model. *Cancer Research*, **56**, 2130–36.

Jackson, A.L. and Loeb, L.A. (1998) On the origin of multiple mutations in human cancers. *Seminars in Cancer Biology*, **8**, 421–29.

Jiricny, J. (1998) Replication errors: cha(lle)nging the genome. *EMBO Journal*, **17**, 6427–36.

Kanaar, R., Hoeijmakers, J.H.J. and van Gent, D.C. (1998) Molecular mechanisms of DNA double-strand break repair. *Trends in Cell Biology*, **8**, 483–89.

Lehmann, A. R. (1998) Dual functions of DNA repair genes: molecular, cellular, and clinical implications. *Bioessays*, **20**, 146–55.

Prives, C. (1998) Signalling to p53: breaking the MDM2–p53 circuit. *Cell*, **95**, 5–8.

Simpson, A. J. G., (1997) The natural somatic mutation frequency and human carcinogenesis. *Advances in Cancer Research*, **71**, 209–40.

Chapter 9

Casey, G. (1997) The BRCA1 and BRCA2 breast cancer genes. *Current Opinion in Oncology*, **9**, 88–93.

Kinzler, K. W. and Vogelstein, B. (1996) Lessons from hereditary colorectal cancer. *Cell*, **87**, 159–70.

Sudbery, P. (1998) *Human molecular genetics*, Longman, Harlow. Good general text plus a section on inherited predisposition to several types of cancer (pp. 114–25).

Zhang, H., Tombline, G. and Weber, B.L. (1998) BRCA1, BRCA2, and DNA damage response: collision or collusion? *Cell*, **92**, 433–36.

Chapter 10

Proliferation

Bouchard, C., Staller, P. and Eilers, M. (1998) Control of cell proliferation by myc. *Trends in Cell Biology*, **8**, 202–6.

Checkpoint controls and cancer (1997) *Cancer Surveys*, **29**. Series of articles.

Chin, L., Pomerantz, J. and DePinto, R.A. (1998) The INK4a/ARF tumor suppressor: one gene – two products – two pathways. *Trends in Biochemical Science*, **23**, 291–96.

Grandori, C. and Eisenman, R.N. (1997) Myc target genes. *Trends in Biochemical Science*, **22**, 177–81.

Hall, M. and Peters, G. (1996) Genetic alterations of cyclins, cyclin-dependent kinases and Cdk inhibitors in human cancer. *Advances in Cancer Research*, **68**, 67–108.

Jonsson, Z.O. and Hubscher, U. (1997) Proliferating cell nuclear antigen: more than a clamp for DNA polymerases. *Bioessays*, **19**, 967–75.

Lavia, P. and Jansen-Durr, P. (1999) E2F target genes and cell-cycle checkpoint control. *Bioessays*, **21**, 221–30.

Martin-Castellanos, C. and Moreno, S. (1997) Recent advances on cyclins, CDKs and CDK inhibitors. *Trends in Cell Biology*, **7**, 95–98.

Prives, C. (1998) Signalling to p53: breaking the MDM2–p53 circuit. *Cell*, **95**, 5–8.

Simpson, A. J. G. (1997) The natural somatic mutation frequency and human carcinogenesis. *Advances in Cancer Research*, **71**, 209–40.

Taya, Y. (1997) Rb kinases and Rb-binding proteins: new points of view. *Trends in Biochemical Sciences*, **22**, 14–17.

Apoptosis

Cory, S. and Adams, J.M. (1998) Matters of life and death: programmed cell death at Cold Spring Harbor. *Biochimica Biophysica Acta*, **1377**, R25–R44.

Green, D. and Kroemer, G. (1998) The central executioners of apoptosis: caspases or mitochondria? *Trends in Cell Biology*, **8**, 267–71.

Reed, J.C. (1999) Mechanisms of apoptosis avoidance in cancer. *Current Opinion in Oncology*, **11**, 68–75.

Tan, X. and Wang, J. Y. J. (1998) The caspase–Rb connection in cell death. *Trends in Cell Biology*, **8**, 116–120.

Differentiation

Bird, A. (1996) The relationship of DNA methylation to cancer. *Cancer Surveys*, **28**, 87–101.

Jacobson, S. and Pillus, I. (1999) Modifying chromatin and concepts of cancer. *Current Opinion in Genetics and Development*, **9**, 175–84. Describes proteins involved in gene regulation with special relevance to leukaemia.

Sieweke, M.H. and Graff, T. (1998) A transcription factor party during blood cell differentiation. *Current Opinion in Genetics and Development*, **8**, 545–51.

Szyf, M. (1998) Targetting DNA methyltransferase in cancer. *Cancer and Metastasis Reviews*, **17**, 219–31.

Telomerase

Shay, J.W. (1999) Towards identifying a cellular determinant of telomerase repression, *Journal of the National Cancer Institute*, **91**, 4–6.

Harley, C.B. and Sherwood, S.W. (1997). Telomerase, checkpoints and cancer. *Cancer Surveys*, **29**, 263–84.

Chapter 11

Signalling from kinase receptors

Heimbrook, D.C. and Oliff, A. (1998) Therapeutic intervention and signalling. *Current Opinion in Cell Biology*, **10**, 284–88.

Garrington, T.P. (1999) Organisation and regulation of mitogen-activated protein kinase signalling. *Current Opinion in Cell Biology*, **11**, 211–18.

Kretzschmar, M. and Massague, J. (1998) SMADs: mediators and regulators of TGF-beta signalling. *Current Opinion in Genetics and Development*, **8**, 103–11.

Leevers, S.J., Vanhaesebroeck, B. and Waterfield, M.D. (1999) Signalling through phosphoinositide-3-kinase: the lipids take centre stage. *Current Opinion in Cell Biology*, **11**, 219–25.

Schwartz, M.A. and Baron, V. (1999) Interactions between mitogenic stimuli or, a thousand and one connections. *Current Opinion in Cell Biology*, **11**, 197–202.

Tzahar, E. and Yarden, Y. (1998) The ErbB-2/Her2 oncogenic receptor of adenocarcinomas: from orphanhood to multiple stromal ligands. *Biochimica Biophysica Acta*, **1377**, M25–M37.

Cell adhesion

Bullions, L.C. and Levine, A.J. (1998) The role of β-catenin in cell adhesion, signal transduction and cancer. *Current Opinion in Oncology*, **10**, 81–87.

Christofori, G. and Semb, H. (1999) The role of the cell-adhesion molecule E-cadherin as a tumour-suppressor gene. *Trends in Biochemical Science*, **24**, 73–76.

Keely, P., Parise, L. and Juliano, R. (1998) Integrins and GTPases in tumour cell growth, motility and invasion. *Trends in Cell Biology*, **8**, 101–106.

Gumbiner, B.M. (1996) Cell adhesion: the molecular basis of tissue architecture and morphogenesis. *Cell*, **84**, 345–57.

Holzmann, B., Gosslar, U. and Bittner, M. (1998) Alpha 4 integrins and tumor metastasis. *Current Topics in Microbiology and Immunology*, **231**, 125–41.

Humphries, M.J. and Newham, P. (1998) The structure of cell-adhesion molecules. *Trends in Cell Biology*, **8**, 78–83.

Polakis, P. (1997) The adenomatous polyposis coli (APC) tumor suppressor. *Biochimica Biophysica Acta*, **1332**, F127–F147.

Sy, M-S., Mori, H. and Lui, D. (1997) CD44 as a marker in human cancers. *Current Opinion in Oncology*, **9**, 108–12.

Schoenwaelder, S.M. and Burridge, K. (1999) Bidirectional signalling between the cytoskeleton and integrins. *Current Opinion in Cell Biology*, **11**, 274–86.

Sheetz, M.P., Felsenfeld, D.P. and Galbraith, C.G. (1998) Cell migration: regulation of force on extracellular matrix–integrin complexes. *Trends in Cell Biology*, **8**, 51–54.

Signalling by hydrophobic molecules

Freedman, I.P. (1999) Increasing the complexity of coactivation in nuclear receptor signalling. *Cell*, **97**, 5–8.

Grimwade, D. and Solomon, E. (1997) Characterisation of the PML/RAR alpha rearrangement associated with t(15:17) acute promyelocytic leukaemia. *Current Topics in Microbiology and Immunology*, **220**, 81–112.

Slack, J.L. (1999) The biology and treatment of acute progranulocytic leukemia. *Current Opinion in Oncology*, **11**, 9–13.

Taketo, M.M. (1998) Cyclooxygenase-2 inhibitors in tumorigenesis (Parts 1 and 2). *Journal of the National Cancer Institute*, **90**, 1529–36 (Part 1) and 1609–20 (Part 2). Part 1 deals with enzymology and Part 2 with biological effects.

Tsujii *et al.* (1998) Cyclooxygenase regulates angiogenesis induced by colon cancer cells. *Cell*, **93**, 705–16.

Xu, L., Glass, C.K. and Rosenfeld, M.G. (1999) Coactivator and corepressor complexes in nuclear receptor function. *Current Opinion in Genetics and Development*, **9**, 140–47.

Zou, A., Marschke, K.B., Arnold, K.E., Berger, E.M., Fitzgerald, P., Mais, D.E. and Allegretto, E.A. (1999) Estrogen receptor *β* activates the human retinoic acid receptor *α*-1 promoter in response to tamoxifen and other estrogen receptor antagonists, but not in response to estrogen. *Molecular Endocrinology*, **13**, 418–30. Technical paper but contains general information on estrogen receptor *β*.

Chapter 12

Blancher, C. and Harris, A.L. (1998) The molecular basis of the hypoxia response pathway: tumour hypoxia as a therapy target. *Cancer and Metastasis Reviews*, **17**, 187–94.

Chambers, A. F. and Matrisian, I. M. (1997) Changing views of the role of matrix metalloproteinases in metastasis. *Journal of the National Cancer Institute*, **89**, 1260–70.

Ferrara, N. (1999) Vascular endothelial growth factor: molecular and biological aspects. In *Vascular growth factors and angiogenesis*, Claesson-Welsh, L. (ed.). Springer, Berlin, pp. 1–30.

Harris, A.L. (1998) Are angiostatin and endostatin cures for cancer? *Lancet*, **351**, 1598–99.

Holzmann, B., Gosslar, U. and Bittner, M. (1998) Alpha 4 integrins and tumor metastasis. *Current Topics in Microbiology and Immunology*, **231**, 125–41.

Tsujii *et al.* (1998) Cyclooxygenase regulates angiogenesis induced by colon cancer cells. *Cell*, **93**, 705–16.

Yancopoulos, G. D., Klagsbrun, M. and Folkman, J. (1998) Vasculogenesis, angiogenesis and growth factors: ephrins enter the fray at the border. *Cell*, **93**, 661–64.

Zetter, B.R. (1998) Angiogenesis and tumor metastasis. *Annual Review of Medicine*, **49**, 407–24.

Chapter 13

Chaney, S.G. and Sancar, A. (1996) DNA repair: enzymatic mechanisms and relevance to drug response. *Journal of the National Cancer Institute*, **88**, 1346–60.

Dougherty, T.L., Gomer, C.J., Henderson, B.W., Jori, G., Kessel, D., Korbelik, M, Moan, J. and Peng, Q. (1998) Photodynamic therapy. *Journal of the National Cancer Institute*, **90**, 889–905.

El-Deiry, W.S. (1997) Role of oncogenes in resistance and killing by cancer therapeutic agents. *Current Opinion in Oncology*, **9**, 79–87.

Gottesman, M.M., Pastan, I. and Ambukar, S.V. P-glycoprotein and multidrug resistance. (1996) *Current Opinion in Genetics and Development*, **6**, 610–17.

Nass, S.J., Hahm, H.A. and Davidson, N.E. (1998) Breast cancer biology blossoms in the clinic. *Nature Medicine*, **4**, 761–62.

New treatments

Cheresh, D.A. (1998) Death to a blood vessel, death to a tumor. *Nature Medicine*, **4**, 395–96.

Fan, Z. and Mendelsohn, J. (1998) Therapeutic application of anti-growth factor receptor antibodies. *Current Opinion in Oncology*, **10**, 67–73.

Flanagan, W.M. (1998) Antisense comes of age. *Cancer and Metastasis Reviews*, **17**, 169–76.

Harris, A.L. (1998) Are angiostatin and endostatin cures for cancer? *Lancet*, **351**, 1598–99.

Klohs, W.D., Fry, D.W. and Kraker, A.J. (1997) Inhibitors of tyrosine kinase. *Current Opinion in Oncology*, **9**, 562–68.

Lobell, R.B. and Kohl, N.E. (1998) Pre-clinical development of farnesyltransferase inhibitors. *Cancer and Metastasis Reviews*, **17**, 203–10.

Nestle, F.O., Burg, G. and Dummer, R. (1999) New prospects on immunobiology and imunotherapy of melanoma. *Immunology Today*, **20**, 5–7.

Rosenberg, S.A., Kawakami, Y., Robbins, P.F. and Wang, R-F. (1996) Identification of the genes encoding cancer antigens: implications for cancer immunotherapy. *Advances in Cancer Research*, **70**, 143–77.

Scott, A.M. and Welt, S. (1997) Antibody-based immunological therapies. *Current Opinion in Imunology*, **9**, 717–22.

Van den Eynde, B.J. and van der Bruggen, P. (1997) T cell defined tumor antigens. *Current Opinion in Immunology*, **9**, 684–93.

Yu, A.E., Hewitt, R.E., Connor, E.W. and Stetler-Stevenson, W.G. (1997) Matrix metalloproteinases: novel targets for directed cancer therapy. *Drugs and Aging*, **11**, 229–44.

Chapter 14

Breast cancer and hormonal contraceptives: collaborative reanalysis of individual data on 53,297 women with breast cancer and 100,239 women without breast cancer from 54 epidemiological studies (1996) *Lancet*, **347**, 1713–27.

Carotenoids. (1998) *IARC Handbooks of Cancer Prevention*, 2. IARC Press, Lyo. Series of articles on the topic.

Fisher, B., Constantino, J.P., Wickerham, L., Redmond, C.K., Kavanah, M. *et al.* (1998) Tamoxifen for the prevention of breast cancer: report of the National Surgical Adjuvant Breast and Bowel Project P-1 study. *Journal of the National Cancer Institute*, **88**, 1371–88.

American Institute for Cancer Research (1997) Food, nutrition and the prevention of cancer: a global perspective. World Cancer Research Fund/American Institute for Cancer Research, Washington DC. Detailed review and conclusions of current data on all foodstuffs implicated in specific cancers.

Non-steroidal anti-inflammatory drugs. (1997) *IARC Handbooks of Cancer Prevention*: Vol. 1, IARC Press, Lyon. Series of articles on each topic.

King, R.J.B. (1997) Endometrial cancer: an introduction. In *Biology of female cancers*, Langdon, S.P., Miller, W.R. and Berchuk, A. (eds), CRC Press, Baton Rouge LA, pp. 183–92.

Nutritional aspects of the development of cancer (1998) *Report on health and social subjects*, Vol. 48 (COMA report). Stationery Office, London. Detailed review and conclusions of current data on all foodstuffs implicated in specific cancers.

Lippman, S.M., Lee, J.J. and Sabichi, A.L. (1998) Cancer chemoprevention: progress and promise. *Journal of the National Cancer Institute*, **90**, 1514–28.

Rubin, S.S. (1998) Chemoprevention of hereditary ovarian cancer. *New England Journal of Medicine*, **339**, 469–71.

Powles, T., Eeles, R., Ashley, S., Easton, D., Chang, J., Dowsett, M. *et al.* (1998) Interim analysis of the incidence of breast cancer in the Royal Marsden Hospital tamoxifen randomised chemoprevention trial. *Lancet*, **352**, 98–101.

Taketo, M.M. (1998) Cyclooxygenase-2 inhibitors in tumorigenesis (Parts 1 and 2). *Journal of the National Cancer Institute*, **90**, 1529–36 (Part 1) and 1609–20 (Part 2). Part 1 deals with enzymology and Part 2 with biological effects.

INDEX

Main entries are indicated in **bold** type. When the cited pages contain relevant figures or tables, an asterisk (*) is included. Where necessary, individual cancers or genes have been classified into clinical, gene or other subcategories. Clinical includes natural history, epidemiology and pathology details. Gene contains references to familial cancers. The sections designated 'other' contain functional (cellular) details.